Review of LABORATORY MEDICINE

Review of
LABORATORY MEDICINE

JOHN S. MEYER, M.D.

Associate Professor of Pathology, Washington
University School of Medicine; Associate
Pathologist, The Jewish Hospital, St. Louis,
Missouri

LAWRENCE S. STEINBERG, M.D.

Clinical Assistant Professor, Department of Pathology,
University of California at San Diego School of Medicine, San Diego;
Director of Laboratories, Mission Bay Hospital.
San Diego, California

LAURENCE A. SHERMAN, M.D.

Associate Professor of Pathology and Medicine,
Washington University School of Medicine;
Director, Blood Bank, Barnes Hospital,
St. Louis, Missouri

SECOND EDITION

with 162 illustrations

The C. V. Mosby Company

Saint Louis   1975

Second edition

Copyright © 1975 by The C. V. Mosby Company

All rights reserved. No part of this book may be reproduced
in any manner without written permission of the publisher.

Previous edition copyrighted 1971

Printed in the United States of America

Distributed in Great Britain by Henry Kimpton, London

Library of Congress Cataloging in Publication Data

Meyer, John S   1930-
    Review of laboratory medicine.

    Includes bibliographies and index.
    1. Medicine, Clinical—Examinations, questions, etc.
I. Steinberg, Lawrence S., 1935-   joint author.
II. Sherman, Laurence A., 1935-   joint author.
III. Title. [DNLM: 1. Diagnosis, Laboratory—Examination
questions. 2. Technology, Medical—Examination questions. QY18 M612r]
RB37.M467 1975   616.07′5′076   75-2456
ISBN 0-8016-3416-4

VH/M/M   9 8 7 6 5 4 3 2 1

PREFACE

This review is intended as an aid to study for the beginner and as a means of self-evaluation and review for those more advanced in the study of laboratory medicine. It can be utilized best by first reading one or several of the suggested references and then answering the questions as thoughtfully as possible. Several persons can review together by scheduling question and answer sessions on specific topics.

We have tried to cover principles that are useful in the routine practice of laboratory medicine, and we believe that the questions appearing in the text are likely to confront the resident or practitioner in real experience as well as on specialty board or national board examinations.

A short bibliography appears at the beginning of most chapters. It usually includes one or more textbooks or monographs and a list of references to newer material that is not adequately covered in textbooks. Bibliographic references are cited in the text only when adequate coverage is not available in current textbooks. The first three books listed below are comprehensive texts of general laboratory medicine with balanced stress on technology and clinical applications. We recommend the text by Davidsohn and Henry because it has recently been updated.

Davidsohn, I., and Henry, J. B., editors: Todd-Sanford clinical diagnosis by laboratory methods, ed. 15, Philadelphia, 1974, W. B. Saunders Co.

Bauer, J. D., Ackermann, P. G., and Toro, G.: Clinical laboratory methods, ed. 8, St. Louis, 1974, The C. V. Mosby Co.

Frankel, S., Reitman, S., and Sonnenwirth, A. C., editors: Gradwohl's clinical laboratory methods and diagnosis, ed. 7, St. Louis, 1970, The C. V. Mosby Co.

Hepler, O.: Manual of clinical laboratory methods, ed. 4, Springfield, Ill., 1973, Charles C Thomas, Publisher.

The texts by Bauer, Ackermann, and Toro and by Hepler are primarily surveys of clinical laboratory methods. *Gradwohl's Clinical Laboratory Methods and Diagnosis* is the definitive compendium of technical methods.

We are grateful for the interest and assistance of our associates and for the encouragement and understanding of LaVerna, Kathy, and Judy.

John S. Meyer
Lawrence S. Steinberg
Laurence A. Sherman

CONTENTS

Review of LABORATORY MEDICINE

CHAPTER 1

Amniotic fluid

The laboratory examination of amniotic fluid for diagnosis of the fetal isoimmunization syndrome and for grading severity of fetal hemolysis has become routine during the last decade. More recently, laboratory examination of chemical and cytologic features of amniotic fluid has achieved success in prediction of fetal maturity. Much of the recently acquired information is not yet fully developed in textbooks. Space does not permit consideration of cyto-biochemical tests for inborn errors of metabolism and genetic defects in the fetus.

Fairweather, D. V. I., and Eskes, T. K. A., editors: Amniotic fluid: research and clinical application, Amsterdam, 1973, Excerpta Medica.
Natelson, S., Scommegna, A., and Epstein, M. B., editors: Amniotic fluid physiology, biochemistry, and clinical chemistry, New York, 1974, John Wiley & Sons, Inc.

■ **What is the volume of amniotic fluid during the last trimester of gestation?**

The volume of amniotic fluid increases rapidly during the first two trimesters until it reaches a mean volume of about 650 ml at the twenty-eighth week. Thereafter the volume increases less rapidly to a mean of about 900 ml at 36 weeks. Little change occurs until the fortieth week, but decreases may be observed in postmature pregnancies. Since the ranges of amniotic fluid volume are broad at all stages of pregnancy, the measurement has little clinical importance.

■ **With what does the amniotic fluid exchange, and at what rate?**

It exchanges with both fetal and maternal plasma. Total exchange rates are 12 mEq Na and 0.6 mEq K/hr. The exchange rate of water is difficult to measure. One estimate is 470 ml/hr.

■ **In isoimmunization of pregnancy, how early in gestation may hemolysis begin?**

Hemolysis may begin at the sixteenth week.

■ **The yellow pigment found in amniotic fluid has a maximum absorbance at what wavelength, and what are its characteristics of reaction with Ehrlich's diazo reagent?**

Maximum absorption is at 450 nm. It reacts as "indirect" bilirubin.

■ **Is amniotic bilirubin conjugated or unconjugated?**

Amniotic fluid bilirubin is almost entirely unconjugated unless the concentration is increased by fetal hemolysis. In the latter circumstances glucuronyl transferase may be activated, and up to 50% of the bilirubin may be conjugated.

■ **Relative to water and electrolytes in amniotic fluid, is the turnover of bilirubin fast or slow?**

The turnover is slow because the albumin to which it is bound has a long turnover time.

■ **From the twenty-eighth week of a normal gestation to term, does the net absorbance of amniotic fluid at 450 nm increase or decrease?**

It decreases from a maximum of 0.06 to a maximum of 0.02 optical density (OD) units with a 1 cm light path.

■ **What precautions need be taken with an amniotic fluid specimen before analysis for pigments?**

It must be protected from light. The half-life of bilirubin pigment in laboratory daylight is 10 hours, and in sunlight it is 12 to 18 minutes. It is stable for months when refrigerated in the dark.

■ **What is the net OD at 450 nm?**

It is the observed OD measured with a 1 cm light path minus the predicted OD. The predicted OD is derived from interpolation, on semilog paper, of the OD curve between 365 and 550 nm. This method of interpolation is necessary because the OD of amniotic fluid increases exponentially as the wavelength decreases between 550 and 365 nm.

■ **Red blood cells are present in a sample of amniotic fluid. What tests may be used for their identification?**

1. Grouping and typing
2. Direct Coombs test
3. Betke-Kleihauer test

■ **What is the Betke-Kleihauer test?**

It is a test for fetal hemoglobin. Fetal erythrocytes can be identified in films of bloody amniotic fluid by resistance of their hemoglobin to elution by an acid (pH 3.2) buffer. After this treatment the fetal erythrocytes stain well, and maternal erythrocytes appear as ghosts.

■ **What are the prognoses for the following Liley groups?**

1. Mild or unaffected zone (net OD less than 0.06 at 28 weeks, less than 0.02 at 40 weeks)
2. Moderately affected zone (net OD 0.06 to 0.25 at 28 weeks, 0.02 to 0.09 at 40 weeks)
3. Severely affected zone (net OD above 0.25 at 28 weeks, above 0.09 at 40 weeks)

Infants in the mild zone are usually unaffected and do not require exchange transfusions. Those in the moderate zone survive but often require one or more exchanges. Infants in the severe zone often die despite exchange transfusions.

■ **If the maternal anti-Rh$_o$ titer is positive to 1:16 dilution and if an amniocentesis produces colorless fluid with a normal scan at a given time in gestation, how soon should amniocentesis be repeated?**

It should be repeated probably with 2 weeks, since the "safe period" based on a normal scan is only 1 to 2 weeks. Hemolytic disease can develop rapidly in 2 weeks or less.

■ **On the spectrophotometric scan, what is the effect of hemorrhage into the amniotic fluid, and how long does the effect last?**

The scan will show the absorption peaks of oxyhemoglobin released by hemolysis of the RBC at 415, 540, and 577 nm. A major hemorrhage will be cleared in about 2 weeks. After a small hemorrhage, only the 415 nm absorbance may be detected.

■ **Interpret the six amniotic fluid scans shown below.**

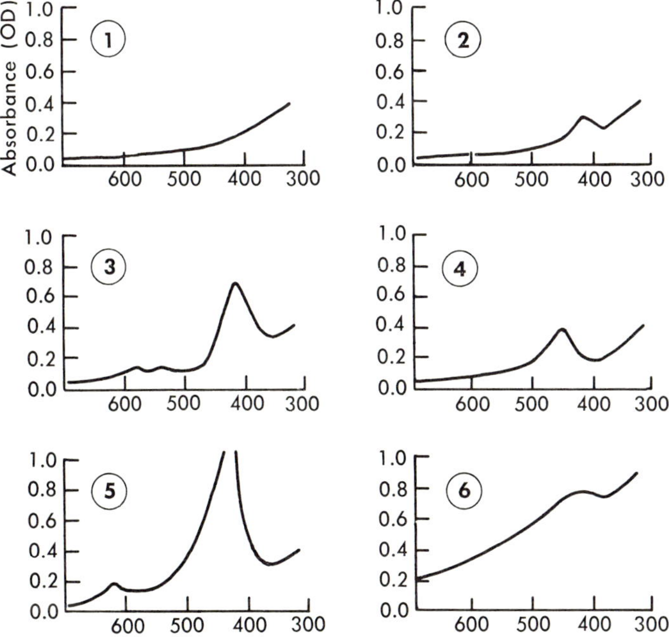

1. Normal amniotic fluid
2. Slight contamination with blood, oxyhemoglobin peak at 415 nm
3. More marked hemorrhage with oxyhemoglobin peaks at 415, 540, and 575 nm
4. Significant bilirubin peak
5. Marked elevation of bilirubin level with shift of absorbance peak to shorter wavelength indicating acidosis, and methemalbumin peak at 620 nm (These findings indicate impending fetal death.)
6. Amniotic fluid lightly contaminated with meconium (Note failure to approach baseline closely at high wavelength and peak at 405 to 410 nm. Meconium contains bilirubin.)

■ **What conditions other than isoimmunization syndrome can produce an amniotic fluid absorbance peak at 450 nm?**

Biliary atresia, anencephaly and duodenal atresia with polyhydramnios (regurgitation of bile), and tetracycline therapy can produce an amniotic fluid absorbance peak at 450 nm.

■ **Name four conditions that may invalidate the Liley 450 nm absorbance determination of bilirubin in amniotic fluid.**

1. Contamination with meconium
2. Contamination with oxyhemoglobin
3. Presence of tetracycline
4. Erroneous sampling (amniotic sac of uninvolved fraternal twin, fetal ascitic fluid, maternal urine)

■ **How can information on the severity of fetal hemolysis be obtained from a bloody amniotic fluid specimen in which the bilirubin peak is badly obscured by oxyhemoglobin?**

1. The titer of antibody to Rh_0 in the amniotic fluid can be determined. Higher titers suggest more severe disease.[5]

2. Ovenstone slope analysis of the bilirubin peak in the spectrophotometric scan can eliminate most of the oxyhemoglobin interference.[4]

■ **Which tests on amniotic fluid are most useful in determining fetal maturity?**

Measurements of lecithin/sphingomyelin (L/S) ratio,[2,7,9] total lecithin,[6] or surfactant[1] are the most useful tests. Less useful tests include measurement of bilirubin, measurement of creatinine and amniotic fluid/maternal serum, creatinine ratio, and count of Nile blue sulfate–positive epithelial cells.[10]

■ **What is the importance of pulmonary surfactant?**

Pulmonary surfactant lowers the surface tension within alveoli from close to the surface tension of water (73 dynes/cm) to approximately 10 to 15 dynes/cm. Without the surfactant, the lungs would collapse or would require such a negative intrapleural pressure for expansion as to cause transudation of fluid into alveoli.

■ **What are the principal pulmonary alveolar surfactants?**

The principal surfactant is dipalmitoyl lecithin (dipalmitoyl-L-α-phosphatidyl choline), but in newborn infants, particularly premature ones, significant amounts of lecithin with β carbon myristic acid are present.[8]

■ **What are the sources of amniotic fluid lecithins?**

Amniotic fluid lecithins are derived from several sources, including urine and surface epithelium, but it is likely that a major component comes from pulmonary secretions because amniotic fluid lecithin content reflects pulmonary alveolar lecithin content.[3,8]

■ **When during gestation does an abrupt rise in amniotic fluid lecithin concentration occur?**

Amniotic fluid lecithin concentration usually increases abruptly at about the thirty-fifth week of gestation, at the time the fetus achieves extrauterine viability.[7]

■ **Explain the prognostic significance of the amniotic fluid lecithin/sphingomyelin (L/S) ratio.**

The concentration of sphingomyelin remains nearly constant in amniotic fluid throughout gestation. Consequently a rise in the L/S ratio reflects an increase in lecithin concentration. When the L/S ratio is low at the time of birth, the respiratory distress syndrome (RDS) is likely to develop in the infant. A high L/S ratio indicates a low likelihood of RDS.[7,9]

■ **What L/S ratio and concentration of amniotic fluid lecithin indicate fetal pulmonary maturity?**

The L/S ratio indicating maturity depends on the method of visualization, for different methods of staining the chromatogram place different emphasis on lecithin and sphingomyelin. By Gluck's method, a ratio of 2 is consistent with maturity and actually reflects a molar ratio of 4.[2,9] A total lecithin concentration of 3.5 mg/dl is consistent with maturity.[14]

■ **What conditions dispose toward development of RDS despite L/S or other surfactant measurements indicative of maturity?**

Perinatal stress (hypoxia, acidosis, hypothermia, maternal diabetes mellitus) may be followed by RDS despite a mature surfactant measurement.[2,8,14]

■ **Describe the foam test of Clements. What property of amniotic fluid does it test?**

The foam test determines the ability of amniotic fluid to generate stable bubbles in presence of ethanol. This property is dependent on surfactant lecithins.[1,13]

■ **What are the levels of the bilirubin peak, creatinine, and Nile blue positive cells in amniotic fluid that indicate a gestational age of at least 36 weeks with a probability of more than 95%?**

Any one of these criteria—absence of the bilirubin peak, creatinine of 2.0 mg/dl or more, and a Nile blue sulfate–positive count of at least 20%—used alone, indicates fetal maturity with a probability of more than 95%, provided that, in the case of creatinine, the maternal serum creatinine is not elevated and the pregnancy is not toxemic. However, in many mature pregnancies these tests give false negative results.[10,11]

■ **What is the principle of the Nile blue sulfate stain on amniotic fluid for determination of fetal maturity?**

The stain is a mixture of dyes, one of which stains fat orange. Anucleate cells with orange-staining globules in the cytoplasm are derived from fetal sebaceous glands and do not appear in the amniotic fluid until the later stages of gestation. Their number increases rapidly after the thirty-seventh week of gestation. Still later in pregnancy the fatty cells degenerate to yield free fat and ghost cells.

■ **What are the levels of lactic dehydrogenase (LDH) and creatine phosphokinase (CPK) in normal amniotic fluid?**

The level of LDH in normal amniotic fluid is approximately the same as in normal blood serum. Normal amniotic fluid has little or no CPK activity—significantly less than in normal serum.[12]

■ **What is the significance of a tenfold or greater elevation of CPK in amniotic fluid?**

Large increases in CPK activity in amniotic fluid signify fetal death.[12]

REFERENCES

1. Clements, J. A., et al.: Assessment of the risk of the respiratory-distress syndrome by a rapid test for surfactant in amniotic fluid, N. Engl. J. Med. 286:1077, 1972.
2. Coch, E. H., et al.: A modified procedure for evaluation of the lecithin/sphingomyelin ratio in amniotic fluid, Clin. Chem. 19:967, 1973.
3. Condroelli, S., Cosmi, E. V., and Scarpelli, E. M.: Extrapulmonary source of amniotic fluid phospholipids, Am. J. Obstet. Gynecol. 118:842, 1974.
4. Connon, A. F.: Improved accuracy of prediction of severity of hemolytic disease of the newborn, Obstet. Gynecol. 33:72, 1969.
5. Dalton, N. T.: The significance of Rhesus antibodies in liquor amnii, Am. J. Obstet. Gynecol. 107:925, 1970.
6. Ekelund, L., Arvidson, G., and Åstedt, B.: Amniotic fluid lecithin and its fatty acid composition in respiratory distress syndrome, J. Obstet. Gynaecol. Br. Commonw. 80: 1973.
7. Gluck, L., et al.: Diagnosis of the respiratory distress syndrome by amniocentesis, Am. J. Obstet. Gynecol. 109:440, 1971.
8. Gluck, L., et al.: Biochemical development of surface activity in mammalian lung. IV. Pulmonary lecithin synthesis in the human fetus and newborn and etiology of the respiratory distress syndrome, Pediatr. Res. 6:81, 1972.
9. Gluck, L., and Kulovich, M. V.: Lecithin/sphingomyelin ratios in amniotic fluid in normal and abnormal pregnancy, Am. J. Obstet. Gynecol. 115:539, 1973.
10. Henneman, C. E., Anderson, G. V., Tejavej, A., Gross, H. A., and Heiman, M. L.: Fetal maturation and

amniotic fluid, Am. J. Obstet. Gynecol. **108**:302, 1970.

11. Roopnarinesingh, S.: Amniotic fluid creatinine in normal and abnormal pregnancies, J. Obstet. Gynaecol. Br. Commonw. **77**:785, 1970.

12. Sarkozi, L., et al.: Biochemical indicators of fetal maturity and intrauterine death in amniotic fluid, Scand. J. Clin. Lab. Invest. **29**(supp. 26):10, 1972.

13. Thibeault, D. W., and Hobel, C. J.: The interrelationship of the foam stability test, immaturity and intrapartum complications in the respiratory distress syndrome, Am. J. Obstet. Gynecol. **118**:56, 1974.

14. Warren, C., Holton, J. B., and Allen, J. T.: Assessment of fetal lung maturity by estimation of amniotic fluid palmitic acid, Br. Med. J. **1**:94, 1974.

15. Whitfield, C. R., Sproule, W. B., and Brudenall, M.: The amniotic fluid lecithin:sphingomyelin area ratio (LSAR) in pregnancies complicated by diabetes, J. Obstet. Gynaecol. Br. Commonw. **80**:918, 1973.

CHAPTER 2

Bacteriology

Because medical bacteriology is a broad field, beginning with well-chosen textbooks will be helpful in reviewing. Bailey and Scott's book will serve as an introductory text. Sonnenwirth's section in *Gradwohl's Clinical Laboratory Methods and Diagnosis* and Blair, Lennette, and Truant's text can be used as supplementary references. Joklik and Smith's *Zinsser Microbiology* is an excellent text integrating microbiologic, clinical, and pathologic features of infectious diseases. The classification of the Enterobacteriaceae, which is potentially confusing, is nicely sorted out in a chart by Ewing that is reproduced in the treatise by Sonnenwirth previously mentioned. The text by Gillies and Dodds contains many color photographs.

Bailey, W. R., and Scott, E. G.: Diagnostic microbiology: a textbook for the isolation and identification of pathogenic microorganisms, ed. 4, St. Louis, 1974, The C. V. Mosby Co.

Blair, J. E., Lennette, E. H., and Truant, J. P.: Manual of clinical microbiology, Bethesda, Md., 1970, American Society for Microbiology.

Davis, B. D., et al.: Microbiology, ed. 2, New York, 1973, Harper & Row, Publishers.

Gillies, R. R., and Dodds, T. C.: Bacteriology illustrated, Edinburgh, 1973, Churchill Livingstone.

Joklik, W. K., and Smith, D. T., editors: Zinsser microbiology, ed. 15, New York, 1972, Appleton-Century-Crofts.

Smith, L. D., and Holdeman, I. V.: The pathogenic anaerobic bacteria, Springfield, Ill., 1968, Charles C Thomas, Publisher.

Sonnenwirth, A. C.: Microbiology. In Frankel, S., Reitman, S., and Sonnenwirth, A. C., editors: Gradwohl's clinical laboratory methods and diagnosis, ed. 7, St. Louis, 1970, The C. V. Mosby Co.

GENERAL PRINCIPLES

■ **Describe the staining characteristics of gram-positive and gram-negative organisms.**

Gram-positive organisms are dark purple, and gram-negative organisms are orange-red.

■ **Why may gram-positive bacteria become gram-negative in old cultures?**

Autolytic enzymes attack the cell wall with resultant increased permeability that permits washout of the crystal violet–I_2 complex by acetone or alcohol.

■ **What is the principle of the methyl red test?**

Methyl red is an acid-base indicator that is red below pH 4.4 and yellow above pH 6.2. Organisms causing the mixed acid type of fermentation produce large amounts of formic, acetic, lactic, and succinic acids, and relatively little ethanol. The resultant acidification turns the indicator red. Organisms causing the butylene glycol type of fermentation produce relatively little acid and much more ethanol and 2,3-butylene glycol. This type of fermentation does not produce sufficient acid to color the indicator red.

■ **What is the principle of the Voges-Proskauer test, and how is it generally related to the methyl red test?**

Organisms causing the butylene glycol type of fermentation produce the intermediate product, acetoin (acetylmethylcarbinol), which is detectable by the Voges-Proskauer reaction. If one of the two tests, methyl red and Voges-Proskauer, is positive, the other usually is negative. However, a few organisms that form butylene glycol may produce sufficient acid to give a positive methyl red test, and a few organisms causing the mixed acid type of fermentation may ferment glucose slowly enough to give a negative methyl red test.

■ **What reagent is used to detect bacterial production of indole, and what precursor in the culture medium is necessary for its formation?**

Ehrlich's rosindole reagent, which is *p*-dimethylaminobenzaldehyde in hydrochloric acid and ethanol, is used. Red in the ether layer indicates presence of indole formed by bacteria from tryptophan.

■ **Describe Christensen's urea medium. What does it detect, and what is the appearance of a positive reaction?**

It is a peptone agar containing glucose, urea, and an acid-base indicator, phenol red. Urease hydrolyzes urea to ammonia and carbonic acid, thereby alkalinizing the medium and turning the indicator red.

■ **How much time is required for total sterilization (including resistant spores) under the following conditions: (1) steam at 15 pounds per square inch (psi) pressure (121° C), (2) dry heat (160° C), (3) boiling water at sea level pressure?**

1. 15 minutes
2. 1 hour
3. 2 hours or longer

■ **What is the appearance of spores stained by the Gram method?**

They appear as unstained holes in the bacteria.

■ **Is the following sequence of bacteriologic agar media arranged in order of increasing or decreasing selectivity for enteric pathogens: eosin-**

methylene blue, MacConkey, *Salmonella-Shigella* (SS), bismuth sulfite (Wilson-Blair), brilliant green?

The arrangement is in order of increasing selectivity.

■ **What is the principle of Simmons' citrate agar?**

The only source of nitrogen is the ammonium ion, and the sole source of carbon is citrate. A positive reaction is indicated by the appearance of colonies usually accompanied by alkalinization that turns the bromthymol blue indicator dark blue.

■ **What is the appearance of a positive reaction for hydrogen sulfide?**

The iron-containing culture medium blackens by formation of iron sulfide, or, by formation of lead sulfide, lead acetate paper suspended over the medium blackens.

■ **Describe the principle of the oxidation-fermentation (O-F) test medium of Hugh and Leifson.**

The medium contains peptone, minerals, 1% glucose, and bromthymol blue. Oxidative or fermentative utilization of glucose acidifies the medium, and the bromthymol blue indicator turns yellow.

■ **What reactions in the O-F medium indicate that a nonfermentative organism is an oxidizer?**

Oxidative acid production by a nonfermentative oxidizer results in a yellow open tube and a blue oil-covered tube.

■ **What is the significance of acid reactions in both open and closed O-F tubes?**

The organism ferments glucose, and the test is meaningless. The test is useful only when applied to nonfermenters.

■ **What are the appropriate media for blood cultures?**

Blood should be cultured both aerobically (brain heart infusion broth) and anaerobically (thioglycollate broth). When *Neisseria gonorrhoeae*, *N. meningitidis*, or *Brucella* organisms are suspected, the stopper of the aerobic bottle should be replaced with a cotton plug and incubated in 5% to 10% CO_2.

■ **How may a 5% concentration of CO_2 readily be achieved? Do anaerobic conditions result?**

The inoculated culture media are placed in a jar with a burning candle, and the jar is closed with an air-tight lid (the candle jar method). This system is not anaerobic; it cannot be used for culture of obligate anaerobes.

■ **What is Stuart's transport medium?**

It is a nonnutrient medium with low oxygen tension for maintaining viability of bacteria before culturing.

■ **Name three bacteria that must be incubated in 2% to 10% CO_2.**

1. *Neisseria gonorrhoeae*
2. *N. meningitidis*
3. *Brucella abortus*

■ **At what level of colony count are complete speciation and antibiotic sensitivity testing justified for bacteria isolated from voided urine?**

Complete speciation and sensitivity testing are justified when the colony count is 10^3/ml or higher in properly collected uncentrifuged specimens. When the colony count is lower than 10^3, the probability of contamination is greater than the probability of infection. A colony count of 10^5/ml or higher indicates infection with near certainty.[1,13]

■ **What test distinguishes bacteria in urine causing pyelonephritis from those causing cystitis only?**

Identification of human globulin on the surface of the bacteria by immunofluorescent technique indicates that the organisms are causing pyelonephritis. Absence of a surface coat of human globulin is consistent with cystitis.[12,21]

■ **What is the significance of a positive result of a cytochrome (indophenol) oxidase test?**

It is useful as a criterion for deciding whether organisms with Enterobacteriaceae-like but not entirely typical reactions actually are members of Enterobacteriaceae. Enterobacteriaceae give a negative cytochrome oxidase reaction, whereas members of the genera of *Aeromonas, Alcaligenes, Pseudomonas,* and *Vibrio* give positive reactions.

■ **What five kinds of bacteria, when contaminating food, are likely to cause food poisoning?**

Clostridium perfringens (live bacilli), *Staphylococcus aureus* (heat-stable exotoxin), *Salmonella* and *Shigella* species (live bacilli), and *C. botulinum* (heat-labile exotoxin) cause food poisoning when contaminating a variety of foods.[1] *Proteus morganii* causes poisoning by histamine production *(thermostable)* when contaminating scombroid fish.[16]

■ **What are the incubation periods of diarrhea secondary to staphylococcal enterotoxin, salmonellae, shigellae, enteropathogenic *Escherichia coli,* and *Vibrio cholerae?***

The incubation period is 4 to 8 hours for staphylococcal enterotoxin, 12 to 36 hours for salmonellae, and 24 to 72 hours for the other three agents.[11]

■ **What three bacteria are most often isolated from neonatal meningitis?**

Escherichia coli causes about 40%, beta-hemolytic streptococci cause about 30%, and *Listeria monocytogenes* causes 5% of cases of neonatal meningitis.[20]

■ **What are the four aerobes and four anaerobes that are most frequently cultured from intraabdominal infections?**

The most frequently cultured aerobes are *Escherichia coli* and aerobes of the genera *Klebsiella, Proteus,* and *Pseudomonas.* The most frequently cultured anaerobes are *Bacteroides fragilis,* clostridia, peptostreptococci, and peptococci.[8]

■ **What organisms are most often isolated from the infected gall bladder and biliary tract?**

The most frequently isolated organisms are *Escherichia coli* and other coliforms, facultative streptococci, *Clostridium perfringens,* and anaerobic streptococci.[8]

■ **Do cultures of intraabdominal infections usually yield a single organism or a mixture of aerobes and anaerobes?**

Cultures of intraabdominal infections yield an average of five organisms: two aerobes and three anaerobes.[8]

■ **What are R factors, and what role do they play in resistance of bacteria to antibiotics?**

R factors are extrachromosomal genetic elements (episomes) that replicate autonomously in host cells. They can be transferred by bacterial conjugation to essentially all members of the Enterobacteriaceae and can thereby transfer resistance to multiple antibiotics.[5]

ANAEROBES

■ **What specimens are appropriate for anaerobic culture?**

Normally sterile body fluids, abscesses, deep aspirates of wounds, and blood are the most frequent appropriate fluids. Saliva, throat swabs, expectorated sputum, vaginal secretions and feces are among the specimens that are unsatisfactory because of contamination with commensal anaerobes, and urine and cerebrospinal fluid are seldom worth culturing because of infrequency of recovery of anaerobes from them.[10]

■ **What proportions of specimens appropriate for anaerobic culture yield anaerobes when thioglycollate broth is the only anaerobic medium and when the GasPak anaerobic jar technic is used?**

With thioglycollate alone, the incidence of recovery of anaerobes is about 3%. With the GasPak anaerobic jar method, the yield is about 25%. It can be increased to 35% with bedside inoculation of prereduced medium and other specialized technics.[10]

■ **Describe a method for developing an anaerobic culture.**

Flushing with nitrogen or hydrogen is one common method. The airtight jar is evacuated to 0.1 atmosphere or less pressure and then filled with nitrogen or hydrogen. This procedure is repeated for a total of five replacements, with the final filling consisting of 10% CO_2 in N_2 or H_2.

Another common method is the Brewer jar with disposable H_2 and CO_2

generator and catalyst (GasPak) for conversion of H_2 and O_2 to H_2O. A methylene blue indicator becomes colorless when anaerobicity is achieved. This method is well suited to the smaller laboratory.

■ **Describe a method for selective culture of anaerobic spore-forming bacilli.**

Inoculate thioglycollate. Destroy vegetative bacteria by placing in 80° C water bath for 10 to 15 minutes. Then incubate at 37° C.

■ **Name four diseases that are caused by clostridia.**

Wound infections with viable organisms, most often *C. perfringens,* cause gas gangrene; ingestion of *C. perfringens* in food causes a severe jejunitis[1]; wound infections with *C. tetani* causes the intoxication known as tetanus; ingestion of food contaminated with *C. botulinum* causes the intoxication known as botulinism.

■ **What is this large, slightly curved, gram-positive anaerobic rod with terminal spore?**

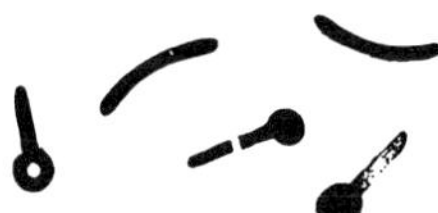

It is *Clostridium tetani.*

■ **What is this anaerobic, gram-positive rod with subterminal and free spores?**

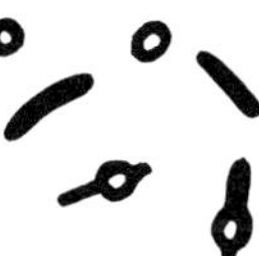

It is *C. botulinum.*

■ **How long must *Clostridium botulinum* be boiled to kill spores?**

It must be boiled several hours at 760 mm Hg pressure.

■ **What is the minimal procedure for culture of clostridia?**

Thioglycollate and anaerobic blood agar controlled with aerobic blood agar must be used.

■ **Which of the clostridia produce stormy fermentation of iron-milk?**

C. butyricum and most strains of *C. perfringens* produce such fermentation, and it occurs within 24 hours of inoculation.

■ **Is the exotoxin of *C. botulinum* destroyed by heating to 100° C for 10 minutes?**

Yes.

■ **Identify the anaerobic organisms shown below that may be seen in gram-stained smears from infected tissues.**

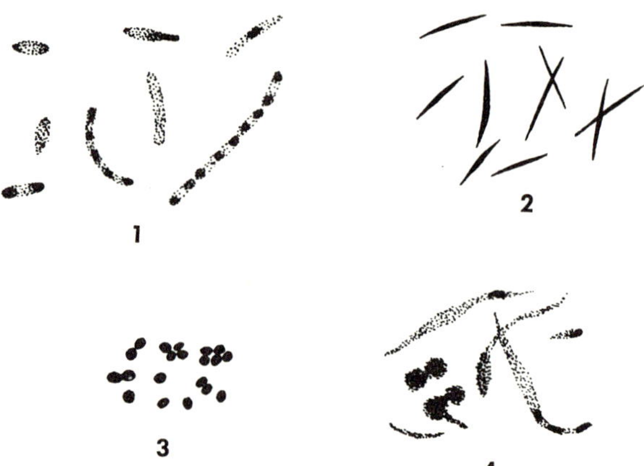

1. *Bacteroides fragilis*
2. *Fusobacterium fusiforme*
3. *Bacteroides melaninogenicus*
4. *Fusobacterium sphaerophorus necrophorus*

■ **To what genus do the most numerous colonic bacteria belong?**

They belong to the genus *Bacteroides*. *B. fragilis* is usually the most numerous, and *B. melaninogenicus* is often present in smaller numbers.

■ **What two atmospheric conditions are necessary for culture of *Bacteroides* species?**

Anaerobicity and 5% to 10% CO_2 are necessary.

■ **What is the role of *Bacteroides* organisms in the blind loop malabsorption syndrome?**

Bacteroides organisms are commonly present in the blind loop in concentrations similar to those in feces (10^9 organisms per gram). This organism is capable of deconjugating bile salts and thereby interferes with absorption of fats. Antibiotic therapy that eliminates the *Bacteroides* organisms from the loop corrects the malabsorption.

■ **How do the growth requirements of "moderate" anaerobes differ from the requirements of "fastidious" anaerobes?**

Moderate anaerobes will grow in the presence of 2% to 8% oxygen concentrations and will survive exposure to atmospheric air for 60 to 90 minutes. Fastidious anaerobes will not grow on artificial media in presence of oxygen levels in excess of 0.5% and are killed by exposure of air for 10 minutes or less. The moderate anaerobes include many strains of *Bacteroides fragilis, B. oralis, B. melaninogenicus, Fusobacterium nucleatum,* and many strains of peptostreptococci. Fastidious anaerobes include certain strains of *Bacteroides fragilis, Bifidobacterium adolescentis,* spirochetes, and some peptostreptococci.[10]

■ **Which are the more important pathogens, the moderate anaerobes or the fastidious anaerobes?**

The moderate anaerobes appear to be the more important group of pathogens.[10]

■ **What are the most abundant organisms in saliva?**

The most abundant organisms in saliva are the anaerobes peptostreptococci, peptococci, *Fusobacterium nucleatum, Bacteroides melaninogenicus, B. oralis, Veillonella* species, and spirochetes.[9]

■ **Which organisms are most commonly isolated from primary lung abscesses?**

The same anaerobes normally found in saliva account for about 85% of primary lung abscesses.[9]

■ **What proportion of bacteremias are anaerobic?**

Anaerobes account for about 10% of bacteremias.[4,9]

■ **Which organism is the most frequent anaerobic pathogen in abdominal and female pelvic infections?**

B. fragilis is the most frequent anaerobic pathogen isolated from these infections.[10]

■ **Why have from 40% to 60% of liver abscesses cultured in the past been reported as sterile?**

They were reported as sterile because they were not cultured adequately for anaerobes. The great majority of liver abscesses harbor anaerobes, frequently in the absence of aerobes.[10]

■ **What accounts for the ability of a normally nonpathogenic, microaerophilic, nonhemolytic streptococcus to produce necrotizing fascitis when infecting wounds in association with *Staphylococcus aureus*?**

The staphylococcus produces hyaluronidase and an unidentified heat-labile growth factor.[10]

■ **Necrotizing lesions of mucous membranes often yield a growth of *B. melaninogenicus*, other strains of bacteroides, and a facultative diphtheroid. What is the role of the diphtheroid?**

The diphtheroid produces vitamin K, which is necessary for the pathogenicity of *B. melaninogenicus*.[10]

■ **Name three sites of infections caused by *Actinomyces israelii*.**

Infections with *A. israelii* usually affect one of three regions: cervicofacial, pulmonary, and ileocecal. Chronic abscesses and fistulas characterize the infection.

■ **How are infections with *A. israelii* acquired?**

They are acquired endogenously. The organisms are found in the normal mouth, tonsils, and intestine, and are opportunistic invaders.

■ **What is the appearance of *A. israelii* in pus from infected tissues?**

Grossly the organisms form small yellowish "sulfur" granules. Microscopically these granules consist of a mat of filaments 1 μm or less in diameter with clubbed ends. They are gram-positive and are not acid-fast.

■ **How should *Actinomyces* species be cultured?**

They will grow only anaerobically. Thioglycollate tubes and brain-heart infusion agar plates incubated anaerobically should be used.

■ **What common anaerobic gram-positive pleomorphic rods are likely to be confused with *Actinomyces* organisms, and how can they be differentiated?**

Anaerobic diphtheroids and *Propionibacterium (Corynebacterium) acnes*. These organisms are widely distributed on human skin. Unlike *Actinomyces* organisms, diphtheroids and *Propionibacterium* species produce catalase and indole.

■ **What organism does *Arachnia propionica* closely resemble in clinical manifestations and cultural characteristics?**

A. propionica resembles *Actinomyces israelii*, but *A. propionica* ferments neither arabinose or xylose (*A. israelii* ferments either or both), contains diaminopimelic acid in its cell wall, and produces large amounts of propionic acid from glucose.[2]

■ **What is Döderlein's bacillus?**

Döderlein's bacillus is any of a variety of strains of *Lactobacillus* isolated from the vagina. Lactobacilli are microaerophilic or anaerobic, fermentative, nonmotile gram-positive rods. They produce lactic acid from glucose and other carbohydrates.

BRUCELLAE

■ **Describe the morphology and gram-staining of brucellae.**

Brucellae are short, slender, pleomorphic, gram-negative coccobacilli.

■ ***Brucella abortus, B. suis,* and *B. melitensis* can each cause acute, subacute, or chronic granulomatous infections (undulant fever) in man. In what animal does each organism characteristically cause disease?**

B. abortus infects cattle, *B. suis* infects pigs, and *B. melitensis* infects goats and sheep. However, a wide variety of animals is susceptible to each organism.

■ **What material ordinarily should be cultured when brucellosis is suspected?**

Blood and bone marrow should be cultured.

■ **Do brucellae grow well on ordinary media?**

They do not usually grow well.

■ **What media should be used to culture *Brucella* organisms?**

Albimi, trypticase soy medium, or a Castaneda bottle should be used.

■ **Which of the *Brucella* species requires a 5% to 10% CO_2 atmosphere for isolation?**

B. abortus requires it. The other *Brucella* species grow better with added CO_2 but do not absolutely require it.

■ **Which of the *Brucella* species are inhibited by 1:50,000 thionine or 1:50,000 basic fuchsin?**

B. abortus is usually inhibited by thionine, *B. suis* by basic fuchsin, and *B. melitensis* by neither.

ENTEROBACTERIACEAE

■ **Which organisms are classified in the family Enterobacteriaceae?**

Gram-negative, nonspore-forming rods that utilize carbohydrates fermentatively, reduce nitrates to nitrites, and lack cytochrome oxidase are classified in the Enterobacteriaceae.

■ **Define the H, O, and K antigens of enteric bacilli. Which are inactivated by heat?**

H antigens are flagellar and are inactivated at 100° C. O antigens are somatic and are not inactivated at 100° C. K antigens are also somatic but cover and obscure the O antigens. K antigens are inactivated at 100° C, and the O antigens then are reactive.

■ **Give the concentrations of sugars and the two indicators in triple sugar iron (TSI) agar.**

The concentrations are lactose and sucrose each 1% and glucose 0.1%; the indicators are ferrous sulfate and phenol red. Organisms fermenting only glucose produce an initially acid (yellow) slant that becomes basic by 24 hours as the glucose is utilized and noncarbohydrate constituents are attacked aerobically. If the organism ferments lactose or sucrose, the slant remains acid for at least 24 hours because of the relatively large amounts of those carbohydrates in the medium. If H_2S is produced, the medium turns black.

■ **Which of the lactose nonfermenting Enterobacteriaceae ferment sucrose?**

Proteus vulgaris, some strains of *P. mirabilis* and *P. rettgeri*, and *Providencia*, *Serratia*, and *Citrobacter* species ferment sucrose.

■ **Name the pathogens that might be responsible for TSI appearances of (1) yellow butt, no gas, red slant, and no blackening; (2) yellow butt, gas, red slant, and no blackening; and (3) yellow butt, gas, red slant, and blackening.**

1. Shigellae, *S. typhi* strains that do not produce H_2S
2. H_2S-negative strains of *S. paratyphi A, S. cholerasuis,* some *Shigella flexneri*
3. Most salmonellae, *Arizona* species

■ **Name the inhibitory agent, the carbohydrate, and the pH indicator in MacConkey agar.**

1. Bile salts
2. Lactose
3. Neutral red (The pH range of neutral red is 6.8 to 8.0. It is red at lower pH and yellow at higher pH. Lactose fermenters will produce red colonies.)

■ **Name four members of Enterobacteriaceae that are slow lactose fermenters.**

1. *Shigella sonnei*
2. *Arizona* species
3. *Citrobacter* species
4. *Serratia* species

■ **How is the *Arizona* group distinguished from the salmonellae?**

Members of the *Arizona* group possess β-galactosidase, liquefy gelatin, and utilize malonate.

■ **What is the pH indicator in brilliant green agar?**

The indicator is phenol red. Its pH range is 6.4 to 8.0. It is red in alkali, yellow in acid.

■ **What color indicates that a colony on brilliant green agar may be that of a pathogen?**

Pink or red is the indication, since salmonellae fail to produce acid from either lactose or sucrose.

■ **Give characteristics of colonies of the following organisms grown on brilliant green agar: (1) *Escherichia coli,* (2) *Salmonella typhi,* (3) *S. paratyphi,* (4) *Klebsiella,* (5) *Proteus vulgaris.***

1. Yellow-green
2. Pink, transparent
3. Transparent to deep fuchsia
4. Yellow-green
5. Small, reddish (usually inhibited)

■ **Which enteric pathogens are most easily inhibited by brilliant green?**

Shigella dysenteriae and *S. boydii* are most easily inhibited. *Salmonella typhi* grows poorly on it.

■ **Explain the rationale of lysine iron agar.**

Lysine iron agar contains 0.1% glucose, 1% L-lysine, ferric ammonium citrate for detection of H_2S, and the pH indicator bromcresyl purple (yellow in acid, purple in alkali). Organisms capable of decarboxylating lysine produce an alkaline slant (purple) and an alkaline or acid (yellow) butt. If H_2S is produced, the medium turns black. *Proteus morganii, P. rettgeri,* and *Providencia* organisms deaminate lysine and do not produce H_2S. This condition results in a characteristic red slant over a yellow butt.

■ **What is the appearance of colonies of *Shigella* and *Salmonella* organisms on the following agar media: eosin-methylene blue, MacConkey, deoxycholate, *Salmonella-Shigella* (SS), and bismuth sulfite (Wilson-Blair)?**

They are translucent and colorless on eosin-methylene blue (EMB), MacConkey, and deoxycholate. On SS agar they are opaque, translucent, transparent and colorless, or centrally black (some salmonellae). *Salmonella typhi* colonies on bismuth sulfite agar typically are black surrounded by a dark halo. Other salmonellae are black, green, or brownish, and shigellae do not grow.

■ **Eosin-methylene blue (EMB), *Salmonella-Shigella* (SS), brilliant green (BG), bismuth sulfite-iron (BS), and xylose-lysine-deoxycholate (XLD) agars are used to isolate gram-negative rods. Which are the best for (1) *Salmonella typhi*, (2) shigellae, (3) most salmonellae other than *S. typhi*?**

1. SS, BS, XLD for *S. typhi*
2. SS, XLD for shigellae
3. BG for most salmonellae other than *S. typhi*

Brilliant green agar is the most inhibitory and for that reason is not suitable for *Shigella* species and *Salmonella typhi*. *S. typhi* grows particularly well on BS agar.

■ **Describe XLD agar and explain the significance of its ingredients.**

Xylose is the fermentable carbohydrate. All enteric pathogens ferment xylose except for shigellae, *Providencia* species, Asakusa group, *Proteus morgani,* and *P. rettgeri*. The excess amino acid is lysine. The xylose/lysine ratio is adjusted so that salmonellae and *Arizona* organisms will exhaust the xylose and attack the lysine within 24 hours, thereby changing the color from yellow to red. The indicators are phenol red for pH (yellow in acid, red in base) and ferric ammonium citrate for H_2S. The inhibitor is sodium deoxycholate.

■ **What types of colonies on XLD agar should be subcultured because they may represent pathogens?**

Red colonies with or without black centers should be subcultured.

■ **Bismuth sulfite and SS agar cultures may be interpreted after 48 hours. Is the same true of XLD agar?**

It is not true, because alkaline reversion and blackening may occur with nonpathogens after 24 hours.

■ **Which organisms of the family Enterobacteriaceae are methyl red positive and Voges-Proskauer negative, and which are methyl red negative and Voges-Proskauer positive?**

1. MR positive, VP negative: *Escherichia coli, Shigella, Salmonella, Arizona, Citrobacter, Proteus, Providencia, Edwardsiella* (Some *P. mirabilis* organisms are VP positive.)
2. MR negative, VP positive: *Klebsiella, Enterobacter cloacae, E. aerogenes, Serratia*
3. Variable reactions: *Enterobacter liquefaciens, E. hafniae*

■ **How is the phenylalanine test performed, and which of the Enterobacteriaceae give a positive result?**

A medium containing 0.2% DL-phenylalanine is inoculated. It is treated with 10% ferric chloride in 0.1N hydrochloric acid 24 hours later. A green color that fades within half an hour indicates deamination of phenylalanine to form phenylpyruvic acid. Note the analogy with the ferric chloride test of urine for phenylketonuria. Only *Proteus* and *Providencia* organisms give positive results, and a positive phenylalanine test result is a prerequisite for their classification.

■ **What is the indicator in urease medium, and which of the following organisms are urease positive: (1) *Escherichia coli*, (2) *Hafnia*, (3) *Serratia*, (4) *Proteus*, (5) *Providencia?***

The indicator is phenol red. *Proteus* species are urease positive (red).

■ **A positive reaction on Cristensen's urease agar within 6 hours indicates that the organism is a member of which genus?**

It is a member of the genus *Proteus*.

■ **Identify a lactose fermenter that is methyl red positive, indole positive, and citrate negative.**

These criteria indicate *Escherichia coli*.

■ **What is the sequence of reactions in an amino acid decarboxylation medium and what is the indicator?**

First the carbohydrate (glucose) is attacked, rendering the medium acid. Then decarboxylation of the amino acid renders it basic. The indicator is bromcresol purple, which has a pH range of 5.2 to 6.8 and is yellow in acid and purple in alkali.

■ **What property distinguishes *Shigella* species, *Klebsiella* species, and the**

Alkalescens-Dispar group from other members of the family Enterobacteriaceae?

They are the only nonmotile members of the family.

■ **Which antigens are used for the serotyping of enteropathogenic *Escherichia coli?***

The O (somatic, heat stable) and K (surface) antigens are used. The K antigen exists as three types: the heat-labile L antigen; the heat-stable A antigen; and the B antigen, which is partially heat stable. Enteropathogenic *E. coli* have the B antigen.

■ **Describe the technic for performing K antigen slide agglutination test for enteropathogenic *E. coli*.**

Emulsify part of a colony from MacConkey agar in a drop of saline. Under a dissecting microscope, mix with a drop of polyvalent antiserum. Clumping during active mixing indicates agglutination.

■ **Which antigen has been found in about 85% of *Escherichia coli* isolates from meningitis in neonatal infants?**

The K1 capsular polysaccharide antigen, immunochemically identical to the meningococcal group B polysaccharide, has been found in nearly 85% of isolates from neonatal meningitis. The K1 capsular polysaccharide seems to be related to invasiveness.[20]

■ **Describe three characteristics of *Shigella* organisms that differentiate them from *Escherichia coli* in the laboratory.**

Shigella organisms are nonmotile, fail to ferment lactose (*S. sonnei* ferments lactose slowly), and produce no gas. (*S. flexneri* may produce gas from glucose.)

■ **What are Alkalescens-Dispar organisms?**

They are nonmotile, nongas-producing *Escherichia coli*. A typing serum for the Alkalescens-Dispar group is useful in differentiating them from shigellae.

■ **How are the four groups of *Shigella* organisms identified?**

They are identified by polyvalent grouping antisera (O antigen). A presumptive grouping can be done biochemically. For example, group A *(Shigella dysenteriae)* failed to ferment mannitol; and group D *(Shigella sonnei)* is indole negative, decarboxylates ornithine, and ferments lactose slowly.

■ **Which species of *Shigella* is the most virulent (up to 15% fatality rate without antibiotic treatment) and grows poorly on SS agar but well on XLD and MacConkey agar?**

S. dysenteriae (shiga bacillus) fits the above description.[7]

■ **A suspected *Shigella* organism is tested with anti-O sera for each of the** four species and the Alkalescens-Dispar group. Saline suspensions of the live organisms are used, and they fail to agglutinate with any of the antisera. What should be done next?

Repeat the typing procedure with saline suspensions of organisms heated for an hour in boiling water to remove interfering surface (K) antigens.

■ **When can positive blood cultures be obtained in the course of typhoid fever?**

They can usually be obtained during the first week of the disease. Organisms disappear from the blood by the end of second week.

■ **When in the course of typhoid fever are stool cultures positive?**

They are positive from the end of the first week until completion of convalescence (and indefinitely in those who become asymptomatic carriers).

■ *Salmonella typhi* **and some other salmonellae may have the Vi antigen. How does it interfere with their agglutinability with O antisera?**

The Vi antigen coats the surface and renders the organism inagglutinable with O antisera. It can be destroyed by heating at 100° C for 15 minutes. The organisms can then be agglutinated with O antisera.

■ **What biochemical properties distinguish** *Citrobacter* **organisms from** *Salmonella* **and** *Arizona* **organisms?**

Citrobacter organisms grow in presence of KCN and fail to decarboxylate lysine.

■ **Identify the organism that has the following characteristics: TSI acid butt with gas, acid slant, indole negative, methyl red positive, H_2S positive, motile, urease negative, decarboxylates arginine and ornithine but not lysine, utilizes citrate, and grows in KCN.**

The organism is a *Citrobacter* species.

■ **1. Identify the organism that has the following characteristics: TSI acid slant, acid butt with gas, no H_2S, indole negative, methyl red negative, utilizes citrate, decarboxylates arginine and ornithine but not lysine, motile.**
   2. If it decarboxylates only lysine and is nonmotile, what is it?

   1. *Enterobacter cloacae*
   2. *Klebsiella* species

■ **Identify the organism that is a nonpigmented lactose nonfermenter or late fermenter that may or may not ferment sucrose, fails to ferment arabinose, rhamnose, and raffinose, decarboxylates lysine and ornithine but not arginine, and otherwise resembles an** *Enterobacter* **organism. It is isolated from the blood of a patient with a chronic, debilitating disease.**

The organism is a *Serratia* species. Most strains are nonpigmented when grown at 37° C. Pigment production may occur when cultures are held at room temperature.

■ **Describe two characteristics of *Proteus mirabilis* that set it apart from other species of *Proteus*.**

It is indole negative and is usually sensitive to penicillin.

■ **Rhinoscleroma, a chronic, tumefactive process involving the nasal and oral mucosae with numerous vacuolated histiocytes that contain bacilli, is caused by what organism?**

Klebsiella rhinoscleromatis causes rhinoscleroma.

■ **Which organisms formerly were classified as paracolons?**

Citrobacter, Arizona, and *Hafnia* organisms were formerly classified as paracolons.

■ **What is the natural host of *Vibrio cholerae*?**

It is found only in the intestine of man.

■ **What media are suitable for culture of *V. cholerae*?**

The organisms grow on ordinary laboratory media, but if a fermentable carbohydrate is present they die as a result of acidification. They grow well at an alkaline pH, up to 9.6 (Ewing's or Monsur's agar).

■ **How may a rapid presumptive diagnosis of cholera be made?**

It may be made by finding gram-negative, comma-shaped organisms 2 to 4 μm long in a watery stool free of fecal matter (rice-water stool).

■ **Describe the cholera red test.**

Grow organisms in tryptone nitrate or peptone broth for 2 to 3 days, and then add concentrated sulfuric acid. Red indicates a positive reaction. This color results from the combination of indole with nitrite.

■ **Is the cholera red test specific for *V. cholerae*?**

No. Other species of *Vibrio* will also give positive test results.

■ **What are the reactions produced by *V. cholerae* on TSI agar?**

Alkaline slant, acid butt, no gas, and no H_2S are the reactions.

■ **How is the diagnosis of *V. cholerae* confirmed?**

Diagnosis is confirmed by slide agglutination using polyvalent antiserum. A serologic diagnosis can be made from the patient's serum in convalescent cases. Antibodies appear on the fourth day and reach a peak on the seventh day after onset of illness.

FRANCISELLA, YERSINIA, AND PASTEURELLA

■ **Describe the morphology of *Francisella (Pasteurella) tularensis*.**

F. tularensis is a short, unencapsulated, markedly pleomorphic gram-negative bacillus.

■ **In a patient with ulceroglandular tularemia, which two of the following procedures are most likely to demonstrate the infectious organism *Francisella tularensis*?**
1. **Direct smear of lesion with Gram stain**
2. **Blood culture**
3. **Culture of lesion on Francis' glucose-cystine blood agar under 10% CO_2 with added penicillin, polymyxin B, and nystatin**
4. **Inoculation of mice and guinea pigs**

Culture of the lesion and inoculation of mice and guinea pigs (3 and 4 above) will provide the most likely demonstration. Ordinary gram-stained smears of exudate are useless, but a diagnosis can be made with specific fluorescent antisera.

■ **In an ordinary bacteriology laboratory, should isolation of *Francisella tularensis* be attempted?**

It should not, because the organism is dangerous and penetrates unbroken skin.

■ **Give characteristics of genus *Yersinia* (formerly included in *Pasteurella*).**

Yersinia organisms are pleomorphic, gram-negative coccobacilli that sometimes form filaments and are catalase positive and methyl red positive. There is no fermentation of lactose; acid but not gas is produced from glucose and mannitol. The three main species are differentiated by fermentation of sugars. There is variable production of H_2S, indole, and urease. All species are nonmotile at 37° C, but *Y. pseudotuberculosis* and *Y. enterocolitica* are motile at 22° C. All species are lethal for laboratory animals on intraperitoneal inoculation.

■ **Can *Yersinia* and *Pasteurella* organisms be distinguished by the oxidase reaction?**

Yes. *Yersinia* organisms are oxidase negative, but *Pasteurella* organisms are oxidase positive.

■ **What is the proper method for making a presumptive diagnosis of plague?**

Aspirate involved lymph node (bubo), and examine for gram-negative rods with bipolar staining.

■ **The terms "beaten copper" and "fried egg" characterize the colonial morphology of which organism?**

These descriptions indicate *Yersinia pestis*.

■ **What is the microscopic morphology of *Y. pestis?***

It is a bipolar staining coccobacillus 0.5 to 0.7 $\times$ 1.5 to 1.75 μm. The capsule can be demonstrated by fluorescent antibody or India ink.

■ **Describe three forms of plague in human beings. What is the rodent-human vector?**

The three forms are bubonic, septicemic, and pneumonic (human-human spread). The vector is any of several *Siphonaptera* (flea) species.

■ **Deoxycholate agar is a good isolation medium for what two species of the genus *Yersinia?***

It is a good isolation medium for *Y. pestis* and *Y. pseudotuberculosis.*

■ **A gram-negative bacillus that grows well on MacConkey agar shows in TSI acid butt, alkaline slant, and no gas or H_2S. If it produces urease (delayed reaction) but does not deaminate phenylalanine, what might the organism be?**

These characteristics probably indicate *Y. pseudotuberculosis.* (An allied organism, *Y. enterocolitica,* differs in that it ferments sucrose and gives acid butt and acid slant with TSI.)

■ **Which organisms are likely to be cultured from benign mesenteric lymphadenitis?**

Y. pseudotuberculosis and *Y. enterocolitica* are the most likely organisms.

■ **From what human sources is *P. multocida* most often isolated?**

It is most often isolated from sputum (bronchiectasis), nasal mucosa (carriers), and animal bites.

GRAM-POSITIVE AEROBIC BACILLI

■ **What type of culture medium is used to isolate *Corynebacterium diphtheriae?* How are the colonies recognized on the medium, and what is the chemical basis for the identifying characteristic?**

Tinsdale or another tellurite-containing medium is used. The colonies are smooth, gray-black, and shiny; and after 24 to 48 hours they are surrounded by a brownish black zone or halo resulting from reduction of tellurite to tellurium. Nonpathogenic diphtheroids lack halos.

■ **What other media are used for culturing *C. diphtheriae?***

Loeffler and Pai media are also used.

■ **Name the three strains of *C. diphtheriae* grown on tellurite-containing medium in order of descending colony size.**

1. Gravis (2 to 4 mm; flat, dry, dull)
2. Mitis (1 to 2 mm; convex, moist)

3. Intermedius (0.5 mm or less; flat, dry)

All three strains can produce toxin, but the gravis strain carries the highest mortality.

■ Describe the typical morphology of *C. diphtheriae*.

The organisms are slender nonsporulating, nonflagellated, pleomorphic gram-positive rods, often with swollen ends (snowshoe forms). They tend to be arranged in palisade or "Chinese letter" formations, and contain metachromatic polyphosphate granules when stained with methylene blue after growth on phosphate-rich Loeffler's medium.

■ Does the pathogenicity of *C. diphtheriae* depend on invasion of the tissues and blood stream or on some other factor?

C. diphtheriae grow only superficially and produce inflammatory cells and a pseudomembrane of fibrin, which can produce serious obstruction of the airway. It does not invade the bloodstream. Its pathogenicity is dependent on a powerful exotoxin that is produced only by strains infected with the B bacteriophage.

■ How can *C. diphtheriae* organisms be tested for virulence?

1. They can be tested in vitro by streaking the organisms perpendicularly across an antitoxin-impregnated strip of filter paper on Elek-King diffusion agar and examining for a precipitin line at an angle of 45 degrees to the streak.
2. They can also be tested by intradermal injection of 24-hour meat infusion broth culture into a guinea pig or rabbit (rats and mice are resistant to the toxin). Two intradermal injections are given spaced 6 hours apart, and 30 minutes before the second injection 500 to 1000 units of diphtheria antitoxin is given intravenously or intraperitoneally. If the strain is toxigenic, necrosis will develop at the site of the first injection.

■ What is the Schick test, and what is the significance of a positive reaction?

One forearm is injected with 0.1 ml of dilute *C. diphtheriae* toxin, and the opposite forearm is injected with a similar amount of heat-activated toxin. Redness and induration appearing after 24 to 36 hours at the first injection site only and reaching a maximum in approximately 5 days constitute a positive reaction and signify susceptibility to diphtheria.

■ What two gram-positive rod-shaped organisms growing aerobically on blood agar can produce beta-hemolysis?

Beta-hemolysis can be produced by diphtheroids and *Listeria monocytogenes*.

■ What gram-positive, aerobic, rod-shaped organisms can cause abortion,

neonatal sepsis, an infectious monocytosis-like illness with negative heterophil antibody test, meningitis, and may complicate malignant disease?

This description indicates *Listeria monocytogenes.*

- **How can *Listeria monocytogenes* rapidly be distinguished from diphtheroids?**

L. monocytogenes is motile, and diphtheroids are nonmotile at room temperature.

- **Name the only species of the genus *Bacillus* that is highly pathogenic for man.**

B. anthracis, a large, spore-forming, gram-positive rod, is the cause of anthrax.

- **Describe two ways of distinguishing *Bacillus anthracis* from *B. subtilis.***

B. anthracis is nonmotile and pathogenic for guinea pigs.

- **Describe a colony of *B. anthracis* seen under the dissecting microscope.**

It is dull and gray with outgrowths of recurved chains of bacilli (Medusa-head).

- **Does *B. anthracis* form spores in vivo?**

It does not, but it forms central spores in vitro and in dead animals.

- **What cultural conditions are suitable for *Nocardia asteroides?***

Blood agar and Sabouraud glucose agar at 37° C and room temperature are suitable.

- **What are the microscopic features of *Nocardia* species and their staining reactions?**

They are gram-positive, branching filaments not more than 1 μm in diameter and may or may not have clubbed ends. *N. asteroides* and *N. brasiliensis* are partially acid fast. To demonstrate acid fastness, they should be decolorized with 1% H_2SO_4 without ethanol. Acid alcohol may be too effective a decolorizing agent.

- **Where are *Nocardia* species normally found? Is nocardiosis contagious?**

They are found in the soil. Nocardiosis is not contagious.

- **Describe three clinical forms of nocardiosis. What type of inflammatory reaction occurs?**

  1. Subcutaneous mycetoma that may extend to deep structures including bone
  2. Pulmonary
  3. Disseminated

Nocardia organisms cause an acute inflammatory response.

■ **How can *Nocardia* organisms be distinguished from atypical acid-fast bacteria?**

Nocardia organisms grow more rapidly than atypical acid-fast bacteria of groups I to III, they branch, and they are less acid fast than the mycobacteria.

HAEMOPHILUS AND BORDETELLA

■ **Describe the morphology of *Haemophilus influenzae*.**

H. influenzae is a small, pleomorphic gram-negative rod. Pathogenic strains have capsules.

■ **Which two growth factor requirements distinguish *H. influenzae* from most other pyogenic bacteria?**

Factors V and X are required in aerobic culture; factor V alone is required in anaerobic culture.

■ **What are factors V and X, and what medium is commonly used to supply them?**

Factor V is nicotinamide adenine dinucleotide (NAD, previously named DPN) or nicotinamide adenine dinucleotide phosphate (NADP, previously named TPN). Factor X is hemin (ferriprotoporphyrin). It apparently is necessary only for formation of heme-containing enzymes used in aerobic metabolism. Both factors V and X are supplied by chocolate agar.

■ **Describe and explain the "satellite" phenomenon of *H. influenzae* growth.**

On media deficient in factor V, *H. influenzae* will grow only around the colonies of *Staphylococcus aureus*, which supply factor V.

■ **What is the most important disease caused by *H. influenzae*?**

It is meningitis in young children and infants.

■ **How can *H. parainfluenzae* be distinguished from *H. influenzae*?**

H. parainfluenzae will exhibit the satellite phenomenon on plain nutrient agar (no blood added) because it does not require factor X for aerobic growth.

■ **What is the organism most commonly causing bacterial meningitis in children 3 to 5 years of age?**

It is *H. influenzae*.

■ **Which organism causes chancroid?**

H. ducreyi causes chancroid.

■ **What is the most practical method for diagnosis of *H. ducreyi*?**

Examine a gram-stained smear of the lesion for small, ovoid gram-negative rods in pairs or chains and grouped like a school of fish. Confirmation by culture requires specialized methods.

■ **How does *H. ducreyi* differ from *H. parainfluenzae?***

H. ducreyi is the only member of *Haemophilus* that does not reduce nitrates. Furthermore, *H. parainfluenzae* requires factor V but not factor X, whereas *H. ducreyi* requires factor X but not factor V.

■ **How does *H. aegyptius* differ from *H. influenzae?***

H. aegyptius agglutinates red blood cells strongly, whereas *H. influenzae* agglutinates them weakly. Both require X and V factors.

■ **What are the distinguishing characteristics of the genus *Bordetella?***

Members of this genus require nicotinamide but not X and V factors. They are gram-negative rods or coccobacilli, nonsaccharolytic, and catalase positive.

■ **Are any members of the genus *Bordetella* likely to be isolated on ordinary laboratory media?**

B. bronchiseptica is likely to be isolated.

■ **How is *B. pertussis,* the cause of whooping cough, cultured and identified?**

Bordet-Gengou (potato-glycerin-blood) agar is used as a cough plate or is inoculated with posterior pharyngeal swab. The inoculum is spread with a drop of penicillin solution to inhibit normal flora. Colonies resembling mercury droplets appear after 4 to 5 days at 35° to 37° C. Identity can be confirmed by agglutination with specific antiserum.

■ **How can a definitive bacteriologic diagnosis of whooping cough be made much more rapidly?**

The diagnosis can be made by staining of the organisms in a nasopharyngeal smear with fluorescein-labeled antibody.

MYCOBACTERIA

■ **Describe the essentials of the acid-fast stain.**

The organisms are stained with the help of heat and/or phenol or detergents to facilitate penetration. In the classic Ziehl-Neelsen technic, carbol fuchsin and heat are used. The organisms are then decolorized with 3% concentrated HCl in 95% ethanol for a few seconds and counterstained (usually with methylene blue). The acid-fast organisms retain the fuchsin dye and appear red.

■ **What causes the beaded appearance of *Mycobacterium tuberculosis* after acid-fast staining?**

M. tuberculosis contains glycogen granules and polymetaphosphate (volutin) bodies that cause irregularity of staining.

■ **Most pathogenic bacteria are facultative aerobes or anaerobes. What is *M. tuberculosis?***

It is an obligate aerobe.

■ **Give distinguishing characteristics of three types of media used to grow mycobacteria, and cite examples.**

1. Liquid medium: Dubos' Tween 80 (polyoxyethylene sorbitan monooleate) albumin medium
2. Solid semisynthetic medium: Middlebrook-Cohn 7H-10 medium
3. Solid egg media: Lowenstein-Jensen and Petragnani media

■ **How long must tubercle bacilli (*M. tuberculosis*) be incubated before colonies appear?**

Colonies usually appear on the solid media by 3 to 4 weeks. Organisms may be found in sediment of liquid media somewhat sooner. The doubling time of tubercle bacilli in optimum cultural conditions is 12 hours, whereas most other bacteria have doubling times of 20 to 30 minutes.

■ **What is the neutral red test?**

It is a test for virulence. Virulent strains take up the dye when colonies are suspended in an alkaline solution of neutral red, whereas avirulent strains fail to be colored.

■ **Describe the colonies of *M. tuberculosis* on solid media as seen with the naked eye.**

The colonies are rough, dry-appearing, and nonpigmented.

■ **Describe the niacin test applied to acid-fast bacteria.**

Take 0.1 ml of heavy growth of AFB incubated 10 days in Dubos' liquid Tween 80 albumin medium and place it in 3 ml of the same medium. Add 1 ml 4% aniline in 95% ethanol and 1 ml 10% aqueous cyanogen bromide. Yellow color indicates presence of niacin.

■ **Which acid-fast bacteria give a positive niacin test?**

Only *Mycobacterium tuberculosis* is strongly positive, but *M. bovis* may be weakly positive.

■ **Which acid-fast bacteria show adherent organisms forming serpentine cords in smears of their colonies? On what is the cord formation dependent?**

M. tuberculosis, *M. bovis*, and *M. ulcerans* show cord formation, which depends on presence of dimycolytrehalose in the bacteria.

■ **What is the purpose of the catalase test in mycobacteriology?**

A negative catalase test identifies some isoniazid-resistant mutants of *M. tuberculosis* and *M. kansasii*. Essentially all other mycobacteria are catalase positive.

■ **How does *M. bovis* differ from *M. tuberculosis* in the laboratory?**

M. bovis does not produce a positive niacin test result, does not reduce nitrates, is more highly pathogenic for rabbits, and grows more slowly on artificial media, producing small (dysgonic) colonies.

■ **Which of the tubercle bacilli forms smooth, nonpigmented colonies and grows optimally at 41° C?**

These criteria identify *M. avium*. *M. tuberculosis* and *M. bovis* do not grow at 41° C.

■ **What are the four groups of atypical acid-fast bacteria?**

They are group I (photochromogens), group II (scotochromogens), group III (nonchromogens or Battey organisms), and group IV (rapid growers).[14,22]

■ **What types of infections are most specifically associated with the atypical mycobacteria?**

Although some of the atypical mycobacteria can cause pulmonary tuberculosis, more typically several of them infect the skin and cervical lymph nodes.

■ **Which of the atypical acid-fast bacteria will produce pigment in darkness or light, and which will produce pigment in light only?**

The scotochromogens will produce pigment in dark or light, and the photochromogens will produce pigment only in light.

■ **How are the rapid growers distinguished from other mycobacteria?**

Their colonies appear within 5 days, whereas the other mycobacteria require 10 days or more for appearance of colonies.

■ **How do atypical acid-fast organisms differ from *M. tuberculosis* as regards animal pathogenicity?**

Atypical acid-fast organisms are not pathogenic for the rabbit or guinea pig but are pathogenic for mice.

■ **Why is it important to differentiate between pathogenic atypical acid-fast bacteria and *M. tuberculosis?***

Most atypical acid-fast bacteria (except a few in the photochromogen group) are resistant to standard antituberculosis therapy.

■ **Name the clinically important atypical mycobacteria of groups I, II, III, and IV.**

Group I: Both members, *M. kansasii* and *M. marinum*, are pathogenic
Group II: *M. scrofulaceum*
Group III: *M. xenopi*, *M. avium*, and *M. intracellulare*
Group IV: *M. fortuitum* and *M. chelonei*[14]

■ **Which organism or group of organisms usually cause scrofula (cervical lymphadenitis)?**

Members of the scotochromogen group of atypical acid-fast bacteria usually cause scrofula.

■ **An acid-fast organism that is cultured from the sputum forms no serpentine cords, does not give a positive niacin test, does not bind neutral red, is avirulent for guinea pigs, and produces nonpigmented colonies in about 3 weeks. What is it?**

It is a group III (Battey) strain.

■ **Identify an acid-fast photochromogen, cultured from a skin lesion in a swimmer or tropical fish fancier, that grows at room temperature but not at 37° C.**

It is *M. marinum.* These organisms produce granulomatous inflammation of the skin but do not invade internal organs. The lesion is often called "swimming pool granuloma."

■ **What characteristic of *M. ulcerans* limits its pathogenicity?**

M. ulcerans cannot grow above 33° C. Therefore, like *M. marinum,* it infects only the cool parts of the body. It resembles *M. tuberculosis* in most other respects.

■ **How is the diagnosis of leprosy made in the laboratory?**

The diagnosis is made by finding intracellular acid-fast bacilli in skin scrapings or biopsied lesions. *M. leprae* cannot be grown on artificial media.

NONFERMENTATIVE GRAM-NEGATIVE BACILLI

■ **How are the nonfermentative gram-negative bacilli recognized in triple sugar agar slants?**

They fail to acidify the butt.

■ **Which of the following (1) are oxidizers, (2) are oxidase positive, (3) utilize citrate, (4) reduce nitrate to nitrite, (5) are rods, (6) are coccobacilli, (7) are motile: *Pseudomonas* species, *Alcaligenes* species, *Acinetobacter (Achromobacter) anitratus (Herellea vaginicola,* bacillus anitratus), *Acinetobacter lwoffii (Mima polymorpha),* and *Bordetella bronchiseptica?***

	Glucose	Nitrate	Citrate	Oxidase	Rods	Coccobacilli	Motile
Pseudomonas species*	Ox	+	+	+	+	−	+
A. anitratus	Ox	−	+	−	−	+	−
Alcaligenes species, B. bronchiseptica	−	+	+	+	+	−	+
A. lwoffii	−	−	−	−	−	+	−

P. maltophilia is usually oxidase negative and fails to oxidize glucose.[17-19]

■ **What is the likely identity of a gram-negative, nonfermentative coccobacillus that is oxidase negative and strongly saccharolytic with lactose?**

It is probably *A. anitratus (Herellea vaginicola).* It is frequently encountered as an opportunistic pathogen.

- **What is an organism that forms large colonies on blood agar and Mac-Conkey agar with diffusion of greenish pigment into the medium and a grapelike odor?**

It is *Pseudomonas aeruginosa.*

- **Give two characteristics of *Pseudomonas* organisms that help identify strains lacking the characteristic odor and pigment production.**

  1. They oxidize gluconate to ketogluconate (commercially available substrate tablets and overnight incubation).
  2. The oxidase test with paraphenylenediamine is positive except for *P. maltophilia.*

- ***Alcaligenes odorans* is isolated from clinical material much more frequently than *A. faecalis.* What are the characteristics of *A. odorans* on blood agar?**

The characteristics are an applelike odor and alpha-hemolysis.

SPIROCHETES AND SPIRILLACEAE

- **Name the genera of Treponemataceae. Which can be cultivated in artificial media?**

The genera are *Leptospira, Borrelia,* and *Treponema.* Of the pathogenic spirochetes, only *Leptospira* species can be cultured, but some nonpathogenic treponemes can be cultured anaerobically on complex media.

- **How is infection with *Borrelia* diagnosed, and how is it transmitted?**

Rat-bite fever caused by *B. recurrentis* is diagnosed by observing spirochetes in Giemsa-stained blood. In some cases the spirochetes are difficult to find, and an immunoenzyme test that in principal resembles the FTA test for syphilis has been developed.[6] Cross reactions with various species of *Borrelia* occur, and some syphilitic sera give positive reactions with the immunoenzyme test. The disease is transmitted by insect vectors: ticks and lice.

- **Describe procedures for the bacteriologic diagnosis of leptospirosis.**

Presumptive diagnosis is made by dark-field examination of blood or urine. Diagnosis can be confirmed by culture in Fletcher's or Stuart's medium.

- **How is *Spirillum minus* infection acquired, and how is it diagnosed?**

It is acquired by rat bite; the incubation period is about 2 weeks. Diagnosis is made by dark-field or phase contract examination of exudate from primary lesion, regional lymph nodes, or blood. Mice or guinea pigs are inoculated after checking to be sure their blood is free of spirochete-like organisms.

- **Match the species with the descriptions following: *Spirillum minus, Borrelia recurrentis, Leptospira icterohemorrhagica, Treponema pallidum.***

  1. Large and long with shallow, coarse, irregular coils; corkscrewlike motility

2. Tightly wound coils, bent at one or both ends to form hook; undulatory, rapid spinning, and lashing movements
3. 5 to 20 μm long, four to fourteen regular spirals spaced at about 1 μm, forward and backward movement, slow bending and twisting
4. Short and thick (0.5 $\times$ 3.0 μm), two or three regular spiral windings, motile by bipolar tufts of flagella

1. *Borrelia recurrentis*
2. *Leptospira icterohemorrhagica*
3. *Treponema pallidum*
4. *Spirillum minus*

■ **What is the significance of finding organisms typical of *T. pallidum* in scrapings from a lesion of the oral cavity?**

The organisms may or may not be *T. pallidum*. Saprophytic treponemes morphologically indistinguishable from *T. pallidum* are ordinarily present in the oral cavity, particularly in the gingivae around the teeth.

■ **A patient has a painless, raised, indurated, flat ulcer of the prepuce that has been present for 10 days. A dark-field examination of the penile lesion is negative, but dark-field examinations of fluid aspirated from an enlarged inguinal lymph node show spirochetes approximately 7 μm long, 0.25 μm in diameter, with about seven regulary spaced coils and slow forward and backward movement with corkscrewlike rotation about the long axis and slow bending and undulation from side to side. What is the diagnosis?**

This description indicates primary syphilis. Occasionally too few organisms may be present in the primary chancre for dark-field detection, but they may be seen readily in aspirate taken with a syringe and needle from an inguinal lymph node.

■ **In a patient with a genital chancre, what studies must be done before syphilis can be excluded?**

At last three dark-field examinations and several serologic examinations must be made, with the last serologic examination at least four months after appearance of the chancre.

■ **What is the incubation period of primary syphilis (time between exposure and appearance of the chancre)?**

It is 10 to 90 days; the mean is 3 weeks. Without treatment the lesion heals in 10 to 40 days.

■ **When do lesions of secondary syphilis (skin and mucous membranes) appear? Are they dark-field positive?**

They appear 2 to 6 weeks after the primary chancre heals. Spirochetes are difficult to demonstrate in macular lesions, but many are present in ulcerated mucous membrane lesions. Mucosal and cutaneous recurrences may occur for as long as 4 years.

- **Is it possible to make a microscopic diagnosis of *T. pallidum* without a dark-field condenser?**

It is possible by the fluorescent antibody technic. Air-dried smears of primary and secondary lesions may be prepared for staining later.

- **A man who has been bitten recently by ticks abruptly develops a fever (40° C) accompanied by chills, albuminuria, leukocytosis, and prostration. After 7 days he suddenly improves, but a relapse lasting 7 days occurs 2 weeks later. During both periods of illness the organisms shown in the drawing are found in Wright-stained blood films. What is the diagnosis?**

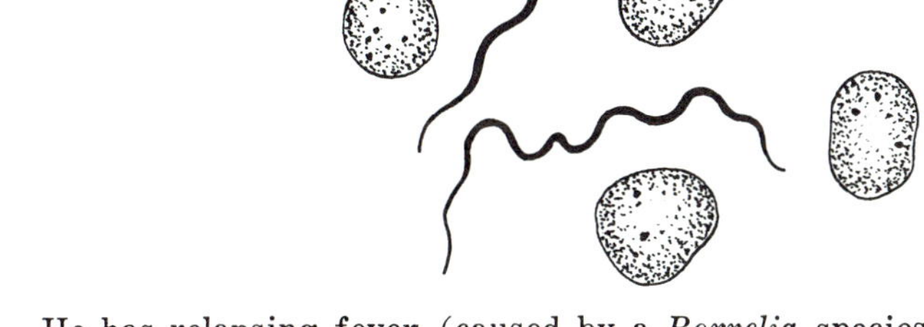

He has relapsing fever (caused by a *Borrelia* species). Note the thickness of spirochetes and their loose coils, which contrast with the tighter coils of treponemes.

- **Dark-field examination of urine from a patient with fever, jaundice, and meningeal symptoms shows organisms with tightly wound spirals and hooked ends 6 to 10 μm long that move with spinning and lashing activity. What is the diagnosis?**

The patient has Weil's disease, for the organism fits the description of a leptospire.

- **Why is 5-fluorouracil used in media for culture of leptospires?**

Leptospires do not incorporate exogenous pyrimidines. Other microorganisms will not grow in presence of the pyrimidine antimetabolite.

PYOGENIC COCCI

- **Which of the pyogenic cocci are gram-positive and gram-negative?**

Staphylococci, pneumococci and streptococci are gram-positive. *Neisseria* organisms (meningococcus, gonococcus) are gram-negative.

- **How are micrococci differentiated from staphylococci?**

Staphylococci occur in clusters and ferment glucose. Micrococci occur in pairs, fours, or small clusters and may utilize glucose oxidatively but fail to ferment it.

■ **Which of the pyogenic cocci can produce a powerful heat-stable entero-toxin when it contaminates food?**

Staphylococcus aureus produces enterotoxin in food. The toxin causes vomiting and diarrhea.

■ **Which organisms are selected by mannitol salt agar?**

Staphylococci are selected.

■ **Describe the substrate and end point of the coagulase test for staphylococci.**

The end point is clotting of citrated or oxalated plasma within 24 hours at 37° C.

■ **What is the significance of the coagulase test in classification of staphylococci?**

Coagulase-positive staphylococci are *S. aureus,* and coagulase-negative "staphylococci" are *S. epidermidis* or *Micrococcus* species. Coagulase-positive staphylococci are pathogenic.

■ **What simple test can be applied to colonies on agar to distinguish staphylococci, micrococci, and *Gaffkya* organisms from streptococci and pneumococci?**

The catalase test can be applied. Catalase is produced by staphylococci, micrococci, and *Gaffkya* species and causes bubbling by conversion of hydrogen peroxide to free oxygen and water.

■ **Should the catalase test be performed on colonies on blood agar?**

It should not, because red blood cells are rich in catalase.

■ **White, nonhemolytic colonies with raised centers and flat margins typical of staphylococci appear on blood agar inoculated with material from a wound. A Gram stain shows gram-positive cocci in clusters. Should they be dismissed as *Staphylococcus epidermidis?***

No. Differentiation between *S. aureus* and *S. epidermidis* is made strictly by the coagulase test. Some strains of *S. aureus* do not form pigment, and *S. aureus* may be nonhemolytic, particularly if the agar contains human rather than sheep blood.

■ **What features distinguish colonies of *Diplococcus pneumoniae* (pneumococcus) on blood agar?**

A tendency to develop a central plateau or depression and alphahemolysis (greening) are the distinguishing characteristics.

■ **Name four types of pneumococcal infection.**

The pneumococcus is the most frequent cause of lobar pneumonia, often causes otitis media, and occasionally causes meningitis and peritonitis.

■ **Describe the appearance of gram-stained pneumococci.**

 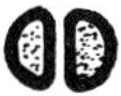

Pneumococci   Neisseria

They are lancet-shaped, gram-positive diplococci (as contrasted to bean-shaped, gram-negative *Neisseria* species).

■ **Name three in vitro differential characteristics of pneumococcus.**

1. Bile solubility
2. Inulin fermentation (by most strains)
3. Optochin sensitivity

■ **Can pneumococci be differentiated from greening (viridans) streptococci by inoculation of mice?**

Yes. Intraperitoneal inoculation of pneumococci (except type 14) kills the mouse, and the organisms can be seen in stained smears of the peritoneal exudate. Viridans streptococci are avirulent for mice.

■ **What structural component of the pneumococcus is closely related to virulence?**

The capsule is related to virulence because it inhibits phagocytosis.

■ **How is the Neufeld-Quellung reaction performed on sputum?**

Air-dry a smear of sputum, and place 0.01 ml antiserum on it with a calibrated loop. Place an equal amount of 0.3% aqueous methylene blue on the cover slip, and place the cover slip on the specimen. The capsular precipitin reaction can be seen immediately with oil immersion magnification and reduced illumination. The Quellung reaction can be used to identify pneumococci and *Neisseria* and *Haemophilus* organisms.[15]

■ **Compare the reliability of diagnosis of pneumococci by examining sputum by the gram stain and by the Quellung reaction with a polyvalent antiserum.**

A 55% correlation with cultural results can be expected with the gram stain, and 90% correlation can be expected with the Quellung reaction.[15]

■ **What proportion of human streptococcal infections are caused by group A streptococci, and what organs are most often infected?**

Group A streptococci causes 85% to 95% of human streptococcal infections. The pharynx and skin are most often infected.

■ **Compare group A streptococcal and staphylococcal skin infections.**

Staphylococci and streptococci both cause superficial (impetigo) and deep (furuncle, carbuncle) infections of the skin. Streptococcal infections more readily spread in the subcutis to cause cellulitis and erysipelas.

■ **What feature on blood agar plates leads to the suspicion that a streptococcus belongs to group A?**

Beta-hemolysis (complete clearing of red cells in the agar adjacent to the colony) indicates that a streptococcus may belong to group A.

■ **Describe the commonly used presumptive test for identification of group A streptococci.**

The test used most often is inhibition of growth by a bacitracin-impregnated disk. (The amount of bacitracin in the disk is crucial.)

■ **Describe three colonial types of group A streptococci that are dependent on capsular hyaluronic acid.**

Mucoid and matt (dull) colonies are formed by organisms that produce abundant hyaluronic acid. The matt colonies are dried mucoid colonies. Glossy colonies indicate lack of production or retention of hyaluronic acid.

■ **How are streptococci grouped serologically?**

An HCl extract containing the C-substance (carbohydrate) from the cell wall is tested with group-specific precipitating antisera.

■ **How are streptococci typed?**

Group A streptococci can be classified into more than fifty-five types on the basis of the M protein. Typing can be done by a precipitin test like that for grouping or by agglutination, since the M antigen is readily accessible as fimbriae on the surface of the organism.

■ **Name five extracellular products of group A streptococci.**

Five such products are erythrogenic toxins, streptolysin O, streptokinases, hyaluronidase, and deoxyribonucleases.

■ **What types of group A streptococcus are often implicated in acute glomerulonephritis and rheumatic fever?**

Type 12 and less often types 4 and 25 cause nephritis, but many different types are involved in rheumatic fever.

■ **Can streptococci be cultured from the lesions of poststreptococcal glomerulonephritis and rheumatic carditis and arthritis?**

Streptococci cannot be cultured from these lesions.

■ **Is alpha-hemolysis truly hemolysis?**

No. The red cells are intact although discolored in alpha-hemolysis.

■ **How are viridans streptococci identified?**

Viridans streptococci produce greening on blood agar and are neither bile-soluble nor optochin-sensitive.

■ **Which of the following four tests for identification of Lancefield group D streptococci (enterococcus, _S. faecalis_) is the most reliable?**

1. Growth in media containing 6.5% sodium chloride
2. Heat resistance: growth at 45° C and survival 62° C for 30 minutes
3. Growth in methylene blue milk with reduction of the dye
4. Positive bile-esculin test result

A positive result of the bile-esculin test is the most reliable.

■ **What organisms most often cause subacute bacterial endocarditis? What organism is most often the cause of acute bacterial endocarditis involving previously undamaged valves?**

Subacute bacterial endocarditis involving valves damaged by rheumatic valvulitis is usually caused by *Streptococcus viridans* or group D streptococci (*S. faecalis*, enterococcus). *S. aureus* most frequently causes acute endocarditis on previously undamaged valves, for example, in heroin addicts.

■ **Describe a simple biochemical test that can help identify colonies of *Neisseria* organisms on agar plates.**

One can test for oxidase reaction. Colonies of *Neisseria* organisms turn dark brown to black within a minute after exposure to a solution of para-phenylenediamine.

■ **What are the proper conditions for culture of *Neisseria meningitidis* and *N. gonorrhoeae?***

Chocolate agar with 3% to 10% CO_2 at 35° to 36° C must be used.

■ **What selective medium is used for cultivation of *Neisseria gonorrhoeae?***

Thayer-Martin, which is chocolate agar with vancomycin, colistin, and nystatin added, is used.

■ **What is the efficacy of a single cervical culture on Thayer-Martin medium for the diagnosis of gonorrhea?**

Ninety percent of women who are positive by isolation of gonococci on any of three successive daily cervical and rectal cultures will have a positive result on a single cervical culture. Another 7% will be detected by a second cervical culture, and the remaining 3% will be detected by a single rectal culture.[3]

■ **Which species of *Neisseria* oxidizes glucose and maltose but not sucrose?**

N. meningitidis oxidizes glucose and maltose.

■ **What site should be cultured to detect asymptomatic carriers of *Neisseria meningitidis?***

The nasopharynx should be cultured.

MISCELLANEOUS BACTERIA

■ **What is the ordinary laboratory approach to the diagnosis of granuloma inguinale?**

Demonstrate the causative organism, *Calymmatobacterium (Donovania) granulomatis,* by staining an air-dried smear or sectioned tissue with Wright's stain or by the Gomori methenamine–silver nitrate method. The organisms are short, gram-negative rods with bipolar staining that occur within cystlike vacuoles in the cytoplasm of large macrophages. They are difficult to culture.

- **What is the appropriate approach to diagnosis of suspected rat-bite fever?**

  1. Examine air-dried, Wright-stained and heat-fixed, gram-stained smears of exudate from the ulcer at the site of the rat bite. *Spirillum minus,* one cause of rat-bite fever, cannot be cultured but will be seen in the Wright-stained smears. It is gram negative, 4 to 7 μm long, and spiral with two to seven regular waves.
  2. Culture the blood. Enough of the patient's blood should be added to result in a final concentration of 20%. *Streptobacillus moniliformis,* the second cause of rat-bite fever, is a gram-negative aerobic rod that will grow on the surface of the sedimented cells.

- **With what disease are *Fusobacterium fusiforme* and *Borrelia vincentii* associated, and how is the bacteriologic diagnosis made?**

The disease is Vincent's angina. The diagnosis is made by finding large numbers of the gram-negative fusiform bacilli and spirochetes in stained smears from the pharyngeal lesion. The fusiform bacilli can be grown anaerobically, but the spirochetes cannot be cultured.

- **Name four diseases caused by members of the genus *Chlamydia.***

Members of the genus *Chlamydia* cause trachoma, inclusion body conjunctivitis, lymphogranuloma venerum, and pneumonitis (ornithosis).

- **How do *Chlamydia* organisms reproduce?**

They reproduce by binary fission within intracellular vacuoles. Therefore they cannot be grown on artificial media.

- **How do mycoplasmas differ from typical bacteria?**

Mycoplasmas are smaller (150 to 300 nm diameter) and lack cell walls.

- **Can mycoplasmas be grown on artificial media?**

They can be grown on artificial media.

- **What important human infection is caused by a mycoplasma?**

Mycoplasma pneumoniae causes primary atypical pneumonia.

REFERENCES

1. Bartlett, R. C.: A plea for clinical relevance in medical microbiology, Am. J. Clin. Pathol. 61:867, 1974.
2. Brock, D. W., et al.: Actinomycosis caused by *Arachnia propionica:* report of 11 cases, Am. J. Clin. Pathol. 56:66, 1973.
3. Caldwell, J. G., et al.: Sensitivity and reproductibility of Thayer-Martin culture medium in diagnosing gonorrhea in women, Am. J. Obstet. Gynecol. 109:463, 1971.
4. Chow, A. W., and Guze, L. B.: Bacteriodaceae bacteremia: clinical experience with 112 patients, Medicine 53:93, 1974.
5. Davies, J. E., and Rownd, R.: Trans-

missible multiple drug resistance in Enterobacteriaceae, Science 176:758, 1972.

6. Felsenfeld, O., and Wolf, R. H.: The indirect immunoenzyme test for the detection of antibodies against North American borreliae. II. Experiments with human sera, Am. J. Clin. Pathol. 61:844, 1974.

7. Friedman, C. T. H., et al.: Shiga bacillus infection: experience in Los Angeles County, 1966-1971, J.A.M.A. 226:1559, 1973.

8. Gorbach, S. L., and Bartlett, J. G.: Anaerobic infections (first of three parts), N. Engl. J. Med. 290:1177, 1974.

9. Gorbach, S. L., and Bartlett, J. G.: Anaerobic infections (second of three parts), N. Engl. J. Med. 290: 1237, 1974.

10. Gorbach, S. L., and Bartlett, J. G.: Anaerobic infections (third of three parts), N. Engl. J. Med. 290:1289, 1974.

11. Grady, G. F., and Keusch, T. G.: Pathogenesis of bacterial diarrheas, N. Engl. J. Med. 285:831, 1971.

12. Jones, S. R., Smith, J. W., and Sanford, J. P.: Localization of urinary-tract infections by detection of antibody-coated bacteria in urine sediment, N. Engl. J. Med. 290:591, 1974.

13. Kass, E. H.: Asymptomatic infections of the urinary tract, Trans. Assoc. Am. Physicians 69:56, 1956.

14. Kubica, G. P.: Differential identification of mycobacteria. VII. Key features for identification of clini-cally significant mycobacteria, Am. Rev. Resp. Dis. 197:9, 1973.

15. Merrill, C. W., et al.: Rapid identification of pneumococci: Gram stain vs. the Quellung reaction, N. Engl. J. Med. 288:510, 1973.

16. Merson, M. H., et al.: Scombroid fish poisoning: outreach traced to commercially canned tuna fish, J.A.M.A. 228:1268, 1974.

17. Pedersen, M. M., Marso, E., and Pickett, M. J.: Nonfermentative bacilli associated with man. III. Pathogenicity and antibiotic susceptibility, Am. J. Clin. Pathol. 54:178, 1970.

18. Pickett, M. J., and Manclard, C. R.: Nonfermentative bacilli associated with man. II. Detection and identification, Am. J. Clin. Pathol. 54:164, 1970.

19. Pickett, M. J., and Pedersen, M. M.: Nonfermentative bacilli associated with man. II. Detection and identification, Am. J. Clin. Pathol. 54:164, 1970.

20. Robbins, J. B., et al.: *Escherichia coli* K1 capsular polysaccharide associated with neonatal meningitis, N. Engl. J. Med. 290:1216, 1974.

21. Thomas, V., Shelokov, A., and Forland, M.: Antibody-coated bacteria in the urine and the site of urinary-tract infection, N. Engl. J. Med. 290:588, 1974.

22. Wayne, L. G., and Runyon, E. H.: Mycobacteria: a guide to nomenclatural usage, Am. Rev. Resp. Dis. 100:732, 1969.

CHAPTER 3

Blood banking

For those who have no previous experience in blood banking, the section on that subject in the chapter by Stern, Lee, and Davidsohn in *Todd-Sanford Clinical Diagnosis by Laboratory Methods* or the *Hyland Reference Manual of Immunohematology* is recommended. The book by Huestis, Bove, and Busch is a good supplement, and Mollison's classic treatise is an exhaustive reference. A battery of instructional aids is available from Ortho Diagnostics, Raritan, New Jersey. The programmed instruction manuals by Jennings, by Stern, and by Davidsohn and Stern provide simulated experience in blood banking situations. Standard methods and procedures and a variety of advanced seminars not listed below are contained in publications of the American Association of Blood Banks.

Davidsohn, I., and Stern, K.: Selected topics in immunohematology, Chicago, 1966, American Society of Clinical Pathologists Commission on Continuing Education.

Huestis, D. W., Bove, J. R., and Busch, S.: Practical blood transfusion, Boston, 1969, Little, Brown & Co.

Hyland reference manual of immunohematology: a concise review of principles and procedures, ed. 3, Costa Mesa, Calif., 1965, Hyland Division of Travenol Laboratories.

Jennings, E. R.: The difficult cross-match, Chicago, 1963, American Society of Clinical Pathologists Commission on Continuing Education.

Mollison, P. L.: Blood transfusion in clinical medicine, ed. 5, Philadelphia, 1972, F. A. Davis Co.

Physician's handbook of blood component therapy, Chicago, 1969, Twentieth Century Press, Inc. Available from the American Association of Blood Banks, Washington, D. C.

Schmidt, P. J., editor: Progress in transfusion and transplantation, Washington, D. C., 1972, American Association of Blood Banks.

Stern, K.: Exercises in immunohematology, Chicago, 1969, American Society of Clinical Pathologists Commission on Continuing Education.

Stern, K., Lee, L.-L., and Davidsohn, I.: Blood groups and their application. In Davidsohn, I., and Henry, J. B., editors: Todd-Sanford clinical diagnosis by laboratory methods, ed. 15, Philadelphia, 1974, W. B. Saunders Co.

Red cell freezing: a technical workshop, Washington, D. C., 1973, American Association of Blood Banks.

Technical methods and procedures of the American Association of Blood Banks,
ed. 6, Washington, D. C., 1974, American Association of Blood Banks.
Vyas, G. N., Perkins, H. A., and Schmid, R.: Hepatitis and blood transfusion, New
York, 1972, Grune & Stratton, Inc.
Zmijewski, C. M., and Fletcher, J. L.: Immunohematology, New York, 1972, Apple-
ton-Century-Crofts.

■ **State the differences between natural and immune antibodies.**

In general natural antibodies (IgM) do not cross the placenta, are active
at a lower temperature, have a larger molecular size (and higher sedimentation
constant), and react in saline. Immune antibodies (IgG) cross the placenta,
are more active at body temperature, have smaller molecular size (and therefore lower sedimentation constant), and agglutinate in albumin but not in
saline.

■ **What are "complete" and "incomplete" antibodies?**

A "complete" antibody is one capable of producing agglutination of red
blood cells in saline media. An "incomplete" antibody is one that attaches to
red blood cells but cannot produce hemagglutination in saline media without
assistance (such as adding bovine albumin or the Coombs test) and can block
the agglutination of red blood cells by "complete antibodies."

■ **What is a "mixed-field" reaction?**

A mixed-field reaction is a positive red cell serologic reaction in which there
are some clumps plus many free cells. Classically it is seen when a patient is
transfused with blood to which he has an antibody. A direct Coombs test will
only clump the antibody-coated incompatible cells. Mixed-field reactions are
also seen when typing for subgroups of A and B or in fetomaternal bleeds.

■ **What is the prozone phenomenon?**

It is a false negative reaction secondary to the presence of too much antibody
for the amount of antigen present.

■ **What are lectins?**

Lectins are substances extracted from the seeds of certain plants capable
of producing hemagglutination. Some important types of lectins in blood banking have anti-A_1, anti-**H**, anti-**M**, and anti-**N** activity.

■ **What is the percentage distribution of the A-B-O groups in citizens of the
United States?**

	O	*A*	*B*	*AB*
White	45%	37%	13%	5%
Black	48%	28%	20%	4%

■ **Which person is likely to have the higher titer of anti-A in his serum,
one whose blood type is B or one whose blood type is O?**

One who is O will probably have the higher titer of anti-A. Anti-AB (group
O) serum is useful for detection of some of the weak subgroups of A.

■ **What are subgroups or variants of A?**

They are inherited antigens that react weakly or not at all with anti-A but whose cells usually react with anti-AB (group O) serum. Some may not react with either anti-A or anti-AB sera, but the cells of these groups will absorb anti-A, as shown by elution procedures.

■ **How can one differentiate A_1 cells from A_2 or other subgroups of A?**

Use anti-A_1 lectin, which reacts only with A_1 cells, or use group B serum after absorption with A_2 cells. Absorbed group B serum reacts only with A_1 cells.

■ **Give the probable subgroups of A for the following test results.**

	Antisera			*Control cells*				*Saliva*
	Anti-A	*Anti-A_1*	*Anti-A,B*	*A_1*	*A_2*	*B*	*O*	
1.	+(mixed-field)	−	+	+	−	+	−	H
2.	−	−	+	+	−	+	−	H
3.	−	−	−	+	−	+	−	A

1. A_3
2. A_x
3. A_m

■ **Blood from an infant 6 weeks old is grouped as O by testing the red cells, but by reverse grouping of the serum it appears to be AB. What explanation can be offered for the apparent discrepancy?**

Isoagglutinins do not appear until 3 to 6 months of age.

■ **Can red blood cells ever convert from O to B or from A to AB in vivo?**

The appearance of a spurious B substance in patients with sepsis or malignancy indicates that they can convert.

■ **Can red cells convert from group O to AB in vitro?**

They can seemingly do so, by bacterial growth with production of the T agglutinogen (Huebener-Thomsen-Friedenreich phenomenon). Reverse grouping of the serum would disclose the discrepancy.

■ **What is the Bombay blood group?**

It is characterized by serum that contains both anti-A and anti-B, but with cells that do not react with anti-H, anti-A, or anti-B. Anti-H is present in the serum. It is caused by a recessive gene, *h*, which in the homozygote results in failure to make H substance.

■ **Can a secretor father and a secretor mother have a nonsecretor son?**

They can, if both are heterozygous for the secretor trait.

■ **About what percentage of white Americans are secretors?**

Approximately 80% are secretors.

■ **The MN blood groups are utilized mostly for what purpose?**

They are utilized for paternity determination.

■ **List the phenotypes of the P blood group system.**

1. P_1
2. P_2
3. p
4. P^k

■ **Which of the above phenotypes would one expect to react with anti-Tj[a]?**

P_1, P_2, and P^k would be expected to react with anti-Tj[a].

■ **Which is the most common genotype found in the Lutheran blood group system?**

Lu^bLu^b (greater than 90%) is the most common genotype.

■ **What is the most common Kell blood group phenotype?**

k (88%) is the most common.

■ **Have the Kell or Lutheran blood groups been associated with hemolytic problems?**

They have been associated with both hemolytic disease of the newborn and transfusion reactions.

■ **What is unusual about the Lewis blood group substance?**

Red cell antigens of the Lewis blood group are acquired by absorption from plasma and do not appear on red cells until several weeks after birth. The Lewis phenotype is influenced by secretor and Hh genes.

■ **Duffy blood groups are found in what percentage of white Americans and black Americans?**

1. Whites: 100%
2. Blacks: approximately 30%

■ **What is the best laboratory technic for demonstrating anti-Fy antibody?**

The indirect Coombs test is the best technic.

■ **Approximately what percentage of white and black Americans have Kidd blood group antigens?**

Approximately 100% (of both) have Kidd blood group antigens.

■ **Define private and public blood factors.**

Private blood factors are low-incidence antigens, generally confined to members of a single family (the corresponding antibodies are relatively common and are usually natural agglutinins). Public blood factors are high-incidence antigens found in nearly everyone.

■ **What do the red cell antigens Js^b, U, and Di^b have in common?**

All are "public" antigens. Js^b and U are rarely lacking in blacks, and Di^b is rarely lacking in persons of the Mongoloid race.

■ **Briefly describe the direct Coombs test.**

Antihuman globulin agglutinates washed red cells coated in vivo with antibody.

■ **Briefly describe the indirect Coombs test.**

Test serum is incubated with reagent red blood cells, which are then washed thoroughly. Antihuman globulin is added, and it agglutinates the red blood cells if they were coated by antibodies from the test serum.

■ **In what conditions is a direct Coombs test of value?**

It is of value in erythroblastosis fetalis, acquired hemolytic anemia, and transfusion reactions.

■ **In what conditions is an indirect Coombs test of value?**

It is of value in testing for incomplete antibodies in the serum, in crossmatching, in isoimmunizations of pregnancy, and in typing some red cell antigens.

■ **What are the components of the Coombs antihuman globulin?**

Good antiserum contains both antigamma globulin and anticomplement.

■ **What is the significance of having the anticomplement component?**

Certain antibodies such as anti-I may initially attach to the red cell antigen and bind complement. Subsequently, the antibody may elute from the cell leaving only complement to indicate an immunologic reaction. Studies of in vivo reactions indicate that the $\alpha_2 D$ fragment of C stays on red cells. Thus anticomplement is useful in a Coombs reagent.

■ **Antibodies to which blood groups are often detected only with antigamma globulin of the Coombs serum?**

Antibodies to Rh, S, s, K, k, and Fy blood groups are so detected.

■ **Which blood group antibodies often fix complement and therefore react with anticomplement antisera?**

A, B, Lewis, Kidd, Lutheran, P, and H blood group antibodies often fix complement and may fail to bind in the absence of complement.

■ **Does the antigamma globulin or antinongamma globulin, or both, require complement for its reactions?**

Only antinongamma globulin requires complement for its reaction.

■ **False positive results of the Coombs tests may be caused by what conditions?**

They may be caused by contamination by Wharton's jelly, dirt, scratched glassware, or the presence of bacteria.

■ **What conditions or factors might produce a false negative result of the Coombs test?**

The wrong incubation temperature, inadequate incubation time, inadequate washing of red cells, insufficient or inactivated complement, or a Coombs serum without sufficient activity against complement might produce a false negative result.

■ **When cross-matching, which method or methods should be utilized to detect the greatest range of possible antibodies?**

Saline, high protein, and indirect Coombs compatibility tests should all be done.

■ **Enzyme treatment of red cells increases the sensitivity for detecting which of the following antibodies and destroys reaction sites for which of the following antibodies: Rh, Lewis, P, M, N, and Duffy?**

Sensitivity is increased for the first three, and the latter three have their reaction sites destroyed by enzyme treatment.

■ **In doing a Coombs test, what controls should be used?**

A tube containing normal cells (O, Rh negative) instead of the patient's cells should be used for a negative control, and a positive control of Rh_o (D) cells with anti-**D** antibodies should be used.

■ **In which condition or conditions might an individual possess antibodies to antigens present in his own cells?**

One may have them in acquired autoimmune hemolytic anemia. Warm or cold reactive antibodies may also be present without hemolytic anemia.

■ **What are the possible explanations for a patient's serum reacting with all cells of a cell panel and with his own cells during a cross-match?**

Cold agglutinins, rouleau formation, acquired hemolytic anemia, or panagglutinins (bacterial contamination) might be the cause.

■ **In antibody identification, why is it better to use R^1R^1 (CDe/CDe) and R^2R^2 (cDE/cDE) rather than R^1R^2 (CDe/cDE) or R^2r (cDE/cde) cells?**

Cells with homozygous factors are more sensitive.

■ **In investigating difficult instances of atypical blood group antibodies, why is it a good idea to type the patient's cells for as many factors as possible?**

It should be done because one can usually rule out the presence in the patient's serum of isoantibodies to any of his own antigens.

■ **Why should one test all cells that are apparently group O with anti-AB (group O) serum?**

Some subgroups or variants of A and B may be detected only with anti-**AB** serum.

■ **When testing for blood group antibodies, what control should always be included?**

The patient's serum should be tested against his own cells.

■ **List the three main types of transfusion reactions.**

1. Hemolytic
2. Allergic
3. Pyrogenic

■ **When multiple transfusions are given over a period of days, should a new sample of the recipient's blood be drawn for cross-matching with each transfused unit?**

Blood should be drawn so that atypical agglutinins that may have resulted from previous transfusions can be detected. Amnestic responses may occur, which would be otherwise missed.

■ **Why is it important to use a pretransfusion specimen for cross-matching (in addition to a freshly drawn sample) in a patient who requires multiple transfusions within 2 to 3 days?**

Antibodies may disappear from the circulation immediately after transfusion of an incompatible unit of blood and thereby be missed.

■ **Name a cause of hemolytic transfusion reactions other than mismatched blood.**

Blood that is already hemolyzed accidentally by improper preparation, such as by excessive warming or freezing during storage, or by bacterial growth may produce hemolytic transfusion reactions.

■ **According to the present regulations, what is the required temperature and what is the maximum temperature variation that blood may have during storage?**

Blood should be stored at 1° to 6° C with a maximal permissible variation of ±2° C.

■ **What is the most common cause of death in hemolytic transfusion reactions?**

Renal failure is the most common cause.

■ **What steps should be taken to confirm a suspected hemolytic transfusion reaction?**

1. Repeat the determination of group and type, and cross-match with pretransfusion blood.
2. Look for hemoglobinuria (benzidine test of spun urine).

3. Look for increased bilirubin level in the blood and urobilinogen level in the urine. Carefully draw an anticoagulated sample of blood and examine the spun plasma for hemoglobin.
4. Perform a direct Coombs test on the patient's cells and look for a mixed-field reaction.
5. Rescreen the patient's serum and the donor's serum for atypical antibodies.

■ **Briefly give the pathophysiology of hemolytic disease of the newborn.**

Small numbers of fetal cells crossing the placenta and entering the maternal circulation may induce the production of antibodies if the fetal red cell antigens are incompatible with the mother. These immune antibodies produced by the mother then cross the placental barrier, enter the fetal circulation, and destroy the fetal red cells.

■ **Are women whose blood groups are incompatible with their husbands' blood groups more likely to have infants with hemolytic disease of the newborn in the first, second, or third pregnancy?**

Hemolytic disease in the newborn is uncommon until *after* the second incompatible pregnancy, and hence is more likely to occur in the third pregnancy. Approximately 17% of Rh-negative mothers of Rh-positive children will develop antibodies with the second such child.

■ **What proportion of Rh-negative women are susceptible to sensitization to Rh_o (D) by experimental or natural transplacental transfusion of Rh-positive blood?**

Approximately 70% of Rh-negative women are susceptible to sensitization. The other 30% fail to respond with antibody-production, and they are evidently incapable of recognizing the antigen.[7]

■ **What is the most useful laboratory test to confirm the diagnosis of hemolytic disease in the newborn?**

A direct Coombs test with the newborn infant's cells should be done. Positive results will confirm the diagnosis.

■ **Are the results of the direct Coombs test more likely to be positive in infants with erythroblastosis secondary to A-B-O or to Rh incompatibility?**

In Rh incompatibility the results are usually positive, whereas they may be only weak or negative in A-B-O incompatibility.

■ **List the steps that should be taken in ruling in or ruling out the presence of A-B-O incompatibility in infants suspected of having this cause of erythroblastosis.**

1. Titrate the mother's serum against saline-suspended group A_1 and group B cells.
2. Neutralize the mother's serum with A and B substances, and then titrate against the same cell suspensions in saline and Coombs systems.

3. Perform a direct Coombs test on the infant's cells. Even if the results are negative, elution of the infant's cells may reveal immune anti-**A** or anti-**B**, which will react with adult group A_1 or group B cells.
4. Test for immune anti-**A** or anti-**B** in the infant's serum. Presence of one or the other is evidence of A-B-O incompatibility.
5. Use the mother's serum to test for hemolysis of cells in the same group as the affected baby's. A positive reaction confirms A-B-O incompatibility.

■ **Most A-B-O hemolytic disease of the newborn occurs in infants of mothers of which blood group, and why?**

This disease occurs, in 90% of the cases, with group O mothers. Group O mothers develop IgG anti-**AB**, which can cross the placenta.

■ **What can be done when an antigen or an antibody cannot readily be identified in a patient with suspected hemolytic disease of the newborn?**

For identification, cross-match the father's red cells with the mother's serum. The results may show an incompatibility secondary to a low incidence factor. For exchange transfusion in extreme situations, maternal red cells, but not whole blood, could be used as the donor.

■ **Can a woman who is Rh_o (D)-negative and whose husband is Rh_o (D)-positive have an Rh_o (D)-negative child?**

She can if the father is heterozygous with respect to the Rh_o (D) factor. This occurs about 30% of the time because more Rh_o (D)-positive people are heterozygous than homozygous.

■ **Can a woman who is AB, Rh_o (D)-positive have a child with hemolytic disease of the newborn?**

Yes. Almost all other known blood factors have been reported to cause hemolytic disease of the newborn. Among these rare forms of the disease, isoimmunization to hr′ (c), rh″ (E), and K are relatively frequent.

■ **Why are the Rh_o antibodies often first detected only a few weeks after delivery in Rh_o (D)-negative mothers who have Rh_o (D)-positive offspring?**

Fetal red cells commonly enter the maternal circulation during delivery, and formation of antibodies to these cells takes several weeks.

■ **Briefly outline the screening procedures for the detection of significant Rh incompatibilities in pregnancy.**

Type all pregnant women when first seen. If the woman is Rh_o (D)-positive, nothing further need be done. If the woman is Rh_o (D)-negative, then the husband should be typed. If the husband is Rh_o (D)-negative, nothing further need be done. If the husband is Rh_o (D)-positive, then a screening test for Rh antibodies should be done. It should be repeated in the sixth month and, if negative, again in the eighth month and, if negative, once again 2 to 4 weeks postpartum if the child was Rh_0-positive. If it is still negative, nothing further need be done.

■ **Is there any significance to be placed on the titer of Rh antibodies in the individual patients?**

Although there is some significance, statistically, the titer is not an absolute indication of the outcome of the pregnancy in any individual patient.

■ **If maternal antibodies are found in the work-up of a pregnant woman, why should aliquots of maternal serum be frozen and stored?**

This procedure should be followed to provide for accuate subsequent comparisons in detecting changes in the antibody titer.

■ **Does an O, Rh_0 (D)-negative woman married to an O, Rh_0 (D)-positive husband have a greater, lesser, or the same chance of producing an infant with hemolytic disease of the newborn secondary to Rh incompatibility as an O, Rh_0 (D)-negative woman married to an A, Rh_0 (D)-positive husband?**

The chance is greater, because in the latter instance the A-B-O incompatibility diminishes the incidence of Rh immunization.

■ **What procedure or procedures should be followed to confirm or negate the diagnosis of hemolytic disease in the newborn?**

A direct Coombs test (if negative, Rh, but not A-B-O incompatibility can be ruled out), hemoglobin or hematocrit, cord blood reticulocyte count and serum bilirubin, and a test for the presence of agglutinin in the serum of the infant (anti-**A** or anti-**B**) should be done.

■ **In addition to the possibility of showing negative results of a direct Coombs test, how else does A-B-O incompatibility differ from Rh incompatibility insofar as hemolytic disease of the newborn is concerned?**

In A-B-O incompatibility, difficulty before birth is uncommon; the anemia is usually less severe; jaundice occurs earlier; spherocytosis is a prominent finding; and the reticulocyte response is usually greater.

■ **What is Rh immune globulin and why is it used?**

Rh immune globulin is a concentrated solution of specific gamma globulin (IgG) containing anti-Rh_0 (D) antibody obtained from human plasma. It is used to prevent the formation of active antibodies in the Rh_0 (D)-negative, D^u-negative mother who has delivered an Rh_0 (D)-positive or D^u-positive infant.

■ **List the indications for the administration of Rh immune globulin.**
  1. The mother must be Rh_0 (D)-negative and D^u-negative.
  2. The mother must not already be immunized to the Rh_0 (D) factor.
  3. The baby must be Rh_0 (D)-positive or D^u-positive.

4. The baby should have a negative reaction to the direct Coombs test (A positive reaction to the direct Coombs test because of anti-**Rh$_o$ (D)** should be considered a contraindication to the administration of Rh immune globulin).

5. It should be administered in a miscarriage, an abortion, or an ectopic pregnancy in an Rh$_o$ (D)-negative mother with an Rh$_o$ (D)-positive or D^u-positive mate.

■ **When would one inject Rh immune globulin into the newborn infant?**

Rh immune globulin should not be injected into a newborn infant.

■ **List the contraindications for the giving of Rh immune globulin.**

1. Rh$_o$ (D)-positive or D^u-positive individual
2. A patient previously immunized to Rh$_o$ (D) blood factor

■ **When should Rh immune globulin be given, and what is the proper procedure to follow in giving it?**

Rh immune globulin should be given within 72 hours of delivery of an Rh-positive infant by an Rh-negative mother with a negative reaction to an indirect Coombs test. Rh immune globulin is first cross-matched with the mother's red cells and, if compatible, is then given to her.

■ **Ideally, what should be the A-B-O group and Rh type of blood for exchange transfusion of an infant with erythroblastosis fetalis secondary to Rh$_o$ (D) isoimmunization?**

The A-B-O group should ideally be compatible with the infant's and mother's bloods, and the blood must be Rh$_o$-negative.

■ **Is group O, Rh-negative blood suitable for exchange transfusion of infants with Rh incompatibility erythroblastosis whose blood groups are A, B, or AB?**

If the saline titer of anti-**A** and anti-**B** is not greater than 1:32, the blood is considered safe. (No hemolytic antibody should be present.)

■ **What compatibility test may be performed before exchange transfusion of an infant?**

The donor's red blood cells may be tested for compatibility with the mother's serum. If the baby's A-B-O group is incompatible with the mother's serum, some authorities recommend using group O Rh-negative blood.

■ **How fresh should citrated blood for exchange transfusion be?**

It should not be more than 4 days old.

■ **What dose of Rh immune globulin is used in fetomaternal bleeds?**

A standard 300 μg dose is suitable for a fetomaternal bleed of up to 15 ml of spun red cells.

■ **What steps are necessary in determining whether a patient has an autoimmune hemolytic anemia?**

The following is a rational plan for the establishment of this diagnosis:
1. Establish the presence of decreased red cell survival time (accelerated destruction).
2. Demonstrate that the cause of the red cell destruction is extracorpuscular.
3. Identify an autoantibody in the patient's serum.

■ **What is the most suitable procedure for the demonstration of autoantibodies?**

A positive direct Coombs test will indicate the presence of antoantibodies.

■ **Does the presence of negative results of a direct Coombs test rule out autoimmune hemolytic disease?**

No. Negative reactions to the Coombs test are occasionally seen in patients who are undergoing intensive steroid therapy or who are seen for other reasons. Sometimes enzyme techniques will be positive when the Coombs test is negative.

■ **What type of antibodies are most often found as the cause of autoimmune hemolytic anemia?**

Incomplete immune antibodies are most often the cause.

■ **What should be done for a patient with autoimmune hemolytic anemia who needs blood, and for whom it is not possible to find any blood that is completely compatible?**

Give A-B-O- and Rh-compatible blood that has the lowest titer of agglutination with the patient's serum.

■ **List the laws of blood group inheritance.**
1. Factors **A** or **B** cannot appear in a child unless present in one or both parents.
2. A parent of group AB cannot have a child of group O, nor can a parent of group O have a child of group AB.
3. A child cannot possess **M** or **N** unless these factors are present in the blood of one or both parents.
4. A parent of type M cannot have a child of type N, nor can a parent of type N have a child of type M.
5. A parent of group A_1B cannot have a child of group A_2, nor can a parent of group A_2 have a child of group A_1B.

■ **Antibodies against which red cell antigens tend to be hemolytic?**

Anti-**Lewis** and anti-**Kidd** tend to be hemolytic.

■ **What must be true of the antiglobulin serum used in recognizing these hemolytic antibodies?**

It must be active against complement, since these antibodies bind complement.

■ **What percentage of Americans are hr′ (c)-positive?**

Eighty percent are hr′ (c)-positive.

■ **Describe cold agglutinins.**

The cold agglutinins are natural IgM antibodies directed against the high-incidence I antigens. Normal persons commonly have a low titer. A pathologically high titer with hemolysis is found associated with mycoplasma pneumonia and lymphomas. The rare I-negative i-positive patients have anti-I. At birth the I antigen is poorly developed and the i antigen is found. By 18 months, I specificity is at adult strength. Another antibody in this system, anti-i, has been transiently found in infectious mononucleosis.

■ **How may one test the presence of cold agglutinins?**

The patient's serum is tested against his own cold agglutinin-free cells at 4° C, room temperature, and 37° C. Agglutination should be strongly positive at 4° C, at room temperature, and there should be no agglutination at 37° C. Additionally, the patient's serum is tested against group O cord cells, which either lack or have weak expression of the I antigen. Therefore serum with cold agglutinins should have either no reaction at 4° C with cord cells or a reaction that is substantially less than that observed with the adult cells.

■ **When the presence of interfering cold agglutinins is suspected, how can a specimen of red cells that is free of absorbed cold agglutinins be quickly obtained?**

Draw blood using a warm syringe; place ten drops of blood in saline warmed to 37° C, and mix vigorously. Wash cells three times in 37° C saline.

■ **After absorption of serum with the patient's own enzyme-treated cells to remove the cold agglutinins, how can the serum be tested to check for their removal?**

Mix two drops of absorbed serum with one drop of 2% saline suspension of the patient's cold agglutinin-free cells and keep it at 4° C for 1 hour. The absence of cold agglutinins is shown by the absence of agglutination.

■ **What are the five most frequently found Rh genotypes in Americans?**

They are R_1r (31%), R_1R_1 (17%), rr (14%), R_1R_2 (13%), and R_2r (12.5%).

■ **What percentage of group A individuals belong to group A_1?**

Approximately 80% belong to A_1.

■ **In a paternity case, the mother is group O, the father is group A_1B, the baby's red cells do not react as A_1, and he is classified as A_2. Does this exclude paternity of the suspected father?**

It does if the baby is more than a year old. But children less than a year old may show imperfect development of the A antigen and may not react with anti-A_1.

■ **If red cells have the phenotype A_1, what are the possible genotypes they may have?**

They may have A_1A_1, A_1A_2, or A_1O genotypes.

■ **Red cells with phenotype A_2 have what possible genotypes?**

They may have A_2A_2 or A_2O genotypes.

■ **What is meant by the "gene interaction" type of Rh_0 variant (D^u)?**

This type occurs in individuals who have received a normal Rh_0 (D) from one parent and an rh′ (C) from the other parent. In some manner the rh′ inhibits expression of Rh_0.

■ **What is the "hereditary" type of Rh_0 variant (D^u)?**

This type is simply a weaker form of Rh_0 (D). Both this type and the "gene interaction" type react with the indirect Coombs technic after sensitization with anti-Rh_0 (anti-D).

■ **The Rh_0 variant (D^u) individuals should be considered as what blood group when they are blood donors and blood recipients?**

They may be considered as Rh_0 (D)-positive blood donors and recipients. Some authorities recommend Rh-negative blood for D^u recipients who lack rh′ (C).

■ **Should an Rh_0 (D)-negative woman anticipate difficulty if married to a D^u-positive man?**

She should not. It has never been definitely proved that isoimmunization induced by D^u occurs as a result of pregnancy.

■ **How might the presence of the "gene interaction" type of D^u in an infant lead to erroneous exclusions of parentage?**

The father may appear to be Rh_0 (D)-negative (if the albumin and anti-globulin tests are not used) and have an Rh_0 (D)-positive offspring.

■ **What percentage of Rh_0 (D)-negative recipients will produce Rh antibodies in response to a single transfusion of Rh_0 (D)-positive blood?**

About half will produce Rh antibodies.

■ **What is a dangerous universal donor?**

The dangerous universal donor is a person of O blood type with high (1:50 or more in saline) titers of anti-A, anti-B, or both.

■ **If the results of a cell grouping and serum grouping do not agree, what should be done?**

Repeat the cell grouping with other lots of serum, and repeat serum grouping with other known cells.

■ **If the repeat grouping, however, agrees with the original results, what could explain this phenomenon?**

These results may be caused by the presence of an atypical agglutinin, a warm or cold autoagglutinin, or a weak subgroup of A or B in the blood from which the serum is obtained.

■ **How should one test for the presence of an autoagglutinin?**

One should test the patient's cells against his own serum.

■ **Explain how one could have agglutination of group O cells as well as group A and group B cells by a patient's serum.**

The presence of a nonspecific warm or cold agglutinin is usually the explanation.

■ **A patient's serum agglutinates A_1 cells but not cells of group B. His own cells react with anti-A and anti-B. What is his most likely subgroup, and what further tests might one do to substantiate this?**

He most likely has A_2B. One can test the patient's cells with anti-A_1 lectin, which would give a negative reaction. In the reverse grouping, a negative reaction with A_2 cells would be expected. About 25% of A_2B subjects have anti-A_1.

■ **What is the most significant characteristic of the B subgroups?**

They have a weak or negative reaction with potent anti-B grouping sera, and may have mixed-field reactions.

■ **People with which blood groups are more likely to have anti-H antibodies?**

People with A_1 or A_1B phenotypes are likely to have anti-H antibodies.

■ **List all the possible phenotypes and genotypes in the MN blood group.**
   1. Phenotypes: M, N, or MN
   2. Genotypes: *MM, MN,* or *NN*

■ **Anti-M and anti-N are most often what type of antibody?**

They are naturally occurring (complete).

■ **What is the approved maximal storage period of both acid citrate dextrose (ACD) and citrate phosphate dextrose (CPD) blood?**

It should not be stored longer than 21 days.

■ **What proportion of the initial intracellular potassium concentration is lost by red cells during storage for 3 weeks?**

Approximately half is lost.

■ **What happens to the potassium level of the plasma of stored blood?**

It gradually increases to approximately 15 mEq/L by 15 days.[6]

■ **What happens to the ammonia level in the plasma of stored blood?**

It increases to as high as 900 μg/dl after 21 days and therefore may be not acceptable for transfusion in patients with liver disease when it is more than 7 days old.

■ **Would blood stored in the blood bank for 3 days be satisfactory to treat a patient for factor VIII deficiency?**

It would not because the half-life of factor VIII in stored blood is approximately 7 days. Replacement by whole blood or plasma necessitates the highest possible concentration because of volume limitation.

■ **What is the hematocrit of a unit of packed red blood cells?**

The hematocrit is about 60% to 70%. (Approximately two thirds of the plasma is removed.)

■ **In what conditions is transfusion of packed red blood cells rather than whole blood indicated?**

It is definitely indicated in cardiac diseases (reduced volume, acidity, and potassium), uremia (reduced ammonia, potassium, and citrate), cirrhosis (reduced ammonia and citrate), acute burns (reduced potassium) aplastic anemia, cachectic or debilitated patients, and patients with slow bleeding in whom it would be advantageous to keep the rise in central venous pressure minimal. There is seldom any indication for whole blood except acute massive bleeding.

■ **What are the other advantages of giving packed red blood cells rather than whole blood?**

Removal of plasma of group O blood (anti-A and anti-B) makes it safer to give to recipients not of group O. Adverse allergic reactions to plasma factors are minimized.

■ **What types of patients are most likely to have antileukocyte antibodies?**

Patients who have received multiple transfusions, multiparous women, and tissue or organ transplant recipients are most likely to have antileukocyte antibodies.

■ **What can be done to minimize leukocyte transfusion reactions?**

Leukocyte-poor blood can be transfused. Adequate removal of leukocytes usually cannot be achieved by preparation of packed red cells. Acceptable techniques in increasing order of effectiveness are removal of the buffy coat, sedimentation in high molecular weight dextran or hydroxyethyl starch, and frozen washed cells.

■ **How does the number of platelets in one unit of platelet-rich plasma or**

one unit of platelet concentrate compare with the number in one unit of whole blood?

One unit of platelet-rich plasma contains approximately 85% as many platelets, and one unit of platelet concentrate contains 70% to 80% as many platelets, as one unit of whole blood.

■ **Which is the preferred anticoagulant for platelets prepared for transfusion, acid citrate dextrose (ACD) with added citrate to lower pH to 6.5, CPD, or ethylenediamine tetraacetate (EDTA)?**

ACD or CPD are preferred. EDTA damages platelets and results in excessive sequestration in the spleen. The acid pH prevents aggregation of platelets in response to small amounts of ADP released from damaged platelets.

■ **How long may platelet concentrates be stored before transfusion?**

Ideally transfusion should be accomplished within 6 hours, but platelets remain viable for 48 to 72 hours when stored in plasma at room temperature.

■ **What are the effects of 4° C and room temperature storage on platelet concentrates?**

Storage at 4° C results in decreased survival when platelet concentrates are subsequently transfused. Room temperature storage results in better survival, but the platelets are less effective hemostatically immediately after transfusion. Room temperature platelets will be hemostatically functional 24 hours after survival.[5]

■ **Why are A-B-O and Rh-compatible platelets recommended when feasible?**

Platelets carry A-B-O antigens, and decreased increments may be noted when incompatible platelets are transfused. Platelets do not have Rh antigens, but red cells frequently contaminate platelet preparations and can sensitize Rh-negative recipients.[3]

■ **How many platelets are present in one unit of platelet-rich plasma, and how great a rise in platelet count should be expected after transfusion of platelets concentrated from one unit of plasma?**

One unit of platelet-rich plasma contains approximately 10^{11} platelets, and a rise of approximately 12,000 platelets/cu mm/m^2 body surface should be noted an hour after transfusion.

■ **What are the life spans of platelets in normal subjects, in thrombocytopenic patients, and in thrombocytopenic patients who are bleeding or who have bacterial sepsis?**

The life span in normal subjects is approximately 8 days; in thrombocytopenic patients it is about 3 days; and it is even shorter in the presence of hemorrhage or sepsis. Consequently, transfusions of platelets two or three times a week may be necessary. Platelet transfusions are rarely indicated in ITP.

■ **How frequently do platelet incompatibility transfusion reactions occur?**

They occur rarely, and no fatal reactions have been reported.

■ **What are the clinical indications for plasmapheresis in treating a patient?**

They are circulatory overload, dysproteinemia with high viscosity, or acute drug or chemical poisoning.

■ **How often may a person be allowed to donate blood?**

A person may donate blood a maximum of five times a year, at least 8 weeks apart.

■ **List the possible uses of plasma obtained by plasmapheresis.**

It can be used for preparation of platelet-rich plasma or platelet concentrates, leukocyte-rich plasma or leukocyte concentrates, factor VIII–rich cryoprecipitate, AHG concentrate, albumin, fibrinogen, immune globulins, and factor II-VII-IX-X concentrate.

■ **What precautions should be taken in collecting and utilizing plasma?**

The donor must meet the requirements for whole blood donation, and the donor's serum protein level must be above 6 gm/dl.

■ **What are the disadvantages of using dextran in treating hemorrhagic or burn shock?**

In large quantities dextran may interfere with cross-match tests (dextran produces pseudoagglutination of red blood cells), cause a coagulation defect (decreased platelet aggregation), and it may cause allergic reactions.

■ **How often can plasmapheresis be performed on a given donor?**

Removal of up to 1 L of plasma per week for as long as 32 months has resulted in no ill effects.

■ **What are the approximate risks of hepatitis to patients receiving transfused blood if the blood is from volunteer donors vs. commercial blood bank donors?**

The risk is lower if the blood is from volunteer donors. One estimate is a carrier rate of 6.3% for blood from commercial donors and less than 0.6% from blood from volunteer donors.[8]

■ **What are the serologic characteristics of the Bombay blood group?**

It is characterized by serum that contains anti-**A**, anti-**B**, and anti-**H**. The cells do not react with anti-**H**, anti-**A**, or anti-**B**. When the Bombay individual is a secretor, only Le[a] substance is secreted.

■ **If a Bombay blood group individual marries a person with ordinary blood group O, what will be the blood groups of the children?**

(1) Children may have blood group O, or (2) the Bombay individual may have the gene for A or B blood group which is unable to express itself because there is no H substance to convert to A or B blood groups. A child of such a marriage may have A and B blood groups because the child will have the gene H from its other parent with which to make H substance.

■ **Describe the HL-A antigen system.**

There are two closely linked loci on an autosomal chromosome, one called the LA (first) locus and the other the FOUR (second) locus. Each locus may contain any one of a number of different antigens that are specific for that locus. Thus each individual will have four HL-A antigens (two antigens on each of a pair of chromosomes).

■ **Describe the principle of the lymphocytotoxicity tests for HL-A antibodies.**

Lymphocytes are added to antisera of known specificity. When the antibody combines with the antigen complement is bound, and membrane alteration and cell death occur. Unlike live cells, dead cells are incapable of excluding a dye such as trypan blue, and when viewed under the microscope will have a blue stain. This is a positive test for the presence of the particular antigen, or conversely when screening serum, it is a positive test for the presence of an HL-A antibody.

■ **What is the mixed lymphocyte culture test?**

Lymphocytes from two individuals are mixed together. Nonidentity of antigens will result in stimulus of DNA synthesis, which can be assayed. There is a close correlation between HL-A matching and lack of mixed lymphocyte stimulation; however, occasionally, HL-A identical lymphocytes will demonstrate stimulation. This is interpreted as showing a lack of identity between the individuals at histocompatibility loci other than LA and FOUR.

■ **What HL-A antigen has been associated with rheumatoid spondylitis?**

HL-A 27 is associated with rheumatoid spondylitis.

■ **What is the significance of the HL-A system in transplantation?**

The number of HL-A antigens wherein donor and recipient differ appears to be directly related to the success of the graft to transplantation. That is, the greater the degree of HL-A identity between donor and recipient, the greater the likelihood of successful transplantation.

■ **What is the significance of the HL-A system in white cell or platelet transfusion?**

Multitransfused patients develop HL-A antibodies that will substantially diminish or completely abolish the anticipated rise in platelet count after platelet transfusion. Similar results occur with white cell transfusions.

■ **Give the H and Lewis and phenotypes of the following genotypes in blood (Bld) and saliva (S).**

Genotype	Bld phenotype	S phenotype
1. *Hh, Lele, sese*	H, Le^a	Le^a
2. *HH, Lele, Sese*	H, Le^b	H, Le^a, Le^b
3. *HH, lele, Sese*	H	H
4. *hh, Lele, Sese*	Le^a	Le^a

■ **Why is CPD preferred over ACD as a preservative?**

Levels of 2,3,DPG are well preserved in CPD blood for approximately a week before decreasing. In ACD 2,3,DPG is virtually gone after a week.

■ **What is meant by a "shift to the left" of the oxygen-hemoglobin dissociation curve of blood, and why is it undesirable?**

The oxygen-hemoglobin dissociation curve relates O_2-saturation of hemoglobin to the dissolved P_{O_2} of the blood. When the curve is shifted to the left, at a given P_{O_2} more O_2 remains bound to hemoglobin than normally, and thus less oxygen can be given up to the tissues.

■ **What shifts the oxygen-hemoglobin curve?**

Aklalosis and decreased 2,3,DPG unfavorably shift it to the left. Acidosis and increased 2,3,DPG shift it to the right, delivering more oxygen for the same hemoglobin concentration and P_{O_2}.

■ **When donor blood is tested for hepatitis-associated antigen (HB$_s$Ag) and antibody to HB$_s$Ag, which is more commonly found?**

Either HB$_s$Ag or antibody to HB$_s$Ag may be more commonly found, depending on the group studied and method of examination. The two appear to occur with about equal frequency, which approaches 1% in lower socioeconomic groups.

■ **What proportion of cases of posttransfusion hepatitis are thought to be caused by hepatitis B?**

Studies with RIA for HB$_s$Ag and its antibody have suggested that less than half of such cases are caused by hepatitis B but are rather caused by hepatitis A, cytomegalic virus, or other agents.[4]

■ **When biologic (in vivo) crossmatch fails to demonstrate incompatibility, are blood transfusions effective in alleviating the anemia in severe cases of autoimmune hemolytic anemia (AIHA)?**

Even when rapid injection of a test dose of donor blood is not followed by elevation of plasma hemoglobin 20 minutes later (compatible biologic crossmatch), transfusions usually offer only transient benefit in patients with AIHA. Unless the autoantibody happens to be directed against hr' (e), and hr"-negative blood is transfused, the blood hemoglobin level usually has returned to pretransfusion level within 4 days, and production of multiple isoantibodies often follows transfusion.[1]

REFERENCES

1. Bell, C. A.: Autoimmune hemolytic anemia; routine serologic evaluation in a general hospital population, Am. J. Clin. Pathol. 60:903, 1973.
2. Carrera, A. E., et al.: Screening of blood donors for hepatitis-associated antigen and antibody, Am. J. Clin. Pathol. 60:445, 1973.
3. Goldfinger, D., and McGinniss, M. H.: Rh-incompatible platelet transfusion-risks and consequences of sensitizing immunosuppressed patients, N. Engl. J. Med. 284:942, 1971.
4. Hollinger, F. B., et al.: Limitations of solid-phase radioimmunoassay for HB Ag in reducing frequency of posttransfusion hepatitis, N. Engl. J. Med. 289:385, 1973.
5. Kattlove, H. E.: Platelet preservation—what temperature? A rationale for strategy, Transfusion 14:328, 1974.
6. Michaels, J. M., et al.: Potassium load in CPD-preserved whole blood and two types of packed red blood cells, Transfusion, 1975. (In press.)
7. Mollison, P. L.: Clinical aspects of Rh immunization, Am. J. Clin. Pathol. 60:287, 1973.
8. Walsh, J. H., et al.: Posttransfusion hepatitis after open-heart operations: incidence after the administration of blood from commercial and volunteer donor populations, J.A.M.A. 211:261, 1970.

CHAPTER 4

Cerebrospinal fluid

The cerebrospinal fluid (CSF) provides mechanical protection for the brain and spinal cord, acts as a sink for metabolites, and furnishes an environment low in potassium and high in sodium and magnesium that is propitious for conduction of nervous impulses. Recently it has become clear that the CSF is formed not only by the choroid plexus, but that significant contributions are made by the ventricular walls and by the subarachnoid pial surface.[1] Exchange between the CSF and the brain extracellular fluid occurs readily for various molecules ranging in size from urea to serum albumin.[2] The flow of CSF is not unidirectional from the choroid plexus through ventricles, aqueduct, foramina of Luschka and Magendie to absorption sites in the arachnoid villi, but during each diastole the flow is reversed, and CSF reenters the ventricles from the subarachnoid space.[1] The choroid plexus has been compared to a miniature kidney because it actively transports substances in both directions, and the analogy is further supported by deposition of circulating immune complexes in the choroid plexus.[5,10] These recent developments promise expanded interest in CSF analysis.

A standard text of laboratory diagnosis of neurology should be consulted. The book by Smith presents a fascinating commentary on the diagnosis of syphilis of the central nervous system, and the chapter by Fishman is unusually complete.

Fishman, R. A.: Cerebrospinal fluid. In Baker, A. B., and Baker, L. H., editors: Clinical neurology, vol. 1, New York, 1973, Harper & Row, Publishers.

Smith, J. L.: Spirochetes in late seronegative syphilis, penicillin notwithstanding, Springfield, Ill., 1969, Charles C Thomas, Publisher.

■ **What is the normal cerebrospinal fluid (CSF) volume and the normal rate of formation of CSF in adult men?**

The normal CSF volume in adult men is between 90 and 150 ml. The normal rate of formation is about 500 ml/24 hr.

■ **What is the normal spinal fluid pressure?**

It is 50 to 200 mm of water, with the patient in the lateral recumbent position.

■ **How is the Queckenstedt test performed?**

Bilateral jugular compression should lead to increase in pressure to at least 300 mm of water within 10 seconds (negative reaction). If it does not (positive reaction), correct placement of the needle should be checked by observing a rise in pressure, which should be prompt when the patient contracts the abdominal muscles with closed glottis.

■ **What is the significance of a positive reaction to the Queckenstedt test?**

A positive reaction is consistent with dural sinus thrombosis or subarachnoid block below the foramen magnum. It is positive in about 80% of all patients with compression of the spinal cord.

■ **What circumstance contraindicates withdrawal of an ordinary volume of spinal fluid or performance of a Queckenstedt test?**

The contraindication is increased intracranial pressure (papilledema).

■ **How much spinal fluid should be withdrawn for analysis?**

Ordinarily, 6 to 8 ml is divided among three sterile tubes, but up to 20 ml may be withdrawn when indicated.

■ **What is xanthochromia?**

Xanthochromia is a yellow or orange coloration of supernatant centrifuged spinal fluid.

■ **How soon does orange xanthochromia appear after subarachnoid hemorrhage, and what is the pigment present?**

It appears in 90% of all patients within 12 hours after the hemorrhage and is present in nearly all patients within 24 hours. The pigment is hemoglobin.

■ **Explain the pathogenesis of yellow xanthochromia.**

Yellow xanthochromia results from bilirubin bound to spinal fluid protein. The bilirubin can be derived from reduction of heme pigment liberated by subarachnoid hemorrhage or by transfer of bilirubin diglucuronide across the blood-brain barrier in jaundiced patients. Xanthochromia also occurs in the absence of hemorrhage or jaundice when the spinal fluid protein concentration is high.

■ **How soon does yellow xanthochromia appear after subarachnoid hemorrhage, and how long does it last?**

It appears after 2 to 4 days and lasts 3 to 4 weeks.

■ **Which of the three tubes of spinal fluid should be used for the cell count?**

Use the third tube, because it is least likely to be contaminated with blood.

■ **How is spinal fluid prepared for a cell count?**

It is mixed and counted undiluted in a hemacytometer chamber. Red blood cells may be lysed by drawing glacial acetic acid to the 1 mark of a white blood cell pipet before filling it with spinal fluid and mixing the contents.

■ **What is the normal spinal fluid cell count?**

The count is 0 to 5 mononuclear cells per cubic millimeter with no polymorphonuclear leukocytes.

■ **What types of pleocytosis are characteristic in the following diseases: pneumococcal meningitis, *Haemophilus influenzae* or meningococcal meningitis, tuberculous meningitis, cryptococcal meningitis, meningovascular syphilis, tabes dorsalis, general paralysis, acute poliomyelitis, and multiple sclerosis?**

Meningitis caused by *Streptococcus pneumoniae, H. influenzae,* and *Neisseria meningitidis* cause a predominantly granulocytic pleocytosis; the cell counts may be high, usually 500 to 10,000/cu mm. Tuberculous meningitis causes a mixed granulocytic and lymphocytic or a predominantly lymphocytic pleocytosis with counts of 10 to 500/cu mm. *Cryptococcus neoformans* usually produces a lymphocytic pleocytosis with counts up to 1000/cu mm, but occasionally the cell count is normal. Acute meningovascular syphilis causes a rather severe pleocytosis (100 to 2000/cu mm) with predominance of either lymphocytes or neutrophils. More common forms of meningovascular syphilis, general paralysis, and tabes dorsalis produce a lymphocytic pleocytosis with counts of 15 to 500/cu mm, but the cell count may be normal in old, untreated cases of tabes. The cell count in poliomyelitis is highest (10 to 500/cu mm) during the first week of illness. At first, granulocytes may predominate, but later most cells are lymphocytes. Approximately 35% of all patients with multiple sclerosis have slight lymphocytic pleocytosis (5 to 50/cu mm), but they rarely have more marked pleocytosis.

■ **How does the spinal fluid glucose level relate to the blood glucose level in the absence of central nervous system disease?**

The spinal fluid glucose level is approximately two thirds of the blood glucose level, but when the blood glucose level is abnormally high, the ratio falls below 0.6. Rapid changes in blood sugar also alter the relationship, since equilibration requires 2 hours.

■ **Which chemical test performed on spinal fluid is most useful in distinguishing bacterial meningitis from other conditions?**

Measurement of glucose concentration is most useful. The glucose concentration usually is less than 40 mg/dl in bacterial meningitis.

■ **What conditions, other than bacterial and mycobacterial meningitis, cause decreased glucose levels in the spinal fluid?**

Fungal meningitis, meningeal neoplasms (carcinomatosis, primary neoplasms of the central nervous system with meningeal implants, and lymphomatous and leukemic meningeal infiltration), meningeal sarcoidosis, and hypoglycemia cause decreased glucose levels. Decreased glucose concentrations occur in about 10% of patients after spontaneous subarachnoid hemorrhage and in occasional cases of viral meningoencephalitis.

■ **What effect does meningeal carcinomatosis have on spinal fluid protein concentration and cellularity?**

The protein concentration is elevated to as high as 500 mg/dl, and a predominantly lymphocytic pleocytosis with counts up to 500/cu mm occurs. Malignant cells can be identified by cytologic methods.

■ **How long a time is required for sudden changes in the blood glucose level to be reflected fully in the spinal fluid glucose level?**

Approximately 2 hours is required.

■ **When cerebrospinal fluid rhinorrhea is suspected, does a positive test with glucose oxidase paper establish the diagnosis?**

A positive test with glucose oxidase paper is not reliable evidence for cerebrospinal fluid rhinorrhea, since normal nasal secretions give positive reactions in 45% to 75% of instances.[3]

■ **Describe a reliable test for cerebrospinal fluid rhinorrhea.**

A radioactive substance is introduced intrathecally, and fluid is collected on cotton pledgets placed within the nose. A pledget saturated with nasal fluid is compared to a pledget saturated with plasma, and a ratio of radioactive counts per minute greatly in excess of 1.3 establishes the diagnosis of a cerebrospinal fluid leak. The pledget closest to the leak has the highest count.[4]

■ **Why is the alkaline copper tartrate (biuret) reaction as used to measure serum proteins inadequate for measurement of spinal fluid protein?**

Normal levels of spinal fluid protein are less than 1/100 those in serum, and the biuret reaction is not sufficiently sensitive.

■ **What three methods of measuring protein are satisfactory for spinal fluid?**

1. Lowry method (Folin-Ciocalteu reaction)
2. Turbidimetric methods (sulfosalicylic acid, trichloroacetic acid)
3. Coprecipitation of dye[9]

■ **Cite deficiencies of the Lowry and turbidimetric methods for measurement of protein in cerebrospinal fluid.**

The Lowry method is not entirely specific for proteins, as a number of nonprotein nitrogenous compounds, particularly free amino acids, produce color. The turbidimetric methods are sensitive to temperature; turbidity increases as temperature increases, and albumin gives more turbidity gram for gram than does globulin when precipitated with sulfosalicylic acid.[9]

■ **What are the normal ranges for protein concentration of the cerebrospinal fluid in children and adults?**

The ranges are 15 to 50 mg/dl in both children and adults. No significant increase occurs in older people.

■ **Comment on the normal values for cell counts and protein in the spinal fluid of neonatal premature and mature infants.**

As many as 5000 red cells per cubic millimeter, 40 white cells per cubic millimeter, and as much as 150 mg protein per cubic millimeter are considered normal in neonatal premature infants. Mature infants have slightly increased cell counts and a protein content that averages 80 mg/dl. The cell count reaches normal adult levels by the third month, and the mean protein content falls to 20 mg/dl by the sixth month.

■ **How does the normal concentration of protein in the intraventricular fluid compare with the concentration in the spinal subarachnoid space?**

The concentration of protein in the ventricular fluid normally is only 5 to 15 mg/dl. In the cisterna magna it is 15 to 25 mg/dl, and it increases as the lumbar sac is approached.

■ **In what conditions do the highest levels of spinal fluid protein occur?**

The highest levels occur in acute bacterial meningitis, spinal subarachnoid block, and infectious polyneuritis (Guillain-Barre syndrome). The protein concentration may be as high as 1000 mg/dl in any of these conditions, but higher levels usually indicate subarachnoid block.

■ **Which primary intracranial neoplasms are most likely to be associated with increased levels of protein in the cerebrospinal fluid?**

Neoplasms in contact with the ventricles and acoustic neuromas are most likely. Almost half of the latter are associated with protein levels in excess of 200 mg/dl.

■ **After subarachnoid hemorrhage, is the protein concentration of the spinal fluid usually greater than, less than, or the same as that calculated on the basis of the plasma protein concentration and the spinal fluid red blood cell count?**

It is usually in excess of the calculated amount.

■ **How do proportions of the various protein fractions in normal spinal fluid as revealed by electrophoresis at pH 8.6 compare with those of serum?**

In spinal fluid, the proportion of beta globulin is about twice and the proportion of gamma globulin is about half that in serum, and a fast prealbumin is present.

■ **Does elevation of the gamma globulin fraction of the CSF necessarily indicate disease of the central nervous system (CNS)?**

Since spinal fluid gamma globulin levels reflect plasma gamma globulin levels, elevation of CSF fluid gamma globulin can reflect plasma elevations (cirrhosis, collagen disease, myeloma, etc.) rather than CNS disease.

■ **Cite three diseases of the CNS in which CSF gamma globulin is often elevated with normal or only slight elevation of CSF total protein.**

The three diseases of the CNS in which selective elevation CSF gamma globulin concentration is most striking are multiple sclerosis, neurosyphilis, and subacute sclerosing panencephalitis.

■ **What are the characteristic features of spinal fluid gamma globulin in patients with multiple sclerosis?**

Agar gel electrophoresis shows multiple discrete bands in the gamma region (oligoclonal IgG). Immunoelectrophoresis demonstrates increases in IgG, IgA, certain complement fractions, and transferrin. The increases are more marked during exacerbations than during remissions.[8]

■ **Are the causative organisms usually demonstrable in gram-stained sediments of spinal fluid from patients with pyogenic bacterial, tuberculous, cryptococcal, and syphilitic meningitis?**

Pyogenic bacteria usually are demonstrable, but tubercle bacilli usually are not demonstrable even with acid-fast stains. Cryptococci are difficult to demonstrate by the gram method, and it will never demonstrate *Treponema pallidum.*

■ **What is the appropriate method for microscopic recognition of *Cryptococcus* in spinal fluid?**

It is recognized by contrast with India ink, which demonstrates the voluminous capsule.

■ **How should spinal fluid be processed in the bacteriology laboratory?**

Centrifuge the specimen, and use sediment for smears (gram stain and India ink) and cultures. Use blood agar, chocolate agar, brain-heart infusion broth at 37° C with added CO_2 (candle jar), and thioglycollate broth at 37° C. If yeasts are suspected (lymphocytic pleocytosis), add Sabouraud's glucose agar at room temperature and at 37° C. Use media appropriate for acid-fast organisms and guinea pig inoculation when indicated.

■ **What volume of spinal fluid should be cultured when acid-fast organisms or yeasts are suspected?**

Use the sediment from a large volume (10 ml), because the organisms may be scarce.

■ **What is the normal range of chloride concentration in cerebrospinal fluid?**

It is 118 to 132 mEq/L.

■ **Why is the cerebrospinal fluid chloride concentration much higher than that of plasma?**

It is higher because of the relative deficit of protein-anions in cerebrospinal fluid.

■ **How does the concentration of calcium in normal cerebrospinal fluid compare with that of plasma?**

The cerebrospinal fluid calcium concentration is approximately half that of plasma because of virtual absence of the protein-bound fraction in cerebrospinal fluid.

■ **An 8-year-old child, who was well the previous day, developed a headache and fever, is now obtunded, has a stiff neck, and has multiple cutaneous petechiae. The spinal fluid opening pressure is 350 mm of water; the cell count is 3500/cu mm with 95% granulocytes; the glucose concentration is 6 mg/dl; and the protein concentration is 620 mg/dl. What would one expect to find in a gram stain of the spinal fluid sediment; what precautions are necessary in culturing the fluid; and what is the presumptive diagnosis?**

The presumptive diagnosis is meningococcemia and meningococcal meningitis. If sufficient numbers of organisms are present, gram-negative diplococci with adjacent sides flattened will be seen. The spinal fluid should not be allowed to cool before it is cultured.

■ **Describe the characteristic spinal fluid abnormalities of infectious polyneuritis (Guillain-Barre syndrome).**

One or 2 weeks after onset, the spinal fluid protein level becomes elevated (usually 100 to 400 mg/dl). The cell count usually is normal, but a minority show a predominantly lymphocytic pleocytosis. The glucose concentration is normal.

■ **A 3-year-old child from the inner city has recently refused to eat, vomited several times, and is obtunded. A generalized convulsion occurs in the hospital emergency room, and bilateral papilledema is noted, but no meningeal or localizing neurologic signs can be elicited. The spinal fluid opening pressure is 250 mm of water; the fluid contains 12 lymphocytes per cubic millimeter; the protein concentration is 60 mg/dl; and the glucose concentration is 70 mg/dl. Routine urinalysis and blood examination are unremarkable except for a slight hypochromic anemia and basophilic stippling of the red blood cells. What presumptive diagnosis could account for all the features of this case?**

This description indicates chronic lead intoxication with acute lead encephalopathy.

■ **What is the significance of a negative result of the complement fixation or flocculation test for syphilis on blood and a positive test result on spinal fluid?

These results are indicative of neurosyphilis.

■ **What is the significance of negative complement fixation or flocculation test results for syphilis on blood and spinal fluid in a patient with physical findings consistent with neurosyphilis?**

The negative serologic test results do not exclude the possibility of syphilis of the central nervous system.

■ **What serologic tests should be done when neurosyphilis is suspected?**

Fluorescent treponemal antibody (FTA-ABS) tests on blood serum and spinal fluid should be done. The FTA-ABS test is more sensitive and reliable than complement fixation or flocculation tests.[12,13]

■ **Can the cerebrospinal fluid examination be completely normal (including negative *Treponema pallidum* immobilization test and FTA-ABS test results) in a patient with neurosyphilis?**

Yes. Spirochetes have been found in the spinal fluid of such patients by staining them with fluorescent anti–*T. pallidum globulin*.[12]

■ ***Herpesvirus hominis* is thought to be the most common cause of fatal viral encephalitis in the United States. What characteristics may samples of cerebrospinal fluid have in this type of encephalitis?**

Cerebrospinal fluid samples from patients with *Herpesvirus hominis* encephalitis may be normal, but they usually show a mild elevation of protein content (up to 250 mg/dl), a monocytic pleocytosis rarely exceeding 1000 nucleated cells per cubic millimeter (occasionally polymorphonuclear leukocytes are predominant), and sometimes increased numbers of red blood cells and xanthochromia.[6]

■ **In diabetic ketoacidosis before treatment, is the CSF pH likely to be normal, decreased, or elevated?**

It is likely to be normal or elevated. (Normal CSF pH is about 7.31, lower than the pH of arterial blood.[7])

■ **What change is expected in the CSF during treatment of diabetic ketoacidosis, and how is it explained?**

The pH tends to decrease below normal, probably because CO_2 diffuses across the blood-brain barrier more rapidly than bicarbonate.[7]

■ **What CSF pH levels are associated with stupor or coma?**

Levels below 7.24 are associated with stupor or coma.[11]

■ **For how long can an osmolar gradient persist between blood and CSF?**

It can persist for several hours.[14]

REFERENCES

1. Bering, E. A., Jr.: The cerebrospinal fluid and the extracellular fluid of the brain, Fed. Proc. **33**: 2064, 1974.
2. Fenstermacher, J. D., Patlak, C. S., and Blasberg, R. G.: Transport of material between brain extracellular fluid, brain cells and blood, Fed. Proc. **33**:2070, 1974.
3. Gradeholt, H.: The reaction of glucose oxidase test paper in normal nasal secretion, Acta Otolaryngol. (Stockh.), 58:271, 1964.
4. McKusick, K. A., et al.: Radionuclide cisternography: normal values for nasal secretion of intrathecally injected ¹¹¹In-DTPA, J. Nucl. Med. 14:933, 1973.
5. Koss, M. N.: The choroid plexus in experimental serum sickness, Arch. Pathol. 96:331, 1973.
6. Nolan, D. C., Carruthers, M. M., and Lerner, A. M.: *Herpesvirus hominis* encephalitis in Michigan: report of 13 cases, including 6 treated with idoxuridine, N. Engl. J. Med. **282**: 10, 1970.
7. Ohman, J. L., Jr., et al.: The cerebrospinal fluid in diabetic ketoacidosis, N. Engl. J. Med. 284:283, 1971.
8. Olsson, J. E., and Link, H.: Immunoglobulin abnormalities in multiple sclerosis: relation to clinical parameters: exacerbations and remissions, Arch. Neurol. 28:392, 1973.
9. Pesce, M. A., and Strand, C. S.: A new micromethod for determination of protein in cerebrospinal fluid and urine. Clin. Chem. 19:1265, 1973.
10. Pollay, M.: Transport mechanisms in the choroid plexus, Fed. Proc. 33:2064, 1974.
11. Posner, J. B., Swanson, A. G., and Plum, F.: Acid-base balance in cerebrospinal fluid, Arch. Neurol. **12**: 479, 496, 1965.
12. Smith, J. L.: Spirochetes in late seronegative syphilis, penicillin notwithstanding, Springfield, Ill., 1969, Charles C Thomas, Publisher.
13. Wilkinson, A. E.: Fluorescent treponemal antibody tests on cerebrospinal fluid, Br. J. Vener. Dis. 49: 346, 1973.
14. Wise, B. L.: Effects on infusion of hypertonic mannitol on electrolyte balance and on osmolarity of serum and cerebrospinal fluid, J. Neurosurg. 20:961, 1963.

CHAPTER 5

Chemistry

To aid review, this broad field is presented in several subsections. The study of acid-base traditionally has been the most confusing, chiefly because of hazy concepts of pH, logarithmic relationships, ionization constants, body fluid compartments, and composition of various body fluids and secretions. Some of the difficulty would be avoided if we spoke of hydrogen ion concentration as nano-equivalents per liter instead of as pH units, but this convention is not likely to change. Nonetheless Gambino has correctly stressed the simplification that results from using the linear Hendersen equation for acid-base relationships rather than the logarithmic Hasselbalch equation. Weisberg's concise review of acid-base, blood gases, and electrolytes in the fifteenth edition of *Todd-Sanford Clinical Diagnosis by Laboratory Methods* presents the essential concepts in as lucid a form as any available. A series of papers by Astrup and other authorities on acid-base appeared in the *Annals of the New York Academy of Science* in 1966, and Siggaard-Andersen's book treats the topic comprehensively.

Henry's *Clinical Chemistry: Principles and Technics* is the most exhaustive treatise on the subject. The sections on clinical chemistry in Gradwohl's text (seventh edition) by Frankel and associates, and *Chemistry for Medical Technologists* by White, Erickson, and Stevens are also excellent technical references. Natelson's text is procedurally oriented with emphasis on microanalysis. Williams' text is a good reference in the general field of endocrinology. Cawley's text should be consulted for current information on isoenzymes and clinical enzymology. Conn's review of aldosteronism is excellent.

Astrup, P., Siggaard-Andersen, O., Van Slyke, D. D., et al.: Definitions and terminology in blood acid-base chemistry, Ann. N. Y. Acad. Sci. 133:Art. 1, 1966.

Batsakis, J. G., Briere, R. O., and Markel, S. F.: Diagnostic enzymology, Chicago, 1972, American Society of Clinical Pathologists.

Bauer, J. D., Ackermann, P. G., and Toro, G.: Clinical laboratory methods, ed. 8, St. Louis, 1974, The C. V. Mosby Co.

Bioscience handbook, Van Nuys, Calif., 1974, Bioscience Laboratories.

Cawley, L. P.: Electrophoresis and immunoelectrophoresis, Boston, 1969, Little, Brown & Co.

Chopra, I. J., et al.: Thyroxine and triiodothyronine in human thyroid, J. Clin. Endocrinol. 36:311, 1974.

Conn, J. W.: Primary aldosteronism and primary reninism, Hosp. Pract. 9:131, 1974.

Fisher, D. A., and Levy, R. P.: Radioimmunoassay manual, San Pedro, Calif., 1974, Nichols Institute for Endocrinology.

Frankel, S., Reitman, S., and Sonnenwirth, A. C., editors: Grenwohl's clinical laboratory methods and diagnosis, ed. 7, St. Louis, 1970, The C. V. Mosby Co.

Henry, J. B., and Krieg, A. F.: Endocrine measurements. In Davidsohn, I., and Henry, J. B., editors: Todd-Sanford clinical diagnosis by laboratory methods, Philadelphia, 1974, W. B. Saunders Co.

Henry, R. J., Cannon, D. C., and Winkelman, J. W.: Clinical chemistry: principles and technics, New York, 1974, Harper & Row, Publishers.

Ingbar, S. H., and Woeber, K. A.: Textbook of endocrinology, Philadelphia, 1974, W. B. Saunders Co.

Natelson, S.: Techniques of clinical chemistry, ed. 3, Springfield, Ill., 1971, Charles C Thomas, Publisher.

Siggaard-Andersen, O.: The acid-base status of the blood, ed. 3, Baltimore, 1974, The Williams & Wilkins Co.

Weisberg, H. F.: Water, electrolytes, acid-base, and oxygen. In Davidsohn, I., and Henry, J. B., editors: Todd-Sanford clinical diagnosis by laboratory methods, ed. 15, Philadelphia, 1974, W. B. Saunders Co., pp. 772-803.

White, W. L., Erickson, M. M., and Stevens, S. C.: Chemistry for medical technologists, ed. 3, St. Louis, 1970, The C. V. Mosby Co.

Williams, R. H., editor: Textbook of endocrinology, ed. 5, Philadelphia, 1974, W. B. Saunders Co.

ADRENAL CORTICAL HORMONES

■ **Which are the three principal hormones produced in the adrenal cortex, and in which zones are they produced?**

1. Aldosterone: zona glomerulosa
2. Hydrocortisone: zona reticularis and zona fasciculata
3. Corticosterone: all three zones

■ **Which zone of the adrenal cortex is most affected by ACTH, and with what result?**

The zona fasciculata is most affected by ACTH and responds by an increase in hydrocortisone production.

■ **How are adrenal cortical hormones carried in the plasma?**

They are chiefly bound to transcortin, an alpha globulin.

■ **Which steroid hormone has the greatest effect on ACTH excretion?**

Hydrocortisone, which acts as a negative feedback to decrease ACTH excretion, has the greatest effect.

■ **What is the effect of ACTH on aldosterone production?**

ACTH is not the primary physiologic regulator of aldosterone production, but exogenous ACTH in pharmacologic doses temporarily causes a marked increase in aldosterone production.[6]

■ **What effect will elevation of the plasma potassium level have on aldosterone production?**

It causes increased aldosterone production.

■ **What are the two most important factors that regulate aldosterone excretion, and how is their effect mediated?**

Serum sodium concentration and extracellular fluid volume are the most important regulators. A decrease in serum sodium concentration (or extracellular fluid volume) causes increased renin release from the kidney, which in turn leads to conversion of angiotensinogen to angiotensin I. Angiotensin II (a powerful pressor) is formed from angiotensin I, and leads to increased aldosterone production.

■ **What is the normal diurnal pattern of hydrocortisone secretion?**

The secretion is maximal at 8 A.M. and decreases by approximately 50% by 4 P.M. to 12 P.M.

■ **Describe the "water loading" test.**

The patient is given 1500 ml of water by mouth, and his urine is collected over the next 4 hours. A normal individual will excrete greater than 50% of this water load within 4 hours.

■ **Which natural adrenal steroids are insulin antagonists?**

Hydrocortisone and corticosterone are insulin antagonists.

■ **What happens to the serum and urine calcium levels in patients with Cushing's disease?**

The serum calcium level remains normal, and the urine calcium level is increased.

■ **How does the normal urine excretion of 17-ketosteroids compare in adult men and women?**

Daily 17-ketosteroid excretion is slightly higher in men than in women.

■ **List the diseases or conditions in which the urine excretion of 17-ketosteroids is increased.**

It is increased in adrenocortical carcinoma, adenoma, or hyperplasia; Sertoli-Leydig and other ovarian tumors; acromegaly; ACTH therapy; severe stress and pregnancy (third trimester); and Leydig cell tumors of the testis.

■ **In which diseases or conditions is there usually a decrease in the urine 17-ketosteroid excretion?**

There is usually a decrease in the excretion in Addison's disease, panhypopituitarism, primary hypogonadism, nephrotic syndrome, gout, diabetes mellitus, chronic illness, and thyroid disease (hypothyroidism and hyperthyroidism).

■ **Describe the Porter-Silber reaction.**

Phenylhydrazine + 17-hydroxysteroid gives a blue color.

■ **How do the normal levels of urine excretion of 17-hydroxysteroids compare in adult men and women?**

Daily 17-hydroxysteroid excretion is slightly higher in men than in women.

■ **Under what conditions should one measure the excretion of 17-ketogenic steroids in the urine?**

It should be measured in those rare cases of Cushing's disease in which the 17-hydroxysteroid excretion is normal and in patients with the adrenogenital syndrome (in whom the 17-ketogenic steroids are more often elevated than the 17-hydroxysteroids).

■ **What is the major abnormality in the adrenogenital syndrome?**

It is the absence of 11-hydroxylase or 21-hydroxylase. This absence leads to decreased production of hydrocortisone (the steroid with by far the most feedback effect on ACTH secretion), an increase in ACTH production, and thereby an increase in the precursors of hydrocortisone and androgenic by-products.

■ **Which of the two types of adrenogenital syndrome is more often associated with hypertension?**

Deficiency of 11-hydroxylase is more often associated with hypertension.

■ **What are the major signs and symptoms of primary aldosteronism?**

They are hypertension, polyuria, weakness, myalgia, and tetany.

■ **What proportion of the urinary 17-ketosteroids is produced by the testes?**

One fourth to one third is produced by the testes.

■ **What are the major serum biochemical abnormalities usually present in primary aldosteronism?**

A decreased plasma potassium level, a normal or slightly increased plasma sodium level, and alkalosis are usually present.

■ **List those diseases or conditions that lead to secondary aldosteronism.**

Cardiac failure, renal failure, cirrhosis, pregnancy, potassium loading, and sodium depletion lead to secondary aldosteronism.

■ **How can one differentiate primary from secondary aldosteronism?**

Serum renin levels are increased in secondary but not in primary aldosteronism.

■ **Physiologic low levels of plasma cortisol are expected in patients with what diseases or conditions?**

Low levels are expected in liver disease and hypothyroidism.

■ **Conversely, physiologic high levels of plasma cortisol are found in patients with what diseases or conditions?**

High levels are found in hyperthyroidism and obesity.

■ **Which of the adrenal cortical hormones is the most potent glucocorticoid? How does it work to elevate plasma glucose concentration?**

Cortisol (compound F, hydrocortisone) is the most potent glucocorticoid. Cortisol stimulates gluconeogenesis and inhibits the effect of insulin.

■ **A patient complaining of weakness and mental confusion is noted to have low blood pressure and low plasma cortisol. What is the presumptive diagnosis and what further test or tests should be performed?**

The presumptive diagnosis is hypoadrenalism. An ACTH stimulation test should be done.

■ **What is the preferred method for assaying cortisol?**

Competitive protein binding is the preferred method. It is specific and virtually unaffected by nonsteroidal substances.

■ **Outline the methodology and interpretation of the ACTH stimulation test for hypoadrenocorticism.**

After a baseline prestimulation urine collection of urine or blood of both, ACTH is injected. The blood or urine or both are then collected after ACTH administration. Normal subjects show an increase in adrenocorticoid production within 24 hours. Patients with hypopituitarism will show an increase in adrenocorticoid production after 2 or 3 days of ACTH injections, whereas patients with destruction of the adrenal cortex show little or no change.

■ **Describe the performance and interpretation of the adrenocortical suppression test.**

After a baseline urine collection, an agent, such as dexamethasone, that suppresses ACTH release is given. Normal persons show a depression of the blood and urinary 17-hydroxycorticoid level. Patients with hyperfunction of the adrenal glands secondary to an autonomous adrenocortical adenoma or carcinoma show little or no suppression. Patients with adrenocortical hyperplasia generally show a decrease of about 50% of their baseline urinary hydroxycorticosteroid output. Patients with adrenocortical hyperplasia secondary to an ACTH-secreting tumor usually do not show suppression. Patients with the adrenogenital syndrome show suppression of their markedly elevated 17-ketosteroid excretions (17-hydroxysteroids are usually already decreased in these patients).

■ **Describe the performance and interpretation of the adrenal inhibition (metyrapone) test.**

A baseline 24-hour urinary collection for corticosteroids or 17-hydroxysteroids is established. Metyrapone, which selectively inhibits 11-hydroxylation, prevents the formation of hydrocortisone and thereby inhibits the negative feedback mechanism blocking ACTH secretion. In the normal individual, the total 17-hydroxysteroid and 17-ketosteroid excretions will be increased after metyrapone administration. In patients with adrenocortical hyperplasia, the already elevated urinary steroids usually are increased further. Patients with adrenocortical carcinoma usually show no change, and patients with adrenocortical adenoma may show a slight decrease or no change in the urinary steroid secretion.

ADRENAL MEDULLARY HORMONES

■ **What is the normal ratio of epinephrine to norepinephrine in the blood?**

The normal ratio is 4:1 to 9:1.

■ **What is the normal ratio of epinephrine to norepinephrine excretion by the adrenal?**

The normal ratio is four parts of epinephrine to one of norepinephrine.

■ **What are the major metabolites of the catecholamines present in the urine?**

Vanillylmandelic acid (VMA) and metanephrines are the major metabolites.

■ **What are the normal limits for daily excretion of total catecholamines and vanillylmandelic acid?**

The normal limits are up to 100 μg of catecholamines and 1 to 8 mg of vanillylmandelic acid.

■ **What diseases or conditions can produce an increase in urinary catecholamine excretion?**

Pheochromocytoma and neuroblastoma, stress, vigorous exercise, myasthenia gravis, muscular dystrophy, and treatment with certain drugs (tetracycline, methyldopa, quinidine, etc.) can increase urinary catecholamine excretion.

■ **Elevated levels of urinary VMA excretion are seen after ingestion of which foods or drugs?**

Coffee, fruits (especially bananas), aspirin, and monamine oxidase inhibitors[11] elevate levels of VMA excretion.

■ **What disease or conditions generally show an increase in homovanillic acid (HVA) excretion?**

Neuroblastoma and ganglioneuroma generally show an increase in HVA excretion.

■ **If a patient has an increase in norepinephrine blood levels without increase in epinephrine, what type of tumor is he most likely to have?**

He is most likely to have extra-adrenal pheochromocytoma.

■ **What is the proper type of specimen to be collected for measurement of catecholamines or their metabolites?**

Acidified 24-hour urine collections are best, but a random sample of urine may be adequate for measurement of catecholamines if the urine output is normal.

CALCIUM AND PHOSPHORUS

■ **By what mechanism or mechanisms is parathyroid hormone thought to produce hypercalcemia?**

1. Resorption of calcium and phosphate from bone.
2. Promotion of calcium absorption from the gastrointestinal tract.
3. Inhibition of phosphate reabsorption, resulting in increased phosphate excretion in the urine.
4. Enhancement of calcium reabsorption from the glomerular filtrate.

■ **Approximately how much calcium is present in a normal adult, and how is it distributed among bone, soft tissue, and extracellular fluid?**

The normal adult contains approximately 1 kg of calcium with 99% in bone, 1% in soft tissues, and less than 0.1% in the extracellular fluid.

■ **What are the normal daily rates of absorption of calcium from the intestine and excretion of calcium in the urine when an adult is eating an ordinary diet containing approximately 700 mg of calcium per 24 hours?**

The amounts of calcium absorbed and excreted in the urine are nearly equal, and each is approximately 150 mg/24 hr.

■ **How do the normal concentrations of calcium and phosphorus in the serum of adults and children compare?**

In adults the normal concentration of calcium is 9.0 to 11.0 mg/dl, and the normal concentration of phosphorus is 3.0 to 4.5 mg/dl. In children the level of phosphorus is higher, and the highest normal levels are in infants (up to 6.0 mg/dl), but the calcium concentration is the same as in adults.

■ **What portion of serum calcium is normally bound to protein?**

Approximately 50% is normally bound to protein, and the remainder is ionized.

■ **What is the concentration of calcium in cerebrospinal fluid (CSF) in relation to the blood?**

The concentration is about half that of the blood. It is almost all ionized and is about equal to the concentration of ionized calcium in the blood.

■ **What happens to the calcium level in the CSF in those conditions in which the CSF protein level is increased?**

The calcium level is increased in proportion to the increase in protein level.

■ **What must be measured to calculate the renal tubular reabsorption of phosphorus (TRP)?**

Glomerular filtration rate, plasma phosphorus, and urinary phosphorus excretion for a given period of time must be measured.

■ **The normal range for the TRP is 75% to 90%. In what conditions is the TRP increased, and in what conditions is it decreased?**

The TRP is increased in hypoparathyroidism and pseudohypoparathyroidism and when the serum phosphorus level is low. It is decreased in hyperparathyroidism, in hypercalcemia secondary to malignant neoplasms, in vitamin D–resistant rickets, in the De Toni-Debre-Fanconi syndrome, and in other impairments of renal tubular function.

■ **Is the serum alkaline phosphatase usually normal, increased, or decreased in patients with osteoporosis, osteomalacia, and Paget's disease of bone?**

Normal alkaline phosphatase activity is characteristic of osteoporosis, but it may be elevated after fractures. Elevated levels usually accompany osteomalacia, and Paget's disease of any appreciable extent invariably is associated with elevated serum alkaline phosphatase, often of a degree unsurpassed in other diseases.

■ **What are the typical abnormalities of serum and urine calcium and phosphorus levels in primary hyperparathyroidism?**

Serum and urine calcium levels are increased; the serum phosphorus level is decreased; and the urine phosphorus level is increased.

■ **In patients with hyperparathyroidism and osteitis fibrosa cystica, what change is noted in serum enzyme activities?**

Increased activity of alkaline phosphatase occurs.

■ **What happens to the serum and urine calcium and phosphorus levels in a fullblown case of hypervitaminosis D?**

Serum, urine calcium, and phosphorus levels are all elevated.

■ **Is the serum calcium normal, increased, or decreased in patients with primary bone tumors?**

The serum calcium level usually is normal.

■ **In patients with acute bone atrophy secondary to immobilization (orthopedic cast), are the serum calcium and phosphorus levels increased, decreased, or unchanged?**

The serum calcium level is usually increased, and in children the increase may be marked. The phosphorus level is usually normal or slightly elevated.

■ **What is the milk-alkali syndrome?**

It occurs in patients who drink large amounts of milk and alkali for peptic ulcer. The serum calcium level is usually elevated with a normal serum phosphorus and normal urine calcium excretion. The patients are usually alkalotic, show decreased renal function, and may have renal calcifications.

■ **Hypercalcemic patients with which of the following conditions would be expected to have normal concentrations of parathormone in plasma: milk-alkali syndrome, malignancy, sarcoidosis, hyperparathyroidism?**

Only in hyperparathyroidism would the level of parathormone be elevated.

■ **What are the serum and urine calcium and phosphorus levels and the serum alkaline phosphatase activity in hypoparathyroidism?**

The serum calcium level is decreased; the serum phosphate level is normal or increased; urine calcium and phosphorus excretion are both decreased; and serum alkaline phosphatase activity is usually normal.

■ **In hypoparathyroidism is the decrease in the serum calcium primarily in the ionized or in the bound fraction?**

It is in the ionized portion.[8]

■ **What is pseudohypoparathyroidism?**

Pseudohypoparathyroidism is a congenital disease secondary to end organ insensitivity to parathormone. Affected individuals have a characteristic appearance with a short stature and short extremities.

■ **What is pseudo-pseudohypoparathyroidism?**

It is a disease in which the patients have a clinical appearance similar to that of patients with pseudohypoparathyroidism but have no metabolic abnormality.

■ **Do patients with nephrosis have a normal, increased, or decreased level of ionized calcium in their blood?**

The level of ionized calcium is normal, but the amount of calcium bound to serum protein is decreased in proportion to the decrease in serum protein.

■ **What effect does blood pH have on the ionized fraction of calcium in the blood?**

The ionized fraction concentration is increased in acidosis and decreased in alkalosis.

■ **Hypocalcemic patients with which of the following conditions would be expected to have increased plasma levels of parathormone: chronic renal disease, postthyroidectomy, intestinal malabsorption, vitamin D–resistant rickets?**

All except those in the postthyroidectomy state may have increased parathormone levels.

■ **Would a patient who is alkalotic and has a normal serum calcium level have an increased, decreased, or normal level of ionized calcium?**

The level of ionized calcium would be decreased. With a given total serum calcium level, the ionized portion varies inversely with the serum pH.

■ **Briefly describe the calcium balance test.**

The patient is placed on a diet containing 0.1 gm of calcium per day for 3 days. A normal individual will decrease his urinary calcium output to approximately 0.1 gm/24 hr, but a hyperparathyroid patient cannot excrete less than 0.15 to 0.20 gm/24 hr.

■ **What are the usual biochemical findings in a patient with vitamin D deficiency?**

The serum calcium level is usually normal in the early stages, but the serum phosphorus level is decreased, and serum alkaline phosphatase activity is increased. After a period of time, the serum calcium level may also decrease, especially if the calcium intake is low.

■ **Briefly outline the biochemical abnormalities seen in patients with renal osteodystrophy.**

When first examined, the patient may show acidosis, an increased serum phosphorus level, increased serum alkaline phosphatase activity, and a decreased serum calcium level. Later the serum calcium level may rise to within the normal range secondary to increase in parathormone production.

■ **What effect, if any, does acute pancreatitis have on the serum calcium level?**

The serum calcium level may be decreased secondary to "soap" formation in areas of fat necrosis in and around the pancreas.

■ **A patient who has a carcinoma of the thyroid gland with extensive metastases to lymph nodes, liver, and bones develops hypocalcemia despite a normal serum protein concentration. How can the hypocalcemia be explained on the basis of the thyroid carcinoma?**

Medullary carcinomas of the thyroid gland secrete calcitonin, a hormone that blocks calcium release from bone and calcium absorption from the intestine.

■ **How can cyclic AMP (adenosine 3′,5′monophosphate) excretion in the urine be of help in the differential diagnosis of hypoparathyroidism?**

Urinary excretion of cyclic AMP is subnormal in both primary hypoparathyroidism and pseudohypoparathyroidism. Patients with the former entity show a marked rise in urinary excretion of cyclic AMP after intravenous injection of parathormone, whereas patients with the latter condition show little if any increase.

CARBOHYDRATES

■ **What is the sensitivity of the Benedict qualitative test or Clinitest for glucose in urine, and what are the appearances of trace and maximal reactions?**

A measure of 0.1 to 0.3 gm/dl gives a trace reaction, which is a change from blue to green with no precipitate, whereas 2.0 gm/dl or more gives a maximal reaction that consists of a brick-red precipitate.

■ **Which of the following sugars are reducing sugars and will give positive Benedict (Clinitest) reactions: arabinose, ribose, xylose, galactose, glucose, mannose, fructose, lactose, maltose, and sucrose?**

All except sucrose are reducing sugars and will give positive Benedict reactions.

■ **What is glycogen, and how does it differ from starch?**

Glycogen and starch are polymers of D-glucopyranose with alpha-1,4 and alpha-1,6 linkages. Glycogen has more 1,6 linkages (branches) than starch.

■ **What is the effect of pancreatic amylase on starch?**

The starch is hydrolyzed to dextrins and maltose.

■ **What are the glycogen storage diseases?**

They are a group of diseases in which abnormal quantities of glycogen are stored in various tissues. The storage results from lack of enzymes participating in the breakdown of glycogen (amylo-1,6-glucosidase, liver phosphorylase, muscle phosphorylase, glucose-6-phosphatase, and lysosomal acid maltase) or from lack of the branching enzyme (amylo-1,4 $\longrightarrow$ 1,6-transglucosylase).

■ **Which of the glycogen storage diseases usually do not become manifest until adulthood and do not produce visceromegaly?**

These characteristics indicate myophosphorylase deficiency (McArdle's disease) and phosphofructokinase deficiency (Tarui's disease).

■ **What biochemical feature of venous blood from muscles during ischemic exercise is typical of McArdle's disease?**

Failure of the normal marked rise in lactic acid content to occur is typical.

■ **Describe the intramuscular glucagon test for glycogen storage disease.**

After blood is drawn from the fasting patient, glucagon is injected intramuscularly in a dose of 100 μg/kg of body weight. Thirty minutes later, a second blood sample is drawn. The glucose concentration in the second sample should exceed that in the first by at least 70 mg/dl. The test is abnormal in forms of glycogen storage disease involving the liver except for lysosomal acid maltase deficiency (Pompe's disease).

■ **What is the likely underlying abnormality in an infant who becomes listless, vomits, develops jaundice, and loses weight when milk feedings are** instituted and whose urine is strongly positive for reducing substances when tested with Benedict's solution or Clinitest tablets but is negative for glucose when tested with glucose oxidase paper?

The infant probably has galactosemia.

■ **Which sugars give positive reactions with Bial's orcinol reagent and Seliwanoff's resorcinol reagent?**

Pentoses give a positive reaction to Bial's reagent tests (green or black color), and fructose gives a positive reaction to Seliwanoff's reagent tests (cherry-red).

■ **What is the clinical significance of essential pentosuria and essential fructosuria?**

The disorders are benign and are important only in leading to mistaken diagnosis of diabetes mellitus by urine testing.

■ **What are the normal ranges of fasting blood and serum (or plasma) glucose levels?**

The range for blood is 65 to 110 mg/dl, and for serum and plasma it is about 12 mg/dl higher.

■ **Which gives higher "blood sugar" values, the Somogyi-Nelson or the Folin-Wu method? Explain why.**

The Folin-Wu method gives the higher values, because tungstic acid fails to precipitate much of the nonglucose-reducing substances.

■ **Compare the concentration of glucose in red blood cells (RBC) with that in plasma.**

The glucose concentration is slightly lower in RBC than in plasma because RBC have a lower concentration of water. Glucose diffuses freely between plasma and RBC.

■ **Most of the nonglucose-reducing substances in blood are contained in what component?**

They are contained in the RBC.

■ **Name three nonglucose-reducing substances that are precipitated by $Ba(OH)_2$ and $ZnSO_4$ more completely than by H_2WO_4 (tungstic acid).**

They are glutathione, creatinine, and uric acid.

■ **Does the orthotolidine method for blood glucose measurement avoid interference from nonglucose-reducing substances, or does it have the same nonspecificity as the Folin-Wu method?**

The orthotolidine method gives values corresponding to the Somogyi-Nelson method, because it is relatively specific for aldohexoses.

■ **What method of measuring blood glucose is the most specific?**

The glucose oxidase method is the most specific.

■ **How soon after drawing must blood be analyzed for glucose?**

It must be analyzed within 30 minutes unless it is collected in fluoride anticoagulant. After separation from the cells, the glucose concentration in serum or plasma stored at 4° C is stable for 24 hours.

■ **List the hormones that have a hyperglycemic effect.**

Growth hormone, ACTH, adrenal corticoids, glucagon, and epinephrine have a hyperglycemic effect.

■ **Which of the following is the best screening test for diabetes mellitus: fasting blood sugar, 1-hour postprandial blood sugar, or 2-hour postprandial blood sugar?**

The 2-hour postprandial blood sugar will have the least number of false positives and will have only slightly fewer positives than the 1-hour postprandial test. The fasting blood sugar will miss many mild diabetics.

■ **Describe the method for performing an oral glucose tolerance test.**

1. The patient should have eaten a diet containing at least 300 gm of carbohydrates daily for 3 consecutive days.
2. A sample of blood should be drawn after an overnight fast.
3. The patient drinks a solution containing 1.75 gm of glucose per kilogram of ideal body weight.
4. Blood should be drawn and urine specimens obtained at intervals of ½, 1, 1½, 2, 3, and 4 hours after ingestion of glucose.
5. The glucose concentrations in the specimens of blood and urine should be measured.

■ **What are the criteria of Fajans and Conn for interpretation of oral glucose tolerance tests?**

The normal response is fasting and 2-hour levels less than 110 mg/dl and a peak level less than 160 mg/dl. Diabetes mellitus is diagnosed when the fasting or 2-hour levels or both are greater than 120 and the peak level is greater than 160 mg/dl.

■ **What is the significance of the 1½-hour blood glucose determination in the glucose tolerance test?**

In cases of borderline abnormal results, the level at 1½ hours should be 140 mg/dl or higher to avoid construing rebound hyperglycemia as diabetes mellitus.

■ **When in the course of a glucose tolerance test does the peak of blood immunoreactive insulin occur in normal subjects and in diabetics?**

The insulin peak occurs at 1 hour in normal subjects and at 2 to 3 hours in diabetics. In both groups, blood insulin levels are near zero by 5 hours after ingestion of glucose.

■ **Describe the cortisone-glucose tolerance test.**

1. The patient eats a 300 gm carbohydrate diet for 3 days and then fasts overnight. If the body weight is less than 160 lb, 50 mg of cortisone should be given orally 8½ hours and again 2 hours before glucose ingestion. Each dose of cortisone is 62.5 mg if the body weight is in excess of 160 lb.
2. Fasting blood is drawn 2 hours after the second dose of cortisone.
3. The patient should then be given orally 1.75 gm of glucose per kilogram of ideal weight.
4. The remainder of the test goes according to the standard glucose tolerance test.

- **How is the cortisone-glucose tolerance test interpreted?**

Normal subjects have 1-hour blood glucose levels of less than 160 and 2-hour levels of less than 140 mg/dl. Higher levels indicate a prediabetic state.

- **Which of the following are diagnostic of diabetes mellitus?**
  1. **Fasting blood sugar in excess of 120 mg/dl**
  2. **Oral glucose tolerance test showing peak level in excess of 160 and 2-hour level in excess of 120 mg/dl**
  3. **Cortisone glucose tolerance test with 1-hour level exceeding 160 and 2-hour level exceeding 140 mg/dl**
  4. **Glucosuria, 4+**
  5. **Glucose tolerance test with peak level exceeding 180 mg/dl**

Numbers 1 and 2 above are diagnostic of diabetes mellitus.

- **What is the significance of an abnormal, diabetes-like glucose tolerance test in a patient with chronic renal failure and a blood urea nitrogen level of 200 mg/dl?**

First, be sure that true glucose values have been measured. Interfering substances in uremic plasma or serum may falsely elevate results by copper reduction methods as much as 35 mg/dl but do not interfere with the glucose oxidase measurement. But even when true glucose is measured, an elevated glucose tolerance curve is commonly found in uremic patients and is usually attributable to the uremic state itself. Glucose tolerance test results revert to normal immediately after correction of the uremia by hemodialysis.[10,14]

- **Are the plasma insulin levels of uremic patients with diabetes-like glucose tolerance test results normal, low, or high?**

Their plasma insulin levels are high, and this observation leads to the supposition that the uremic state is a result of insulin-antagonism.[14]

- **Describe the tolbutamide (Orinase) tolerance test.**

The patient should be prepared as for a standard glucose tolerance test with a 300 gm carbohydrate diet for 3 days. Salicylates should be withheld for 3 days before the test. After a 12-hour overnight fast, a blood specimen is drawn. Then 1.0 gm of tolbutamide dissolved in 20 ml of distilled water is injected intravenously over 2 to 3 minutes. Blood is drawn 5, 10, 20, 30, 60, and 120 minutes after the tolbutamide has been administered.

■ **Describe the criteria for interpretation of the tolbutamide (Orinase) tolerance test.**

Diabetes is indicated by a 20-minute blood sugar level of not less than 90% of the pretest value. Levels of 75% or less rule out diabetes, but values between 75% and 90% are inconclusive. A 30-minute level of 77% or more confirms diabetes. Patients with insulin-secreting tumors reveal a profound depression of blood glucose values below 50 mg/dl at 2 hours associated with increased blood insulin levels.

■ **List six causes of glucosuria other than diabetes mellitus.**

1. Altered renal threshold (congenital tubular defects, nephrosis)
2. Pregnancy and lactation (lactosuria also may occur during lactation)
3. Hyperthyroidism
4. Cushing's disease or adrenal cortical tumor
5. Pheochromocytoma
6. Intracranial injury

■ **The patient with acromegaly who has glucosuria probably also has what disease?**

He probably has diabetes mellitus.

■ **What is the response of patients with insulin-secreting tumors or islet cell hyperplasia to the tolbutamide test?**

The response is profound hypoglycemia with levels of glucose persisting below 50 mg/dl at 2 hours.

■ **List six conditions that can be associated with hypoglycemia.**

1. Starvation
2. Decreased hepatic glucogenesis (hepatic failure, glycogen storage diseases)
3. Decreased hormonal insulin antagonism (Addison's and Simmonds' diseases)
4. Hypersecretion of insulin (islet cell hyperplasia, adenoma, or carcinoma or heterotopic insulin-secreting tumor)
5. Galactosemia
6. Exogenous insulin or insulin-releasing compounds

■ **In the insulin tolerance test, 0.1 unit per kilogram of insulin given intravenously has what effect on the blood sugar?**

It falls to 50% to 60% of the fasting level in 30 minutes and is normal by 2 hours.

■ **What does an insulin tolerance test with less than the normal fall in blood sugar indicate?**

It indicates insulin resistance, which can be a result of excessive circulating levels of glucocorticoids, or growth hormone, or of the presence of antibodies to the injected insulin.

■ **Would the insulin tolerance test be recommended for diagnosis of either Addison's disease or panhypopituitarism?**

It would not, because of the likelihood of inducing severe hypoglycemia.

■ **What component of plasma or serum is measured by treating a protein-free filtrate with $CuSO_4$ and $Ca(OH)_2$ to remove interfering substances, oxidation with concentrated H_2SO_4, and reaction with *p*-hydroxydiphenyl to give a purple color?**

Lactic acid is so measured.

■ **What is the upper limit of normal for lactic acid concentration in the serum of subjects at rest?**

It is 1.25 mEq/L.

COPPER

■ **To what plasma protein is most copper bound?**

It is bound to ceruloplasmin, an alpha-2 globulin.

■ **What proportion of the whole blood copper is bound to ceruloplasmin, and how is most of the remainder carried?**

Two thirds is bound to ceruloplasmin, and most of the remainder is carried in the red blood cells.

■ **What proportion of the plasma copper is not bound to ceruloplasmin?**

Five percent, which is loosely bound to albumin, is not bound to ceruloplasmin.

■ **What property of ceruloplasmin permits its chemical measurement in serum or plasma?**

It is an oxidizing enzyme capable of oxidizing aromatic diamines. One procedure for its measurement uses paraphenylenediamine.

■ **In what diseases or conditions may an increase in the serum copper level be found?**

An increase may be found in pregnancy or estrogen therapy, acute and chronic infections, cirrhosis, hyperthyroidism, leukemia, pernicious anemia, and multiple sclerosis.

■ **Is the concentration of copper in tissues increased, decreased, or normal in Wilson's disease?**

It is increased, especially in the brain, liver, and kidneys.

■ **What is the characteristic circulating ceruloplasmin level in Wilson's disease?**

It is decreased, almost always to less than 20 mg/dl.

■ **Is the major defect in Wilson's disease one of copper absorption or copper transport?**

It is a defect in copper transport secondary to a decrease in synthesis of ceruloplasmin.

■ **What is the hematologic effect of hypocupremia?**

The effect is anemia and neutropenia.

■ **In addition to Wilson's disease, what other diseases or conditions may be associated with a decrease in ceruloplasmin?**

A decrease in ceruloplasmin is found in the nephrotic syndrome, in severe malabsorption, and normally in the first 3 to 6 months of life.

ELECTROLYTES, ACID-BASE, AND BLOOD GASES

■ **How soon after blood is obtained should determinations of P_{O_2} be done?**

They should be done within 5 minutes (P_{O_2} decreases rapidly on standing). But determination of pH and P_{CO_2} can be delayed for 20 minutes if the blood is kept at 25° C.

■ **What anticoagulant should be used for blood gas and pH work?**

Heparin should be used. The lithium salt is best if sodium or ammonia determinations are to be done on the same sample.

■ **What differences exist between plasma and whole blood in pH and gas pressures?**

None exist if the plasma is separated from the cells anaerobically (in Vacutainer) at body temperature and if measurements are conducted at body temperature. Separation at a different temperature will induce variances.

■ **How much does the addition of 1 gm molecular weight of a nondissociable solute to a kg of water depress the freezing point?**

The addition depresses the freezing point 1.86° C.

■ **What is the normal plasma and urine osmolality?**

It is 280 to 295 mOsm/kg in plasma and 500 to 800 mOsm/kg in urine.

■ **Is the measurement of plasma sodium levels as sensitive an indicator as urinary sodium excretion in the diagnosis of hypoadrenalism?**

No. Sodium levels in plasma tend to remain within the normal range, whereas levels of urinary excretion are increased if salt intake is adequate.

■ **What are the normal ranges for serum sodium concentration?**

They are 136 to 142 mEq/L before age 65 and 132 to 140 mEq/L after age 65.

■ **Under what circumstances must osmotic pressure effects of nonelectrolytes in plasma not be ignored in evaluating plasma osmolality?**

In patients with alcoholism, hyperglycemia, or uremia, nonelectrolytes contribute significantly to plasma osmolality.[12]

■ **Describe the following in patients with inappropriate secretion of ADH: plasma osmolality, urine/plasma osmolality ratio, urine sodium excretion, plasma sodium level.**

Plasma osmolality and plasma sodium level are decreased, urine/plasma osmolality ratio is greater than 1, and urine sodium concentration is high.

■ **What effects does potassium deficiency have on intracellular and extracellular pH?**

It leads to intracellular acidosis and extracellular alkalosis.

■ **Is potassium citrate given orally a good replacement for potassium deficit?**

It is not, because chloride must also be supplied. Otherwise, isoosmolar reabsorption of sodium by the proximal renal tubule may be decreased, with the result of an increase in the amount of sodium presented to the distal tubular exchange sites. Increased sodium in the distal tubular lumen leads to increased loss of potassium through sodium and potassium exchange.

■ **What is the normal serum potassium level?**

It is 3.8 to 5.0 mEq/L.

■ **What is the effect of acidosis (uncompensated diabetes mellitus, for example) on serum potassium levels?**

Potassium shifts from cells to extracellular fluid in acidosis. This shift causes a rise in serum potassium concentration of approximately 0.6 mEq/L for each 0.1 unit fall in blood pH. Thus in diabetic acidosis with severe potassium depletion, the serum (plasma) potassium level may be deceptively normal.

■ **Although most potassium measurements are made on serum, what is the advantage of using heparinized plasma?**

Potassium concentration of plasma separated from cells is constant. During clotting, potassium is released from leukocytes and platelets, which can result in spuriously high measurements, particularly in patients with high white blood cell and platelet counts.

■ **What are the minimum daily excretions (and the approximate daily dietary requirements) of sodium and potassium in the urine of adults?**

Approximately 15 mEq of sodium and 40 mEq of potassium are the minimum daily excretions.

■ **What is the approximate sodium:potassium ratio in the urine of patients with classical Addison's disease and hyperaldosteronism?**

It is 10:1 in the former and 1:2 in the latter.

■ **How is serum magnesium best quantitated?**

It is best quantitated by atomic absorption spectrophotometry or fluorometry.

■ **What is the normal serum magnesium concentration, and what is the minimum daily requirement of magnesium?**

They are 1.5 to 2.5 mEq/L and 5 mEq/24 hr, respectively.

■ **Define base deficit.**

It is the amount of base that must be added to bring the pH of blood to 7.40 in the presence of P_{CO_2} of 40 mm Hg and a temperature of 37° C.

■ **Define buffer base.**

It is the sum of whole blood bicarbonate and base contributed by hemoglobin and plasma proteins.

■ **What is the normal whole blood buffer base level?**

The normal level is 40.8+ (0.36 × hemoglobin concentration in gm/dl) mEq/L.

■ **What are the normal values for total base excess in arterial and in venous blood?**

1. Arterial and capillary blood: −3 to +2 mEq/L
2. Venous blood: −1 to +5 mEq/L

Note that base excess is greater in venous than in arterial blood.

■ **What is the normal arterial blood value for base excess in neonatal infants?**

Neonatal infants normally have a base deficit of 3.6 mEq/L because of bicarbonate redistribution.

■ **At what pH would plasma proteins contribute nothing to the buffering capacity of blood?**

They would contribute nothing at pH 5.08 (isoelectric point of proteins).

■ **In acute hypercapnia, base deficit is increased more than expected because of the shift of bicarbonate out of plasma. How can this false impression of base deficit be avoided in using the Siggaard-Andersen nomogram?**

It can be avoided by using the curve for a hemoglobin level of 5 gm/dl regardless of the true hemoglobin concentration. The slope of the in vivo CO_2 titration curve is approximately the same as for a blood sample with a hemoglobin level of 5 gm/dl.

■ **What is normal arterial P_{CO_2}?**

It is 31 to 45 mm Hg.

■ **What is normal venous P_{CO_2}?**

It is 34 to 50 mm Hg.

■ **What is normal capillary P_{CO_2}?**

It is the same as arterial (31 to 45 mm Hg).

■ **How should venous blood be drawn for gas and pH measurements?**

Use the ordinary technic with a tourniquet and a Vacutainer (with heparin). It is important not to release the tourniquet before withdrawal of blood.

■ **What is the factor that relates the P_{CO_2} to the concentration of carbonic acid?**

The factor is $0.03 \times P_{CO_2}$ = carbonic acid concentration as mEq/L.

■ **What is the apparent K_a for carbonic acid in blood?**

It is 797×10^{-9}.

■ **What is the apparent pK_a for carbonic acid in blood?**

It is 6.1.

■ **Write the Henderson equation.**

$$[H^+] = K_a \frac{[H_2CO_3]}{[HCO_3^-]} \text{ or } [H^+] = 797 \times 10^{-9} \frac{(0.03)\ (P_{CO_2})}{[HCO_3^-]}$$

■ **Write the Hasselbalch equation.**

$$pH = pK_a + \log \frac{[HCO_3^-]}{[H_2CO_3]}$$

■ **What is the principle of CO_2 determination by P_{CO_2} electrode?**

It is the pH measurement in a solution of bicarbonate separated from the blood by a membrane impermeable to ions but permeable to CO_2.

■ **Does blood pH make a difference in determining P_{CO_2} by a membrane-shielded pH electrode?**

Blood pH does not affect the determination, because hydronium ions cannot diffuse across the membrane.

■ **What is the solubility of oxygen in plasma?**

The solubility is 0.003 ml/dl/mm Hg P_{O_2}.

■ **What is the oxygen-binding capacity of hemoglobin at normal pH?**

It is 1.34 ml O_2/gm hemoglobin.

■ **What is the effect of pH on dissociation of oxygen from hemoglobin?**

Dissociation is increased by increased acidity.

■ **What is the effect of hypothermia on oxygen dissociation from hemoglobin?**

It is decreased because of alkalosis.

■ **Do temperature and pH both affect determination of P_{O_2}?**

Yes. Variances from 37° C and pH 7.4 must be corrected one at a time by the Severinghaus-Astrup nomogram. This nomogram consists of the following scales: temperature and pH, P_{O_2} observed, P_{O_2} corrected, and O_2 saturation.

■ **Name two causes of failure of the Astrup nomogram to relate P_{O_2} to hemoglobin saturation accurately.**

Hemoglobinopathy is one cause. Hemoglobin Barts and hemoglobin H hold O_2 too tenaciously and would give low P_{O_2} when fully saturated. Hemoglobin Seattle releases O_2 readily at high saturation and would give an abnormally high P_{O_2} when near full saturation.

Another cause is presence of carbon monoxide. This gas bound to hemoglobin would result in a low real O_2 saturation relative to a given P_{O_2}.

■ **What is the isobestic point of hemoglobin?**

It is 805 nm, the wavelength at which oxyhemoglobin and unsaturated hemoglobin have equal absorbances.

■ **How is the isobestic point of hemoglobin used in determining oxygen saturation?**

Measure absorbances at 805 and at 650 nm. At 650 nm, absorptivity of oxyhemoglobin is less than that of reduced hemoglobin. Determine the ratio of the two absorptivities, and read the saturation level from a linear calibration curve. The extremes are ratios of 0.44 at 100% saturation and 4.5 at 0% saturation for 650 nm and 805 nm.

■ **What are the effects of short-term (minutes) and long-term (days) hyperventilation on blood pH and bicarbonate concentration?**

Short-term hyperventilation results in uncompensated respiratory alkalosis with an elevated pH and in little change in bicarbonate concentration. Long-term hyperventilation (as seen in patients with pulmonary diffusion barriers) results in a compensated respiratory alkalosis with a lesser elevation of pH but in a decrease in bicarbonate concentration (base deficit) because of loss of bicarbonate by the kidney.

■ **How do the effects of vomiting compare with the effects of loss of similar volumes of body fluids by diarrhea?**

Vomiting ordinarily leads to alkalosis if the gastric fluid contains free acid. Diarrhea results in acidosis because of loss of bicarbonate. Both conditions cause loss of sodium and potassium.

■ **What are the major causes of respiratory acidosis?**

The major causes are rebreathing air (anesthesia) and decreased elimination of CO_2 through the lungs (obstructive emphysema or decreased respiratory rate as seen with morphine).

■ **What mechanisms tend to compensate for the above condition?**

The increased P_{CO_2} stimulates the respiratory center to increase the respiratory rate, and the kidney responds by excreting more acid (NH_4^+) and thereby generating more bicarbonate.

■ **What are the conditions or diseases that may frequently lead to metabolic acidosis?**

They are diabetes mellitus, renal failure, starvation, ketosis, dehydration, renal tubular acidosis, anesthesia, toxemia of pregnancy, and shock (lactic acid acidosis).

■ **What are the basic causes of acidosis in diabetics?**

They are mainly ketosis caused by an inability to utilize carbohydrates properly plus an excessive loss of water with an associated loss of base.

■ **How does the body compensate for metabolic acidosis?**

Compensation is made by increased CO_2 removal through the lungs and by increased acid excretion by the kidney.

■ **Briefly describe renal tubular acidosis.**

It is a syndrome in which there is a tubular defect in acid excretion leading to excretion of increased amounts of Na^+, K^+, Ca^{++}, and $PO_4^{\equiv}$.

■ **Clinically significant lactic acidosis is seen under what conditions?**

It occurs in patients with circulatory failure, shock, myocardial infarction, and gram-negative septicemia.

■ **Following a severe hemorrhage, a patient with advanced liver disease is in shock, and the following observations are made in the laboratory: serum Na^+ 130, K^+ 4.5, Ca^{++} 4.0, Cl^- 90, HCO_3^- 5 mEq/L. A nitroprusside test result on the serum is negative for acetoacetic acid, and the blood pH is 7.11. What might be causing the acidosis?**

The combination of shock, liver disease, and a serum "anion gap" strongly suggests lactic acidosis. Note that the concentrations of measured cations should approximately equal the concentration of measured anions plus 16 mEq/L of protein anion. In the patient described above, there is a difference of 27.5 mEq/L that is attributable to excess lactate. The suspicion of lactic acidosis should be confirmed by measurement of blood or serum lactate.

■ **List the major causes of metabolic alkalosis.**

The major causes are excess alkali intake (i.e., peptic ulcer therapy), pyloric or high intestinal obstruction with vomiting, and K+ depletion (digitalis or diuretic therapy, Cushing's syndrome).

■ **How does the body compensate for metabolic alkalosis?**

There is a decrease of acid excretion by the kidney (except in presence of a K+ deficit).

ENZYMOLOGY

■ **Define international units (I.U.) for measuring enzyme activities as defined by the International Union of Pure and Applied Chemistry.**

One I.U. represents 1 μmol of substrate converted per ml of fluid tested per minute at 37° C. Where this represents too low a number to be convenient, the I.U. may be defined as 1 μmol/L/min, which is equivalent to 1 nmol/ml/min.

■ **The Somogyi unit is 1 mg glucose generated per deciliter of serum in 30 minutes. Convert 100 Somogyi units to I.U.**

$$\frac{1 \text{ mg glucose}}{100 \text{ ml} \times 30 \text{ min}} \times \frac{1 \text{ mmol glucose}}{180 \text{ mg glucose}} \times \frac{1000 \text{ }\mu\text{mol}}{1 \text{ mmol}} \times 100 = \frac{0.185 \text{ }\mu\text{m}}{\text{ml} \times \text{min}} = 0.185 \text{ I.U.}$$

Using the alternative definition of I.U.:

$$100 \text{ Somogyi units} = \frac{185 \text{ nm}}{\text{ml} \times \text{min}} = 185 \text{ I.U.}$$

■ **Why is it preferable to use a zero-order enzyme reaction rather than a first-order one in measuring serum enzyme levels?**

Zero-order enzyme reactions are independent of substrate concentration.

■ **What are the various mechanisms postulated to account for elevated serum enzyme levels in various states?**

Elevated serum enzyme levels may be caused by increased production, impaired disposal and increased release from tissue due to cell necrosis, or increased cell wall permeability.

■ **In what diseases or conditions are less than normal serum enzyme levels of diagnostic significance?**

Low serum enzyme levels occur in chronic pancreatitis (low amylase), hypophosphatasia (low alkaline phosphatase), and Wilson's disease (low ceruloplasmin).

■ **In most individuals, what is the major source of the plasma amylase?**

The liver is the major source.

■ **What are the usual sources when the plasma amylase level is elevated?**

The salivary glands, the pancreas, or both are the usual sources.

■ **A patient gives a history of three days of abdominal pain that is now gone. Pancreatitis is suspected. How might one check this possibility?**

Measure the urine amylase, because the urine level may remain elevated for several days after the serum levels have returned to normal.

■ **Compare serum lipase and amylase levels with regard to elevation and disappearance after pancreatitis.**

Lipase levels begin to rise later, rise more slowly, and remain elevated longer than amylase levels.

■ **List six diseases or states in which there might be an increase in the serum amylase level.**

An increase might occur in pancreatitis, sialadenitis, perforated duodenal ulcer, ectopic pregnancy, strangulated intestinal obstruction, and hyperamylasemia (a rare condition with an abnormal amylase bound to globulins in the blood).

■ **A 55-year-old man develops abdominal pain, tachycardia, hypotension, and acute abdominal signs after a bout of heavy alcoholic intake. The serum amylase on admission to the hospital 12 hours after onset of illness is only slightly elevated (200 Somogyi units per deciliter), but the serum is lactescent. Should a diagnosis of acute, hemorrhagic pancreatitis be made despite the relatively low amylase activity?**

The serum of up to 30% of patients with acute pancreatitis is lactescent, and their amylase values often are unexpectedly low. The lactescence clears as the pancreatitis subsides, and as the lactescence clears the serum amylase activity may rise. Therefore some authors believe that lactescent serum constitutes corroborative evidence for acute pancreatitis that is just as strong as elevation of serum amylase.[1,5]

■ **What drugs may produce an elevation in serum amylase values?**

Morphine and meperidine, presumably by causing contraction of the sphincter of Oddi, may produce an elevation.

■ **In what diseases does one generally find the greatest elevation in the level of serum transaminase?**

Elevation is found in those diseases in which there is hepatocellular necrosis (most often viral hepatitis).

■ **In patients with hepatocellular disease, which enzyme level is usually elevated to a greater degree, glutamic-oxalacetic transaminase (GOT) or glutamic-pyruvic transaminase (GPT)?**

The GPT level usually is more elevated than the GOT level in patients with infectious hepatitis, serum jaundice, and infectious mononucleosis, but in cirrhosis the reverse usually is true.

■ **Which tissues are especially rich in creatine phosphokinase (CPK)?**

The heart, skeletal muscle, and brain are rich in CPK.

■ **What precautions should be taken in determining the serum CPK level?**

The analysis should be performed within a few hours after the blood is drawn, because serum CPK is labile and does not withstand storage.

■ **What proportion of CPK activity remains in serum after 12 hours of storage at 25° C?**

After storage, the activity level is 65% that of normal activity.

■ **In addition to myocardial infarction, in what diseases or conditions may an elevated CPK level be found?**

It may be found in various diseases of skeletal muscle including muscular dystrophies, polymyositis, and rhabdomyolysis, after trauma to muscle including electrical shock and multiple injections, in some instances of myxedema, and only occasionally in lesions involving the brain.

■ **Serum LDH is derived predominantly from what source or sources in normal subjects?**

It comes from red blood cells.

■ **What are isoenzymes?**

Isoenzymes are enzymes having multiple molecular forms but similar chemical functions (that is, acting on the same or similar substrates to catalyze the same chemical reaction).

■ **If one arbitrarily assigns the fastest-moving electrophoretic fraction the designation of LDH-1 and the slowest LDH-5, which of the isoenzymes are associated with heart diseases and which are associated with liver diseases?**

1. Heart disease: LDH-1 and LDH-2
2. Liver disease: LDH-5

■ **What fairly simple technic can be utilized in separating LDH-1 from the other LDH isoenzymes?**

Heat denaturation at 65° C for 30 minutes destroys the activity of LDH-2 through LDH-5.

■ **Under what circumstance might one expect to find an increase in the LDH-5 in a patient with myocardial infarct?**

An increase might be found if congestive heart failure is present.

■ **What happens to the LDH levels in patients with angina pectoris, dissecting aortic aneurysms, and pericarditis?**

There is no significant alteration in the LDH enzymes in any of these conditions.

■ **List four diseases or conditions in which the LDH-5 level is usually elevated.**

It is usually elevated in acute viral hepatitis, shock, and other conditions with hepatocellular necrosis, infectious mononucleosis, metastatic cancer in the liver, and necrosis of skeletal muscle.

■ **Which of the LDH isoenzyme levels are predominantly elevated in pernicious anemia and hemolysis?**

The LDH-1 and LDH-2 levels are greatly elevated.

■ **Which of the LDH isoenzyme levels is elevated in patients with lymphomas, leukemias, and infectious mononucleosis?**

The LDH-3 level is elevated.

■ **What other enzyme fairly closely mirrors LDH-1 (myocardial) levels in patients with myocardial infarcts?**

Alpha-hydroxybutyrate dehydrogenase (αHBD) is the enzyme.

■ **Which of the LDH isoenzyme levels are elevated in renal tubular necrosis or renal infarcts?**

The LDH-1 and LDH-2 levels are elevated.

■ **Which of the LDH isoenzyme levels are elevated in skeletal muscle disease?**

In the inflammatory myopathies the LDH-5 level is elevated, whereas the LDH-1 and LDH-2 levels are elevated in muscular dystrophies.

■ **In what disease or diseases does one find the greatest elevation in the serum LDH level?**

The greatest elevation is found in pernicious anemia and metastatic carcinomatosis.

■ **Under what circumstances might an alcoholic patient have elevated LDH and CPK levels with liver disease?**

If the patient is having delirium tremens or alcoholic myopathy, LDH and CPK levels might be elevated.

■ **Which of the following types of leukemia, in relapse, is not likely to be accompanied by abnormally high levels of LDH activity in the serum: acute lymphoblastic, chronic lymphocytic, monocytic, acute myeloblastic, or chronic myelocytic?**

Chronic lymphocytic leukemia will probably not show an abnormally high level of LDH activity.

■ **Name the feature of the leukemias (other than chronic lymphocytic) with which the serum LDH activity level correlates best.**

The white blood cell count correlates best with the serum LDH activity levels.

■ **What is the significance of elevations of serum LDH level several months or years after "curative" surgery for carcinoma?**

It is suggestive of metastases, especially in the liver.

■ **What is meant by isomorphic LDH isoenzyme abnormality?**

The LDH isoenzyme distribution is normal, but all isoenzymes are present in greater than normal amounts.

■ **In what diseases or conditions is the above pattern most frequently seen?**

It is seen mostly in polycythemia vera or disseminated neoplasm.

■ **What hematologic abnormality is also frequently associated with an isomorphic elevation of LDH isoenzyme activity levels?**

Isomorphic elevation is frequently associated with thrombocytosis.

■ **A patient has a moderately severe myocardial infarct while in the hospital. Describe the changes most often seen in the following enzymes: SGOT, SGPT, LDH, and CPK.**

The CPK level increases by 8 hours after onset of pain, peaks at 36 hours, and is normal by 3 to 4 days. The LDH level increases within 12 hours, reaches a maximum at 2 to 3 days, and decreases to normal at 10 to 14 days. The SGOT level increases within 6 to 12 hours and reaches the maximum in 24 to 48 hours; it then returns to normal within 6 to 7 days. The SGPT level remains normal or is slightly elevated.

■ **Describe the "delayed peak" or "secondary rise" of SGOT seen in patients with coronary artery pain.**

Patients with coronary arterial insufficiency pain may show mild SGOT elevations of 40 to 60 U on the third to sixth day after the pain without any other evidence of myocardial infarction. This is the so-called "delayed peak" of Resnik.[7]

■ **Which of the following enzyme levels is more likely to be moderately to markedly elevated in pulmonary infarcts: SGOT, SGPT, LDH-5, CPK?**

The LDH-5 level is likely to be elevated.

■ **Which of the following enzyme levels are more likely to be moderately to markedly elevated in myocardial infarcts: SGOT, SGPT, LDH-1, CPK?**

All but the SGPT level are likely to be elevated.

■ **What do the following enzymes have in common: ornithine transcarbamylase, leucine aminopeptidase, 5'-nucleotidase, sorbital dehydrogenase, and guanase?**

They are highly specific for the liver.

■ **Serum levels of alkaline phosphatase are normally elevated in healthy patients who are _________ or _________ .**

Serum levels are elevated in patients who are growing or pregnant (third trimester).

■ **Which alkaline phosphatase is associated with the liver, and what value is there in measuring it?**

The alkaline phosphatase is 5'-nucleotidase. Its level is increased in intrahepatic and extrahepatic obstructive disease and is not usually increased in hepatocellular diseases or in bone disease.[4,17]

■ **Which other enzymes are of value in determining whether elevations of alkaline phosphatase levels are caused by bone or liver disease?**

Leucine amino peptidase, 5'-nucleotidase, and γ-glutamyl transpeptidase are elevated most by biliary obstruction and significantly less with hepatocellular damage.

■ **What are the sources of the heat-stable fraction of alkaline phosphatase?**

The liver, placenta, and intestine are the sources.

■ **Give the probable organ sources of alkaline phosphatase in the following circumstances in which serum alkaline phosphatase activity is elevated: (1) Alkaline phosphatase activity reduced below 12% after heat treatment of serum (56° C for 10 minutes), γ-glutamyl transpeptidase activity normal. (2) Alkaline phosphatase activity reduced to between 12% and 48% after heat treatment, γ-glutamyl transpeptidase activity elevated. (3) Alkaline phosphatase activity not reduced below 52% after heat treatment, γ-glutamyl transpeptidase activity not elevated.**

Case 1: bone. Case 2: liver. Case 3: placenta.[4]

■ **What is the half-life of alkaline phosphatase in the plasma?**

The half-life is approximately 7 days.

■ **Why are measurements of acid phosphatase in King-Armstrong, Bessey-Lowry-Brock, and Bodansky units not precisely interconvertible?**

The methods use different substrates that vary in affinity for the various acid phosphatase isoenzymes. Phenylphosphate (King-Armstrong method) will often detect moderate phosphatase rises in pneumonia, hepatitis, and various malignant neoplasms, whereas betaglycerophosphate (Bodansky method) is much more specific for prostatic adenocarcinoma.

■ **What is the Regan isoenzyme?**

The Regan isoenzyme is a heat-stable, L-phenylalanine-sensitive isoenzyme of alkaline phosphatase present in significant concentrations in about 12% of patients with cancer. Physically, chemically, and immunologically it appears to be identical to placental alkaline phosphatase.[16]

■ **Prostatic massage may produce iatrogenic elevation of the serum acid phosphatase activity. How much time must elapse before the effects of massage have become negligible?**

Only 25% of the iatrogenic rise persists after 24 hours, so 48 hours should be enough time.

■ **What is the prostatic fraction of acid phosphatase?**

It is the portion of the acid phosphatase that is inhibited by L-tartrate and 40% ethyl alcohol.

■ **In addition to carcinoma of the prostate, what other diseases or conditions may occasionally be associated with an elevated serum acid phosphatase level?**

An elevated level may be associated with Paget's disease of the bone, Gaucher's disease, osteosarcoma, carcinoma metastatic to bone, hepatitis, and pneumonia.

■ **An acid phosphatase level of 5 Bodansky units or 10 King-Armstrong units or greater is highly suggestive of what disease or condition?**

It suggests metastatic carcimona of the prostate.

■ **What is Sullivan's test?**

Elderly men suspected of having carcinoma of the prostate may have a normal level of serum acid phosphatase. Sullivan's test consists of administering androgens that stimulate metastatic adenocarcinomas to release acid phosphatase.

■ **Measurement of serum or red blood cell cholinesterase levels or both has been most useful for what purpose?**

The measurement has been useful to determine overresponse to organophosphorus insecticides, which are potent inhibitors of cholinesterase activity.

■ **Which of the glycolytic enzymes is the most sensitive reflector of muscle disease?**

Aldolase is the most sensitive glycolytic enzyme, but CPK is the most sensitive of all enzymes for muscle injury.[9]

■ **Is serum aldolase activity significantly elevated in any other diseases or conditions?**

Aldolase, like LDH, is elevated in carcinomatosis, granulocytic leukemia, megaloblastic anemias, and instances of hepatocellular injury.

LIPIDS

■ **In which serum lipoprotein fractions are triglycerides chiefly found?**

They are chiefly found in the chylomicrons and low-density or prebeta lipoproteins.

■ **Which serum lipoprotein fraction carries most of the cholesterol?**

The low-density or beta lipoproteins carry most of the cholesterol.

■ **Which serum lipoprotein fraction carries most of the phospholipids?**

The high-density or alpha lipoproteins carry most of the phospholipids.

■ **What proportion of the chylomicron fraction consists of cholesterol?**

Approximately 5% consists of cholesterol.

■ **Give the order of migration of serum lipid fractions in electrophoresis at pH 8.6.**

The alpha lipoproteins advance the farthest toward the anode and are followed by the prebeta lipoproteins and the beta lipoproteins. The chylomicrons remain at the point of application.

■ **List four diseases in which there is usually an increase in the level of serum cholesterol.**

An increase is usually found in hypothyroidism, nephrotic syndrome, obstructive biliary tract disease, and idiopathic hypercholesterolemia.

■ **List five diseases or conditions in which there is generally a decrease in a serum cholesterol level.**

A decrease is usually found in hepatocellular disease, hyperthyroidism, cachexia, systemic infections, and certain hematologic diseases (i.e., pernicious anemia, iron deficiency anemia, and hemolytic anemia).

■ **What percentage of cholesterol in the blood is esterified?**

About 60% to 80% is esterified.

■ **Define four classes of plasma lipoproteins in terms of electrophoretic mobility at pH 8.6 in paper, agarose, or cellulose acetate, and in terms of density.**

Chylomicrons have density <1.006 and remain at the origin on electrophoresis. Very–low-density lipoproteins (VLDL) also have density <1.006 but migrate toward the anode behind the high-density lipoproteins (HDL) in the prebeta position. Low-density lipoproteins (LDL) have a density range of 1.006 to 1.063 and migrate behind the VLDL in the beta position. HDL migrate far ahead of the prebeta (VLDL) lipoproteins in the alpha band. HDL are alpha lipoproteins, VLDL are prebeta lipoproteins, and LDL are beta lipoproteins.

■ **Describe an important difference between lipoprotein electrophoretic mobility in the above media and in polyacrilamide gel.**

In polyacrilamide gel, the positions of the VLDL and LDL bands are reversed from the positions in paper, agarose, or cellulose acetate.

■ **Hyperlipoproteinemia is not uncommonly seen as a secondary manifestation of many diseases or conditions. Name at least ten.**

Alcoholism, diabetes mellitus, porphyria, biliary obstruction, nephrosis, glycogen storage diseases, pancreatitis, hypothyroidism, hypercalcemia, liver disease, hyperestrogenism, certain dysglobulinemias, and gout may be associated with hyperlipoproteinemia.

■ **How can one differentiate between alimentary hyperlipemia and hyperlipidemia secondary to endogenous production?**

Differentiation can be made by measuring blood lipids after a 12-hour fast.

■ **What is the best type of specimen on which lipoprotein electrophoresis may be performed?**

Fresh plasma anticoagulated with EDTA is preferred.

■ **What are the inheritance patterns of the familial hyperlipoproteinemia types I-IV?**

They are autosomal recessive or dominant with variable penetrance.

■ **In type I hyperlipemia (rare inherited disease), are the triglyceride and cholesterol levels normal, increased, or decreased?**

The triglyceride level is greatly increased, and the cholesterol level is normal or increased to a much lesser degree than the triglyceride level.

■ **Is there any predisposition to coronary artery disease in type I hyperlipidemia?**

There is probably no predisposition.

■ **In type II familial hyperlipoproteinemia, are the triglyceride and cholesterol levels normal, increased, or decreased?**

The triglyceride level is normal, and the cholesterol level is much increased.

■ **What is the major difference electrophoretically between type IIa and type IIb hyperlipoproteinemia?**

Type IIb shows a prebeta as well as a beta band.

■ **What is the characteristic pattern in the lipoprotein electrophoresis in type III familial hyperlipoproteinemia?**

There are increases in both the prebeta and beta lipoprotein fractions, or an abnormal single lipoprotein band occupies the beta lipoprotein and prebeta lipoprotein positions.

■ **Describe the lipoprotein electrophoretic pattern in type IV familial lipoproteinemia.**

The prebeta lipoproteins are increased.

■ **What is the lipoprotein electrophoretic pattern in type V familial hyperlipemia?**

The chylomicron and prebeta lipoprotein levels are elevated.

■ **Which of the five types of hypolipoproteinemia are fat sensitive, and which are carbohydrate sensitive?**

Types I and II are fat sensitive, and types III, IV, and V are carbohydrate sensitive.

■ **Which of the familial hyperlipoproteinemias have eruptive xanthomas?**

Typically type I and occasionally types III, IV, and V have eruptive xanthomas.

■ **Tuberous and tendinous xanthomas are associated with elevation of the level of which lipoprotein (and lipid) fractions?**

They are associated with an elevation in the level of beta lipoproteins (cholesterol).

■ **Which hyperlipoproteinemias are associated with fasting chylomicronemia?**

Types I and V are associated with fasting chylomicronemia.

■ **Which types of familial hyperlipoproteinemic patients have foam cells in the bone marrow and spleen?**

Types I and V have these characteristics.

■ **Among the hyperlipoproteinemic syndromes, glucose intolerance and carbohydrate inducibility correlate with elevation of which serum lipoprotein (and lipid) fractions?**

They correlate with an elevation of prebeta lipoproteins (triglycerides).

■ **What type of hyperlipoproteinemia is usually associated with hypothyroidism?**

Type II (increased beta lipoproteins) is usually associated with hypothyroidism.

■ **What types of hyperlipemia most often occur in patients with diabetes mellitus?**

Those most often occurring are types III, IV, and V (these have in common increased triglyceride levels).

■ **Which types of hyperlipoproteinemia may be seen in relation to heavy alcohol intake?**

Type IV (increased prebeta lipoproteins) and type V (increased prebeta lipoproteins and chylomicrons) are related to heavy alcoholic intake.

■ **How can the comparison of electrophoresis on paper or cellulose acetate** versus polyacrylamide gel help in the diagnosis of type III hyperlipoproteinemia?

In type III hyperlipoproteinemia there is a broad beta-migrating band on the former media, but on the polyacrilamide gel the band migrates as VLDL (crossover). This presumptive test is about 95% accurate, and definitive diagnosis requires ultracentrifugation followed by electrophoresis of the supernatant demonstrating a "floating beta" lipoprotein.

■ **Which of the four major lipid fractions are elevated in patients with biliary obstruction?**

The phospholipid and cholesterol levels are elevated.

■ **A child who has grown poorly has retinal degeneration and malabsorption, and 50% of his red blood cells have long, spinous projections. Autohemolysis is virtually complete after 48 hours of incubation at room temperature. What is the name of his disease, and what abnormalities would be expected in the serum lipids and lipoprotein electrophoresis?**

The disease is acanthocytosis. Total serum lipid, cholesterol, and phospholipid levels are decreased, and beta lipoproteins are absent.

PITUITARY HORMONES

■ **Why is measurement of plasma growth hormone (GH) levels alone insufficient to establish the diagnosis of acromegaly?**

GH levels in normal individuals vary greatly with the state of wakefulness, degree of activity, state of alimentation, etc.

■ **How, then, does one establish a diagnosis of acromegaly?**

The diagnosis can be established by measuring the effect of hyperglycemia on the plasma GH levels. Acromegalics fail to show the normal decrease in GH levels to less than 1 ng/ml an hour after 100 gm of glucose orally.

■ **How can the diagnosis of pituitary dwarfism be established?**

It can be established by measuring the effect of hypoglycemia or intravenous arginine on the plasma GH level. Little if any of the normally expected elevation is noted.

■ **What are the physiologic functions of follicle-stimulating hormone (FSH)?**

In women it induces enlargement and maturation of the ovary and initiates development of the ovarian follicle during the menstrual cycle. In men it stimulates spermatogenesis.

■ **What is the physiologic function of luteinizing hormone (LH)?**

In women it causes ovulation and estrogen and progesterone production by the corpus luteum. In men it stimulates the Leydig cells to produce androgens and estrogens.

■ **Why is it frequently not possible to distinguish hypopituitarism on the basis of single LH and FSH measurements?**

Both hormones are produced normally in pulsatile fashion, and pituitary disease usually causes partial deficiencies. Therefore normal and hypopituitary LH and FSH levels overlap.

■ **How can this overlap usually be overcome?**

By the clomiphene stimulation test. After administration of 50 gm of clomiphene two or three times a day for 7 days, the normal adult will show LH and FSH increases to more than 50% of baseline levels.

■ **What usually happens in levels of FSH and LH in patients with primary gonadal deficiency (i.e., Turner's or Klinefelter's syndrome, orchiectomy, or oophorectomy)?**

They are elevated with FSH levels higher than LH levels.

■ **Under what circumstances will gonadotropin levels be extremely high (greater than 10,000 times normal)?**

Certain tumors (trophoblastic carcinoma, teratocarcinoma, oat cell carcinoma of lung, etc.) elaborate these hormones and cause these high levels.

PROTEINS AND OTHER NITROGENOUS COMPOUNDS

■ **Name four physical conditions that will precipitate globulins from serum.**

1. Increased salt concentration—one-half saturation with $(NH_4)_2SO_4$
2. Decreased salt concentration—dilution with distilled water or ethanol
3. Adjustment of pH to isoelectric point
4. Heat (near 100° C)

■ **Name two hormones that effect increased protein catabolism and two that have anabolic effects.**

1. Catabolic effects: 11-oxysteroids of adrenal cortex, excess thyroid hormone
2. Anabolic effects: androgens, growth hormone

■ **What are the half-lives of plasma albumin and gamma globulins?**

Their half-lives are 4 weeks and 1 to 2 weeks, respectively.

■ **What is the standard procedure for measuring total serum proteins in the clinical laboratory?**

The standard procedure is the alkaline cupric (biuret) method, which gives a blue color with protein.

■ **What are two deficiencies of the biuret reaction for determination of protein in fluids other than serum or plasma?**

1. Low sensitivity (not satisfactory for spinal fluid)
2. Lack of specificity (Ammonium ion is chromogenic with the biuret re-

agent, and the procedure can be applied to urine only if the protein is first isolated by precipitation.)

■ **Do albumin and globulins show approximately equal chromogenicity with biuret reagent?**

Yes. Globulin gives about 2% more color per gram than albumin.

■ **What is the clinical significance of the albumin/globulin (A/G) ratio, and how important is it in clinical diagnosis?**

The A/G ratio has been shown to correlate poorly with electrophoretic protein fractionation and is of little use clinically.

■ **Describe the phenol method of Folin and Ciocalteu for protein. What is its principal advantage?**

Lithium salts of phosphomolybdotungstic acid are reduced to a blue form by tyrosine in an alkaline medium. The principal advantage is high sensitivity that makes it suitable for spinal fluid.

■ **What substances may give false reactions with the Folin-Ciocalteu reagent?**

A variety of easily oxidized substances—streptomycin, sulfanilamide, salicylates, phenacetin, and phenothiazines—may give false reactions.

■ **Which of the protein fractions migrates the fastest electrophoretically at pH 8.6 and why?**

Albumin migrates fastest because it is a relatively small molecule with a large number of negatively charged anionic groups.

■ **Designate serum protein bands resolvable by cellulose acetate, agar gel, or paper electrophoresis at pH 8.6 in order of increasing distances from the anode.**

The serum protein bands are albumin, alpha-1 globulins, alpha-2 globulins (haptoglobin may be resolved as a band closely following the faster alpha-2 globulins), beta globulins (certain fractions of complement may be resolved as slower, beta-2 globulins), and gamma globulins.

■ **What are the normal ranges of the serum protein fractions measured by cellulose acetate electrophoresis?**

Measured as gm/dl of serum, they are: albumin 3.2 to 5.6, alpha-1 globulins 0.1 to 0.4, alpha-2 globulins 0.4 to 1.2, beta globulins 0.5 to 1.1, and gamma globulins 0.5 to 1.6.

■ **What are the normal concentrations of the various immune globulins in serum?**

Normal concentrations are IgG 800 to 1500 mg/dl, IgA 50 to 200 mg/dl, IgM 40 to 120 mg/dl, IgD 1 to 40 mg/dl, and IgE probably 1 mg/dl.

■ **List six causes of decreased total proteins in the serum.**

Six causes are starvation, liver disease, protein-losing gastroenteropathy, massive proteinuria, posthemorrhage, and idiopathic hypoproteinemia (rare, associated with hypocalcemia).

■ **In general, is the alpha globulin level raised or lowered in presence of hypoproteinemia?**

It is raised.

■ **In bisalbuminemia, does the abnormal albumin move more rapidly or more slowly than normal albumin at pH 8.6?**

It moves more slowly.

■ **Where do orosomucoid, ceruloplasmin, transcortin, TBG, and haptoglobin migrate in pH 8.6 electrophoresis?**

They migrate with the alpha globulins. Haptoglobin is separable as a band immediately following alpha-2 globulins by agarose gel electrophoresis at pH 8.6.

■ **Where do complement and transferrin migrate in pH 8.6 electrophoresis?**

They migrate with the beta globulins.

■ **Where does antitrypsin migrate? Can severe (homozygous state) deficiency be ruled out by electrophoresis?**

Antitrypsin migrates with the alpha-1 globulins. The homozygous deficiency state is unlikely if the alpha-1 globulin level exceeds 20 mg/dl.

■ **What is the significance of alpha-1 antitrypsin deficiency?**

Deficiency in alpha-1 antitrypsin disposes toward development of destructive pulmonary emphysema in adulthood and progressive hepatic cirrhosis in childhood.

■ **What are the two major functions of albumin?**

Osmotic effect in the blood and transportation of bound substances (cortisol, thyroxin, and certain drugs) are the major functions.

■ **List eleven causes of hypoalbuminemia.**

The causes are infections, myeloma, malnutrition, nephrosis, liver disease, intestinal malabsorption, protein-losing enteropathy, uremia, pregnancy (all trimesters), eclampsia, and congenital analbuminemia.

■ **Name conditions causing elevation and depression of serum alpha globulin levels, and mention the specific proteins involved.**

Elevations occur in metastatic tumors, acute myocardial infarction, and infections because of C-reactive protein, and in the nephrotic syndrome because of alpha-1 lipoprotein. Depressions occur in acute hepatic necrosis and also in subacute and chronic liver disease because of decreased orsomucoid (glyco-proteins), in intravascular hemolysis because of removal of haptoglobin bound to hemoglobin by reticuloendothelial cells, and in hereditary alpha-1 antitrypsin deficiency.

■ **List diseases that cause alterations in beta globulin levels, and explain the bases of the alterations.**

Elevations occur in iron deficiency (increased transferrin) and pregnancy. Other causes of increased beta lipoproteins are obstructive jaundice, nephrotic syndrome, diabetes mellitus, hypothyroidism, and congenital hyperlipoproteinemia. Depressions may reflect decreased levels of transferrin (hepatitis, infections, neoplastic disease).

■ **Give four causes of acquired hypogammaglobulinemia.**

The causes are nephrotic syndrome, malignant lymphomas, scleroderma, and idiopathic.

■ **Briefly describe the so-called "immediate response" pattern of protein electrophoresis. Under what circumstances is it seen?**

The pattern consists of a slight decrease in albumin with a prominent increase of alpha-1 and alpha-2 globulins. It is seen with acute tissue injuries, acute infections, and malignancy.

■ **Briefly describe the "delayed response" pattern of protein electrophoresis. Under what circumstances is it seen?**

It is similar to the above pattern, but in addition it shows a greater decrease of albumin with an increase of gamma globulin as well as the alpha globulins. It is seen in chronic infections.

■ **Briefly describe the electrophoretic pattern commonly seen with cirrhosis.**

Decreased albumin, increased alpha-2 globulin with polyclonal gamma elevation, and beta-gamma bridging are commonly seen.

■ **What are the criteria generally accepted for the diagnosis of congenital agammaglobulinemia?**

Absence of plasma cells in the reticuloendothelial system, IgG concentration less than 100 mg/dl, and IgA and IgM concentrations less than 1% of normal adult levels are the criteria.

■ **Elevation of which gamma globulin component is most commonly found in patients with multiple myeloma?**

IgG is most commonly elevated, then IgA.

■ **What is the most sensitive method for the detection of Bence Jones protein in the urine?**

Immunoelectrophoresis is the most sensitive method, and it is significantly more sensitive than zone electrophoresis.

■ **What diseases or conditions may be associated with cryoglobulinemia?**

Leukemia, multiple myeloma, macroglobulinemia, autoimmune diseases, polycythemia vera, syphilis, infectious mononucleosis, cytomegalovirus infections, hepatitis, cirrhosis, subacute bacterial endocarditis, and acute glomerulonephritis may be associated with cryoglobulinemia.

■ **List seven diseases that are associated with polyclonal elevation of gamma globulin.**

The diseases are cirrhosis, infections, autoimmune diseases (Hashimoto's thyroiditis, rheumatoid arthritis, Sjogren's syndrome, lupus erythematosus), myelocytic and monocytic leukemias, Hodgkin's disease, carcinomas, hypothyroidism, kwashiorkor, sarcoidosis, and certain allergic states.

■ **What are the various conditions associated with a monoclonal globulin peak *("M spike")* on serum electrophoresis?**

An unselected group of monoclonal peaks will represent the following conditions in roughly the proportions given: plasma cell myeloma (70%), macroglobulinemia (3%), carcinoma (5%), idiopathic causes (11%), associated with various diseases, such as arteriosclerotic heart disease (11%).

■ **Asymptomatic elevations of M-component in patients with "benign" monoclonal gammopathy have been associated with occult infections or malignancies or both of what organ or organs of the body?**

The gastrointestinal and biliary tracts, in particular, have been involved.

■ **What is the probable significance of a band between albumin and alpha-1 globulin on cellulose acetate, pH 8.6 electrophoresis of serum from a patient with an enlarged liver and hepatic functional deficit?**

These characteristics probably indicate the presence of alpha fetoprotein, indicative of primary hepatic carcinoma. It is electrophoretically detectable when in concentration of 50 mg/dl or more.

■ **What major components make up the nonprotein nitrogen of serum?**

NPN consists of urea (55%); amino acids (20%); uric acid (20%); and creatinine, creatine, ammonia, and other substances (5%).

■ **What are the normal limits of urea nitrogen concentration in whole blood, plasma, and serum?**

The normal range for all three fluids is approximately 5 to 25 mg/dl.

■ **What is the principle of urea nitrogen measurement that is common to the nesslerization and alkaline phenate hypochlorite (Berthelot) methods?**

Urea in a protein-free filtrate is converted quantitatively to ammonia and carbon dioxide by urease, and the ammonia is measured by a colored reaction product.

■ **What are the advantages and disadvantages of the diacetyl monoxime method for measurement of urea?**

It does not require hydrolysis with urease and is readily adaptable to continuous-flow automated equipment (AutoAnalyzer). The reaction is not entirely specific for urea; the color develops and fades rapidly; the timing of maximum color development is dependent on the concentration of urea; and the color is photosensitive.

■ **What is the normal range of the serum creatinine concentration?**

The normal range is 0.5 to 1.5 mg/dl.

■ **How are urine and serum creatinine concentrations determined?**

They are determined by the Jaffe reaction, which produces a red color with creatinine and an alkaline picrate reagent.

■ **Name four noncreatinine Jaffe chromogens.**

They are ascorbic acid, diacetic acid, acetone, and pyruvate.

■ **Does the protein precipitant affect recovery of creatinine?**

It does, because recovery is 85% to 90% in pH range 3.5 to 4.0 (tungstic acid), but it is 100% below pH 2.0 (trichloroacetic acid), because low pH prevents adsorption of creatinine to protein.

■ **How is creatine determined in urine and serum?**

It is determined by conversion to creatinine by boiling in presence of picric acid and then by using the alkaline picrate method (Jaffe reaction). Preformed creatinine is determined separately and subtracted from the total determination of creatinine plus creatine.

■ **In addition to those with significant renal impairment, elevated BUN levels are seen in patients under what condition or conditions?**

Gastrointestinal bleeding and conditions with decreased renal blood flow (dehydration, hypotension, congestive heart failure, etc.) may cause elevated BUN.

■ **Generally the BUN level does not begin to rise in patients with chronic renal disease until how much functioning renal parenchyma remains?**

Only 30% to 40% functioning renal parenchyma remains when the BUN rises.

■ **What is the significance of an elevated serum creatinine concentration?**

It indicates a decrease in glomerular filtration, which may result from disease of the kidneys, postrenal obstruction, or decreased renal blood flow.

■ **Why is the serum creatinine level in the blood a better screening test of renal function than the BUN level?**

Serum creatinine is virtually independent of protein metabolism and state of hydration.

■ **What is the significance of an elevated serum creatine level?**

The creatine level of serum is elevated above normal (0.6 mg/dl in men and 1.0 mg/dl in women) in a variety of diseases affecting skeletal muscle, including dystrophies, atrophies, myositis, and hyperthyroidism.

■ **What is the normal daily excretion of creatinine in the urine?**

It is 0.5 to 1.5 gm in women and 0.9 to 2.2 gm in men.

■ **Is the creatinine content of a timed urine specimen useful in determining whether the collection was complete?**

It is at best a rough guide, for daily creatinine excretion varies considerably from one subject to another and varies by as much as onefold from one day to another in the same subject.

■ **What are the sources of uric acid in the blood?**

Uric acid is formed by deamination and oxidation of adenine and guanine. It is a catabolic product of nucleic acids.

■ **How much uric acid is excreted daily by normal adults?**

The amount excreted is 0.4 to 0.8 gm.

■ **What happens to uric acid in the glomerular filtrate of a normal kidney?**

Most or all of it is reabsorbed by the tubules. The uric acid in the urine chiefly represents uric acid actively secreted by the renal tubules.

■ **What are the normal ranges of serum uric acid in men and women?**

The normal ranges are 2.1 to 7.8 mg/dl in men and 2.0 to 6.4 mg/dl in women.

■ **How do serum uric acid levels vary with age in men and women?**

They are constant with increasing age in men, but they increase with age in women.

■ **What conditions other than gout cause elevation of the serum uric acid level?**

Elevation is caused by starvation, acidosis, conditions in which destruction of cells is accelerated (lobar pneumonia, polycythemia vera, leukemias and malignant lymphomas, particularly under effects of cytotoxic therapy), renal failure, and eclampsia.

■ **What is the effect of allopurinol on the urinary excretion of purine catabolites?**

Allopurinol blocks oxidation of hypoxanthine to xanthine and of xanthine to uric acid. Consequently, urinary excretion of uric acid is diminished, and urinary excretion of hypoxanthine and xanthine is increased.

SEX HORMONES

- **What is the most important estrogen secreted by the ovary?**

It is estradiol.

- **What are the principal metabolic products of estradiol and progesterone that are measurable in the urine?**

They are the glucuronides of estriol and pregnanediol.

- **What are the relative potencies of estradiol, estrone, and estriol?**

Estradiol is five times more potent than estrone and 100 times more potent than estriol.

- **Do patients receiving oral diethylstilbestrol therapy have an increase, a decrease, or no change in the urinary excretion of estriol?**

They have a decrease in estriol excretion, because diethylstilbestrol inhibits pituitary secretion of gonadotropin without contributing to urinary estriol.

- **How can one differentiate between pituitary insufficiency and ovarian failure in a woman by measuring estrogen excretion?**

Administer FSH (follicle-stimulating hormone). If the patient has pituitary insufficiency, estrogen secretion will occur. If the problem is caused by ovarian failure, there will be no increase in estrogen release.

- **List three diseases or conditions that are associated with a decrease in urinary estriol excretion.**

They are hypopituitarism, oral synthetic estrogen and progestational therapy (these are not excreted as estriol and are not measured), and ovarian failure.

- **In patients with a hydatidiform mole, are the urinary levels of estriol and total estrogen usually increased or decreased relative to normal pregnancy levels?**

They are decreased below normal pregnancy levels.

- **What happens to the urinary pregnanediol level of pregnant women with placental insufficiency?**

It is significantly decreased below normal pregnancy levels.

- **What happens to the urinary estrogen level of the pregnant woman in the "fetal distress syndrome?"**

It decreases progressively.

- **In which of the following is the testosterone production decreased: Klinefelter's syndrome, adrenogenital syndrome, Stein-Leventhal syndrome, or Sertoli-Leydig cell tumors?**

Testosterone production is decreased in Klinefelter's syndrome.

- **Describe the blood testosterone levels and LH levels in primary and secondary hypogonadism.**

Testosterone levels in both are low. LH levels are high in the former, low in the latter.

- **What effect will HCG (human chorionic gonadotropin) or clomiphene have on blood testosterone levels in primary and secondary hypogonadism?**

No effect is seen in primary hypogonadism. They will increase testosterone levels at least twofold in secondary hypogonadism.

- **Which organs produce progesterone?**

The ovary, adrenals, and placenta produce progesterone.

- **Briefly outline changes in the urinary excretion of pregnanediol during the menstrual cycle.**

In the preovulatory phase, pregnanediol excretion is low. It then increases after ovulation and rapidly decreases approximately 3 days before menstruation.

- **List those diseases or conditions in which urinary pregnanediol excretion is increased.**

It is increased in granulosa-thecal cell tumors, diffuse thecal cell luteinization, adrenal hyperplasias, ACTH therapy, and pregnancy.

- **Briefly outline the pattern of progesterone secretion during pregnancy.**

Beginning at about 12 weeks, there is a gradual increase of progesterone production until about 25 weeks of pregnancy, at which time the increase becomes more rapid and continues until about 37 weeks. Then just before delivery, there is a slight decrease.

THYROID HORMONES

Measurement of thyroid hormones has undergone rapid improvement during the last few years. The application of radioimmunoassay methods in measuring thyroxine (T4) and triiodothyronine (T3) have all but eliminated indirect measurements, i.e., PBI, T4 by column, etc., and enable us to measure what we really wanted to know all along, the levels of free T3 and free T4, the metabolically active hormones. To understand thyroid pathology, a good knowledge of thyroid physiology is almost mandatory. This can be obtained from several good textbooks including Davidsohn and Henry's *Todd-Sanford Clinical Diagnosis* and Williams' *Textbook of Endocrinology*. The most concise reference on thyroid testing is Fisher and Levy's *Radioimmunoassay Manual*. The Bioscience Handbook is a handy and concise reference with numerous "pearls" scattered throughout. It seems rather obvious that several of the frequently performed tests of thyroid function that were popular until recently, such as PBI, T4 by column, and Murphy-Pattee T4, soon will have historical interest only. An excellent recent journal article on thyroid is that of Chopra and associates.

■ **To which serum proteins are triiodothyronine (T3) and thyroxine (T4) bound?**

T3 is bound to albumin and thyroid-binding globulin (TBG). T4 is bound to prealbumin, albumin, and TBG.

■ **What percentage of T3 and T4 are bound by the above proteins, and what percentage is free (unbound)?**

The bound portions are 99.8% of T3 and 99.98% of T4, with 0.2% of T3 and 0.02% of T4 free. Only the free portion is thought to be metabolically active.

■ **What are the major differences between thyroxine (T4) and triiodothyronine (T3) regarding their activity?**

Triiodothyronine has a shorter latent period and a shorter duration of action.

■ **Which of the two thyroid hormones is the most active metabolically?**

T3 is about three to four times more active metabolically than T4.

■ **What are the two major pathways for iodide clearance from the plasma in euthyroid patients?**

Approximately 70% is excreted in the urine, and most of the remainder is extracted by the thyroid gland.

■ **What factor or factors increase iodide trapping by the thyroid?**

Thyroid-stimulating hormone (TSH), long-acting thyroid stimulator (LATS), and decreased iodide stores increase iodide trapping.

■ **What drugs or chemical compounds can inhibit iodide trapping by the thyroid?**

Iodate, thiocyanate, nitrate, perchlorate, chlorate, and hypochlorite can inhibit iodide trapping.

■ **What drugs or chemicals are capable of blocking the organification of iodides by the thyroid?**

Certain sulfa drugs, cobalt, propylthiouracil, phenylbutazone, para-aminosalicylic acid (PAS), iodide, and imidazole drugs can block the organification of iodides.

■ **What is the effect of thyroid hormone on protein metabolism?**

In physiologic amounts, it produces an anabolic effect (positive nitrogen balance). In excess, it exerts a catabolic effect (negative nitrogen balance).

■ **What is the effect of thyroid hormone on carbohydrate metabolism?**

Thyroid hormone increases the rate of monosaccharide absorption by the gastrointestinal tract. It decreases glycogen stores in the liver, heart, and skeletal muscle, and it increases gluconeogenesis.

- **What is the range of normal circulating plasma thyroxine concentration?**

  It is 5 to 12 μg/dl.

- **What is the range of normal circulating plasma T3 concentration?**

  It is 70 to 200 ng/dl.

- **Compare the serum level of T3 and T4; then, taking into consideration their binding by protein and metabolic activity, compare the overall metabolic effect of each.**

  There is about twenty times more T4 than T3 in the serum, but since T3 is bound only 10% as much and has three to four times more activity, T3 exerts a greater influence hormonally than T4.

- **Where is thyrotropin-releasing hormone (TRH) formed and what is its effect?**

  It is formed in the hypothalamus and leads to the release and production of thyroid-stimulating hormone (TSH) by the anterior pituitary.

- **What effect or effects does TSH have on the thyroid gland?**

  TSH increases iodide trapping, coupling of iodotyrosines in thyroglobulin, hydrolysis of thyroglobulin, the T3/T4 ratio, and size and vascularity of the thyroid gland.

- **In addition to TRH, TSH release from the anterior pituitary is controlled by what factor or factors?**

  The levels of circulating free T3 and T4 have a reciprocal effect on TSH release.

- **What does the T3 resin uptake test actually measure?**

  It measures the unbound binding sites of TBG.

- **List those diseases or conditions associated with elevated TBG levels (increased binding capacity).**

  Pregnancy, estrogen therapy, perphenazine (Trilafon) therapy, acute intermittent porphyria, infectious hepatitis, and rare congenital excess of TBG are the diseases and conditions.

- **List those diseases or conditions associated with decreased TBG levels or decreased thyroid hormone binding capacity.**

  Androgen and steroid therapy, salicylate or diphenylhydantoin (Dilantin) therapy (normal TBG but decreased binding sites), nephrotic syndrome, acromegaly, major stress, and rare congenital deficiency of TBG comprise the list.

- **In euthyroid patients with elevated TBG levels, will the levels of total T4 and T3 resin uptake and free T4 be increased, decreased, or normal?**

Total T4 will be increased and T3 resin uptake will be decreased, but the free T4 will be normal.

■ **Describe the principle of the free thyroxine (free T4) test.**

The patient's serum is diluted and mixed with a tracer dose of thyroxine ^{125}I, which equilibrates with the thyroxine naturally present. Next, the proportion of dialyzable ^{125}I-labeled thyroxine is determined. The free thyroxine concentration in nanograms per deciliter of serum is the serum thyroxine concentration (total T4) multiplied by the fraction of added labeled thyroxine that is dialyzable.

■ **What are the indications for a free T4 test?**

A free T4 test is indicated when the measurement of total T4 may not accurately reflect the free T4.

■ **In what circumstances should one suspect that the total T4 does not accurately reflect the free T4?**

A discrepancy in the free T4 to total T4 ratio may be suspected in circumstances that alter the levels of thyroxine-binding globulin and prealbumin or when exogenous substances compete for thyroxine-binding sites.

■ **Describe the T3 resin uptake test.**

The radioactivity of a known amount of triiodothyronine tagged with ^{125}I is measured by scintillation counting, and aliquots are added to measured volumes of the patient's serum and a standard serum. The unbound added T3 is then removed on a resin. The radioactivity bound to the resin divided by the radioactivity in the added T3 is the fraction of the added T3 bound to the resin and, therefore, not bound to the serum proteins. The result on the patient's serum is evaluated by comparison with that from the standard serum. The test is a measurement of unoccupied binding sites on thyroxine-binding proteins.

■ **In the T3 resin uptake test, why is ^{125}I preferable to [131]I?**

The half-life of ^{125}I is 60 days as compared with approximately 8 days for [131]I.

■ **Is the T3 resin uptake normal, increased, or decreased in hypothyroidism?**

It is decreased.

■ **How is a radioactive iodine (RAI) uptake test performed?**

The patient is given an oral tracer dose of radioactive iodine, and the percentage of the dose present in the thyroid gland at some later time (ordinarily 24 hours) is determined by scintillation counting with appropriate correction for isotopic decay.

■ **What effect will the administration of iodine in various chemical forms have on the RAI uptake in a normal individual?**

It will decrease the uptake (the effect will last for up to 60 days).

■ **What are the effects of cortisone, ACTH, and para-aminosalicylic acid (PAS) on the RAI uptake in a normal individual?**

All three decrease the RAI uptake.

■ **What effect does iodine-containing X-ray contrast media have on the RAI uptake?**

They all decrease it. The effects last from 1 to 2 weeks with diatrizoate (Hypaque) or iodopyracet (Diodrast) to 30 years or more with iodized oil (Lipiodol) or iophendylate (Pantopaque).

■ **What effect will the following have on the RAI uptake by the thyroid gland: T3 therapy, propylthiouracil therapy, Graves' disease, and acute renal failure?**

The first two will decrease and the latter two will increase the RAI uptake.

■ **What effect will administration of thyroid hormone (T3 supression test) have on the RAI uptake in euthyroid and hyperthyroid patients?**

It will decrease the RAI uptake in euthyroid but not in hyperthyroid patients.

■ **How are circulating levels of TSH measured?**

They are measured by radioimmunoassay.

■ **How will TSH measurements help distinguish between primary and secondary hypothyroidism?**

TSH levels greater than 20 μU/ml occur in patients with primary hypothyroidism, and levels are less than 10 μU/ml in patients with secondary hypothyroidism.

■ **How is the thyrotropin-releasing hormone (TRH) stimulation test used to confirm the diagnosis of hyperthyroidism?**

The stimulation of TSH release by TRH is inhibited by increased levels of free T3 and T4 present in hyperthyroidism.[13]

■ **What is the most definitive test available to diagnose hypopituitarism as a cause of hypothyroidism?**

The TRH stimulation test is the most definitive test. TSH levels will either not increase or increase to less than 10 μU/ml after TRH administration.

■ **What are the typical levels of circulating thyroid hormones and TSH in hypothyroidism that is (1) secondary to pituitary or hypothalamic failure and (2) secondary to primary disease of the thyroid gland?**

In the first set of cases levels of circulating thyroid hormones and TSH are both low. In the second case circulating thyroid hormone levels are low, but TSH levels are elevated.

■ **Describe the levels of TSH, T4 and T3 in Graves' disease.**

The T3 and T4 are elevated, with the T3 increased more than the T4. TSH is decreased.

■ How is Graves' disease different from Plummer's disease?

Plummer's disease is toxic nodular goiter and is not associated with exophthalmos or with presence in the plasma of long-acting thyroid stimulator (LATS).

■ Describe the levels of TSH, T4, and T3 in Plummer's disease.

Both T4 and T3 are usually elevated although on rare occasions only one or the other is elevated. TSH is decreased.

■ Describe the above parameters in Hashimoto's thyroiditis.

They are usually within normal limits, but occasionally patients may be hypothyroid with decreased T3 and T4 levels and increased TSH.

■ Would one expect the T3 suppression test result to be positive, negative, or equivocal in Graves' disease or in Plummer's disease?

One would expect it to be negative in both conditions, because thyroxine secretion has escaped regulation by TSH.

■ What is T3 thyrotoxicosis?

It is a form of thyrotoxicosis in which T3 levels are elevated with normal or low T4 levels.[15]

■ Which of the various forms of hormone replacement therapy utilized in the treatment of hypothyroid individuals usually results in normal total T4 and T3 levels if the patient is maintained in the euthyroid state?

Dessicated thyroid and combination thyroxine triiodothyronine drugs with a T4/T3 ratio of about 4:1 result usually in normal T4 and T3 levels. Thyroid extract contains a low T4/T3 ratio and gives a low total T4. Synthroid (T4) gives a high total T4 and low T3. Cytomel (T3) gives a low total T4.

■ If a patient has been on long-term thyroid therapy and her physician desires to obtain a true picture of her thyroid status, how long should she be off medication before obtaining thyroid hormone studies?

At least a month without thyroid medication is necessary.

REFERENCES

1. Cameron, J. L., et al.: Acute pancreatitis with hyperlipemia: the incidence of lipid abnormalities in acute pancreatitis, Ann. Surg. 177: 483, 1973.
2. Chopra, I. J., et al.: Thyroxine and triiodothyronine in human thyroid, J. Clin. Endocrinol. 32:311, 1974.
3. Conn, J. W.: Primary aldosteronism and primary reininism, Hosp. Pract. 9:131, 1974.
4. Ewen, L. M.: Separation of alkaline phosphatase isoenzymes and evaluation of the clinical usefulness of this determination, Am. J. Clin. Pathol. 61:142, 1974.
5. Fallat, R. W., Vester, J. W., and

Glueck, C. J.: Suppression of amylase activity by hypertriglyceridemia, J.A.M.A. 225:1331, 1973.

6. Horton, R.: Aldosterone—a review of its physiology and diagnostic aspects of primary aldosteronism, Metab. Clin. Exper. 22:1525, 1973.

7. Krauss, K. R., Hutter, A. M., Jr., and DeSanctis, R. W.: Acute coronary insufficiency: course and follow-up, Ann. Intern. Med. 129:808, 1973.

8. Low, J. C., et al.: Ionic calcium determination in primary hyperparathyroidism, J.A.M.A. 223:152, 1973.

9. Munsat, T. L., et al.: Serum enzyme alterations in neuromuscular disorders, J.A.M.A. 226:1537, 1973.

10. Powell, J. B., and Djuh, Y.: A comparison of automated methods for glucose analysis in patients with uremia before and after dialysis, Am. J. Clin. Pathol. 56:8, 1971.

11. Rayfield, E. J., et al.: Influence of diet on urinary VMA excretion, J.A.M.A. 221:704, 1972.

12. Robinson, A. G., and Loeb, J. N.: Ethanol ingestion—commonest cause of elevated plasma osmolality? N. Engl. J. Med. 284:1253, 1971.

13. Snyder, T. J., and Utiger, R. D.: Response to thyrotropin releasing hormone (TRH) in normal man, J. Clin. Endocrinol. 34:380, 1972.

14. Spitz, I. M., et al.: Carbohydrate metabolism in renal disease, Quart. J. Med. 39:201, 1970.

15. Sterling, K., Refetoff, S., and Selenkow, H. A.: T3 thyrotoxicosis, J.A.M.A. 213:571, 1970.

16. Usategui-Gomez, M., Yeager, F. M., and Fernandez de Castro, A.: A sensitive immunochemical method for the determination of the Regan isoenzyme in serum, Cancer Res. 33:1574, 1973.

17. Winkelman, J., et al.: The clinical usefulness of alkaline phosphatase isoenzyme determinations, Am. J. Clin. Pathol. 57:625, 1972.

CHAPTER 6

Coagulation

The clinical pathologist not specializing in coagulation should secure an understanding of the most important basic principles and a few simple tests. The pathologist should have a schematic concept of the intrinsic and extrinsic pathways of coagulation and should understand how a deficiency of each of the established coagulation factors affects each of a simple battery of tests. We suggest the following tests for inclusion: Ivy bleeding time, platelet count, thrombin time, quantitative fibrinogen assay, one-stage prothrombin time, activated partial thromboplastin time, urea solubility test for factor XIII, and euglobulin clot lysis. The pathologist should know which plasmatic factors are removed by absorption with barium sulfate and how to use mixes of test plasma with barium sulfate–absorbed plasma and normal, fresh, or aged plasma to investigate prolongations of the thrombin, prothrombin, and partial thromboplastin time tests. Finally, the pathologist should understand the clinical and laboratory features of the more common acquired and inherited abnormalities of coagulation. Thrombocytopenia, disseminated intravascular coagulation and fibrinolysis, liver disease, uremia, and administration of coumarins and heparin account for most of the hemorrhagic disorders seen in ordinary hospital practice. The hemophilias and von Willebrand's disease are seen on occasion, but the other genetically determined deficiencies are rare. The book by Harker is concisely written and is current. Those by Ratnoff and by Owen and associates are excellent texts. A new edition of *The Diagnosis of Bleeding Disorders* is available. The book by Bowie and associates is a good guide to methodology. Biggs' book is the standard exhaustive reference. The symposium on intravascular coagulation is a recent discussion of a range of clinical and laboratory problems, albeit from the viewpoint of a single group.

Biggs, R.: Human blood coagulation, haemostasis and thrombosis, Oxford, 1972, Blackwell Scientific Publication, Ltd.
Bowie, E. J. W., et al.: Mayo Clinic laboratory manual of hemostasis, Philadelphia, 1971, Little, Brown & Co.
Harker, L. A.: Hemostasis manual, ed. 2, Philadelphia, 1974, F. A. Davis Co.
Owen, C. E., Jr., et al.: The diagnosis of bleeding disorders, ed. 2, Boston, 1974, Little, Brown & Co.

Ratnoff, O. D.: Treatment of hemorrhagic disorders, New York, 1968, Harper & Row, Publishers.
Symposium on the Intravascular Coagulation-Fibrinolysis (ICF) Syndrome, Mayo Clinic proceedings, vol. 49, no. 9, Rochester, Minn., 1974, Mayo Clinic.

■ **What are the initial events in intravascular thrombosis secondary to endothelial damage?**

Platelets immediately adhere to naked collagen fibers and release adenosine diphosphate (ADP), which leads to further aggregation of platelets. Activation of factor XII by the collagen begins the series of enzymatic reactions resulting in generation of thrombin. Thrombin is also an aggregator of platelets.

■ **What are the meanings of the terms "extrinsic system" and "intrinsic system"?**

These terms can be defined accurately only under in vitro conditions. Blood can clot either by a pathway involving only components of the blood itself (intrinsic) or by a second pathway (extrinsic), which is triggered by a nonblood element, tissue thromboplastin.

■ **Which of the plasmatic coagulation factors are not involved in the extrinsic system?**

Factors VIII, IX, XI, and XII are not involved. Deficiencies in these factors (and in factor XIII) will not prolong the prothrombin time.

■ **Which of the coagulation factors is not involved in the intrinsic system?**

Factor VII is not involved. Deficiency of this factor and factor XIII will not prolong the partial thromboplastin time.

■ **Which coagulation factors are involved in the extrinsic system?**

Tissue thromboplastin and factors X, VII, V, II, I, and IV (calcium) are involved in the extrinsic system.

■ **For which steps in the intrinsic coagulation pathway is calcium required?**

It is required for activation of factors IX and X and for conversion of prothrombin to thrombin.

■ **Which coagulation factor activities are lost in platelet-free plasma by aging?**

Factors V and VIII are the most labile with storage.

■ **Which coagulation factors are adsorbed by barium sulfate?**

Barium sulfate adsorbs factors II, VII, IX, and X.

■ **What are the *approximate* half-lives of the plasmatic clotting factors?**

The half-lives are VII, 5 hours; V and VIII, 12 hours; IX, 24 hours; X and XII, 40 hours; II, 60 hours; and I and XIII, 90 to 100 hours.

■ **What questions should be asked a patient suspected of having a hemorrhagic diathesis?**

1. Have there been previous episodes of bleeding (bruises unaccountable for by trauma, nosebleeds requiring medical attention, excessive bleeding after tonsillectomy or with menses)?
2. Does the patient have any relatives with bleeding tendency?
3. Has the patient had any diseases that are associated with bleeding (liver disease, tumor, uremia, thrombocytopenia, lupus)?
4. Has the patient had any recent drug ingestion (aspirin, phenylbutazone, diphenylhydantoin, coumarins)?

■ **What are the basic screening tests for each stage of coagulation?**

1. Hemostatic plug: platelet count, Ivy bleeding time
2. Intrinsic system: partial thromboplastin time (PTT)
3. Extrinsic system: prothrombin time (PT)
4. Fibrinogen and split products: thrombin time (TT)
5. Fibrin stabilization: urea (5M) solubility of clot

■ **How is the Ivy bleeding time determined?**

It is determined by using a blood pressure cuff around the arm inflated to 40 mm Hg, then making two slits 1 mm deep and 1 cm long in the volar forearm. Blotting should be done at 30-second intervals until bleeding ceases. A useful modification using a template for better standardization has been described by Mielke.[7]

■ **Why should the prothrombin time determination be performed promptly after collection of blood?**

Deterioration of factor V (proaccelerin) on standing *may* prolong the prothrombin time.

■ **In deficiencies of prothrombin components or factors VIII, IX, XI, or XII, what is the approximate amount of normal plasma that needs to be added to the deficient plasma to give normal prothrombin or partial thromboplastin times?**

One should add at least enough to give 30% final concentration of normal plasma, depending on the sensitivity of the reagents. A 50:50 mixture is commonly used.

■ **What is the significance of a prolonged thrombin time that is not corrected by a 50:50 mix with normal plasma or a prolonged prothrombin or partial thromboplastin time that is not corrected by a 50:50 mix with fresh normal plasma?**

Presence of a circulating anticoagulant (for example, heparin or fibrin-split products) is indicated.

■ **Using determinations of prothrombin time (PT), partial thromboplastin** time (PTT), and barium sulfate-adsorbed plasma, explain how deficiencies of coagulation factors V, VII, VIII, IX, and X can be differentiated.

Deficiencies in factors VIII and IX prolong the PTT but not the PT. Deficiency of factor VII prolongs the PT but not the PTT. Deficiencies of factors V and X prolong both the PT and the PTT. Deficiencies of factors V and VIII are corrected by addition of barium sulfate-adsorbed plasma, but deficiencies of factors IX and X are not corrected.

■ **What is the source of Stypven, and what is the principal role of the Stypven time in diagnosis of coagulation defects?**

The source is Russell's viper (Sir Arthur Conan Doyle's speckled band). Its principal role is differentiation of deficiencies of factors VII and X. Factor X deficiency prolongs the Stypven time, whereas factor VII deficiency does not prolong it.

■ **What is the mode of action of heparin?**

The chief effects of heparin are to neutralize thrombin and activated factor X. In the blood this occurs with a potent cofactor, antithrombin III, which is the same as anti-X_a.[11]

■ **Describe the anticoagulant action of ancrod (Arvin).**

Ancrod (Arvin) is an intravenously administered snake venom that has a proteolytic effect on fibrinogen, converting it to an unstable form of microfibrin that is rapidly cleared from the circulation. The result is to induce hypofibrinogenemia, which has an anticoagulant effect.

■ **How do the coumarin drugs exert their effect?**

Coumarin derivatives depress hepatic synthesis of the vitamin K–dependent factors II, VII, IX, and X.

■ **What is the effect of alcoholism on metabolism of oral anticoagulants (coumadin, for example)?**

The metabolism of coumadin (Warfarin) and a number of other drugs that are handled by the microsomal system is accelerated in alcoholics. Conversely, patients with severe alcoholism and cirrhosis may be sensitive to coumadin drugs because of decreased synthesis of the prothrombin complex.

■ **What is the half-life of the anticoagulant effect of injected heparin?**

It is approximately 1½ hours.[3]

■ **How can bleeding from heparin excess be differentiated from bleeding due to other causes by one simple test?**

Heparin excess causes marked prolongation of the thrombin time, and the thrombin time is corrected to normal by addition of 1 drop of protamine sulfate, 10 mg/ml, to 1 ml of patient's plasma, only when the prolongation is caused by heparin excess.[8] This will be a dramatic change such as from 90 seconds to 15 seconds. A shortening of 1 or 2 seconds may occur with protamine addition to normal plasma and should be ignored.

■ **How can most carriers of classical hemophilia (hemophilia A) be detected?**

Factor VIII can be detected in plasma by both immunologic and functional activity methods. In classical hemophilia, immunoreactive functionally inactive factor VIII is present. Carriers have disproportionately more immunoreactive than functionally active factor VIII, as compared with normal individuals.[1]

■ **What is the normal range for the platelet count?**

The normal range is 140,000 to 440,000 (phase contrast or Coulter counter).

■ **What is the coefficient of variation (C.V.) of platelet counts when done automatically and by phase contrast microscopy?**

The C.V. will usually be ±10% to ±20% by phase contrast microscopy and ±5% to ±10% by Coulter counter unless the platelet count is low. The C.V. increases with low platelet counts.

■ **Above what level of the platelet count is thrombocytopenia unlikely to be the sole cause of bleeding?**

A level of approximately 60,000/cu mm or higher indicates that thrombocytopenia is probably not the sole cause of bleeding.

■ **What is the normal life span of platelets?**

It is approximately 8 days.

■ **What is the productive life span of megakaryocytes?**

It is approximately 4 days. The platelet count begins to fall 4 days after total bone marrow irradiation.

■ **List the various platelet coagulation factors.**

Platelet factor 1 is absorbed plasmatic factor V, 2 is a fibrinoplastin, 3 is a thromboplastin, and 4 is an antiheparin.

■ **Outline a classification of thrombocytopenias.**

    I. Decreased platelet production
        A. Megakaryocytic population normal or increased (uremia, vitamin B_{12} or folate deficiency)
        B. Megakaryocytic population reduced (amegakaryocytic thrombocytopenia of infancy, myelophthisis, aplastic anemia, including drug-induced aplastic anemia)
    II. Sequestration of platelets in spleen
    III. Increased destruction of platelets
        A. Nonimmune (disseminated intravascular coagulation, microangio-

pathic processes, bacterial and viral infections, cardiac bypass operations)
   B. Immune
      1. Isoimmunization (mother-fetus, posttransfusion purpura)
      2. Autoimmunization (idiopathic thrombocytopenic purpura)
      3. Passive transfer of antibodies (blood transfusion, infant born of mother with ITP)
      4. Drug-induced immune destruction, as with quinidine

■ **Name three disorders with increased mean platelet volume and three with decreased volume.**

1. Increased volume: autonomous thrombocytosis, immune destruction of platelets, hypoproliferative disorders of megakaryocytes (irradiation, chemical or drug damage, neoplastic marrow replacement, myelofibrosis), or a predominance of young platelets
2. Decreased volume: reactive thrombocytosis in response to hemorrhage, infection, or iron deficiency

■ **In what common way do the following conditions and substances affect blood coagulation: uremia, increased levels of macroglobulins, fibrin-split products, acetylsalicylic acid?**

They inhibit aggregation of platelets.

■ **How does acetylsalicylic acid (ASA) modify the events that take place when platelets are exposed to collagen?**

ASA prevents release of ADP by platelets and thereby interferes with platelet aggregation. The defect appears to persist for the life of the platelet.

■ **What defects do platelets show in Glanzmann's thrombocytopathy?**

They fail to aggregate in response to ADP or thrombin.

■ **Give three indications for platelet transfusions.**

Platelet transfusions are necessary, first, in patients with severe thrombocytopenia and who are bleeding; second, to bring the platelet count up to a safe level when a surgical operation is necessary on a severely thrombocytopenic patient; and third, as prophylaxis against hemorrhage during temporary severe depression of the platelet count, particularly during chemotherapy of leukemia and other neoplastic diseases.

■ **Name three conditions with severe thrombocytopenia in which platelet transfusions are usually impractical.**

They are usually impractical in aplastic anemia without bleeding, idiopathic thrombocytopenia purpura (except immediately preoperatively), and patients who have developed antiplatelet antibodies secondary to multiple transfusions.

■ **Describe the intravascular fibrinolytic system.**

The splitting of polypeptides from plasminogen by an activator results in the appearance of an active fibrinolytic agent, plasmin. Active factor XII, thrombin, urokinase (in the urinary tract), and streptokinase (a streptococcal product) are activators of plasminogen activator.

■ **Which coagulation factors and products are attacked by plasmin?**

Factors I, V, VIII, and XIII are attacked by plasmin.

■ **Name two activators of plasminogen that arise during coagulation.**

The active form of factor XII and thrombin arise during coagulation.

■ **List three conditions with increased fibrinolysis.**

1. Large, denuded body surface in presence of normal fibrinolytic system (example: transurethral resection of prostate gland or suprapubic prostatectomy)
2. Disseminated intravascular coagulation (DIC) (The fibrinolytic activator is generated in increased amounts in the microvasculature and is activated by factor XII.)
3. Increased circulating plasminogen activator occurring in some patients with metastatic carcinoma of prostate and liver disease (decreased clearance of activator)

■ **What is fibrinogen-related antigen (FRA)?**

Fibrinogen-related antigen is nonclottable protein found in serum, presumably fibrinogen split products, which reacts with antisera to fibrinogen in hemagglutination inhibition (TRCHII) or similar assays.

■ **What are the relative sensitivities of tanned red cell hemagglutination inhibition immunoassay (TRCHII), staphylococcal clumping, immunodiffusion, and the Fi test for fibrinogen/fibrin degradation products?**

The TRCHII and staphylococcal clumping tests are more sensitive than the other two tests. Both the former detect early, large degradation products well, but TRCHII is better for the late fragments.[6]

■ **What is the principle of the staphylococcal clumping test?**

Certain strains of staphylococci will clump in the presence of fibrinogen and its derivatives (fibrin and split products). When performed on serum it is similar in results to the TRCHII for FRA.

■ **What is the significance of a positive protamine paracoagulation test?**

The protamine paracoagulation test is positive when coagulable fibrin lysis products are present in the blood plasma. Positive tests suggest active intravascular coagulation. Only early fibrin lysis products, presumably complexed with fibrinogen, are coagulable by this test. Late fibrin lysis products and fibrinogen lysis products are not coagulable.[5] In performing this test it is important to distinguish between strand or gel formation (positive) and precipitates (negative).

■ **In which circumstance can a false negative euglobulin lysis test result occur in the presence of excessive circulating plasminogen activator?**

It can occur when plasminogen is depleted.

■ **Describe abnormalities that often appear in the blood film in disseminated intravascular coagulation.**

Such abnormalities are schistocytes, burr and helmet red blood cells, and thrombocytopenia.

■ **List five causes of the disseminated intravascular coagulation syndrome.**

The causes are obstetrical complications (abruptio placentae, amniotic fluid embolism), endotoxin in bacterial sepsis, severe intravascular hemolysis, carcinomatosis, and certain snake venoms.

■ **Which clotting factors are most often decreased in the disseminated intravascular coagulation syndrome?**

Platelets and factors I, II, V, VIII, and XIII are most often decreased.

■ **What are the modes of inheritance of hemophilias A and B and of von Willebrand's disease?**

The inheritance of both hemophilias is sex-linked recessive. Inheritance of von Willebrand's disease is autosomal dominant. The remainder of the coagulation protein deficiencies are, in general, autosomal recessive.

■ **Are the hemophilias inherited deficiencies or dysproteinemias?**

The hemophilias are dysproteinemias. Recent work on inherited disorders of factors I, VIII, and IX would suggest that most such disorders involve functionally inactive proteins rather than actual deficiencies.

■ **What is the component of choice in treating bleeding in Christmas disease (hemophilia B)?**

Fresh frozen plasma is the component of choice. Major bleeding may require use of concentrates containing factors II, VII, IX, and X, but these materials have a high risk of hepatitis.

■ **What two plasma factors are deficient in von Willebrand's disease?**

A "bleeding factor" (von Willebrand's factor) that affects aggregation of platelets, and factor VIII (AHF) are deficient.

■ **Are VWF activity and antihemophilic factor (AHF) activity normally contained in the same molecule?**

VWF and AHF normally are contained in the same macromolecular complex. In hemophilia A the VWF activity and antigenic reactivity are intact, but the AHF activity is deficient. It is possible in vitro with gel chromatography to separate these activities.[9]

■ **What is "factor VIII antigen," and how does it differ from AHF?**

Factor VIII antigen plays a role in aggregation of platelets and is immuno-logically similar to AHF. The antigen is present in hemophiliacs, who show normal platelet aggregation and have normal Ivy bleeding times, but it is decreased in von Willebrand's disease. Patients with von Willebrand's disease have a defect in platelet aggregation and prolonged bleeding times. Factor VIII antigen and von Willebrand's factor may be identical.

■ **What abnormal laboratory findings typify classical von Willebrand's disease?**

Prolonged bleeding time, decreased platelet adhesiveness, decreased platelet aggregation with ristocetin, and decreased plasmatic factor VIII level typify classical von Willebrand's disease.[10]

■ **Which factors are defective in hemophilias A and B?**

Factor VIII is defective in hemophilia A, and factor IX is defective in hemophilia B.

■ **Will hemophilic plasma correct the defect in von Willebrand's disease in vivo?**

It will, because hemophilic plasma evidently contains a precursor from which the patient with von Willebrand's disease can form factor VIII.

■ **How do patients with von Willebrand's disease differ from those with factor VIII deficiency in their response to factor VIII transfusions?**

Both have an immediate rise in factor VIII proportional to the amount of infusion. The level in hemophiliacs then falls rapidly ($t\frac{1}{2}$:12 hours). In contrast in von Willebrand's patients, the factor VIII rises further, reaching a peak 6 to 18 hours after transfusion, and then it declines.

■ **Which of the following conditions will benefit from cryoprecipitate: (1) hemophilia A, (2) hemophilia B, or (3) von Willebrand's disease?**

Hemophilia A and von Willebrand's disease will benefit from cryoprecipitate.

■ **Can factor VIII concentrates transmit hepatitis?**

Yes. The risk is particularly high with concentrate prepared from pooled plasma.

■ **Give a simple "rule of thumb" for factor VIII dosage for treatment of hemorrhage in a hemophiliac or in preparing one for an elective surgical operation.**

A factor VIII level of 20% of normal or more will effect hemostasis under ordinary circumstances, but the level should be at least 30% before undertaking a surgical operation. Taking 1 unit of factor VIII as the amount present in 1 ml of fresh plasma, infusion of 50 units per kilogram of body weight will give a 100% level in a severe hemophiliac. The half-life of transfused factor

VIII is approximately 12 hours. Levels of factor VIII approaching 100% can be obtained in severe hemophiliacs only by use of concentrates (cryoprecipitate or glycine-precipitated factor VIII).

■ **Antibodies to factor VIII may be found in what types of patients?**

1. Patients with classical hemophilia A
2. During pregnancy and postpartum
3. Diseases of an immunologic nature (drug reactions, bullous impetigo, etc.)
4. Otherwise healthy elderly[4]

■ **How may the antifactor VIII antibody be distinguished from the circulating anticoagulant found in some patients with systemic lupus erythematosis (SLE)?**

The SLE anticoagulant inhibits at the factor X_a, factor V, phospholipid, Ca^{++}-complex stage. This is where intrinsic and extrinsic pathways join, and, as a result, both PT and PTT will be abnormal. The anti-VIII antibody affects only the intrinsic system (PTT), and the PT will be normal.

■ **A 57-year-old man who previously was well had a sudden onset of severe epistaxis, hematuria, and ecchymoses. The following studies were done:**

Platelet count 300,000/cu mm

	Prothrombin times
Patient's plasma	34 sec
Control plasma	12 sec
1:1 mixes	
Patient's plasma + normal plasma	12 sec
Patient's plasma + aged normal plasma	12 sec
Patient's plasma + barium sulfate–absorbed normal plasma	35 sec
Patient's plasma + normal serum	14 sec

What is the probable cause of the bleeding?

The patient has probably been poisoned with a dicumarol-like drug. Note that the studies are consistent with deficiencies of any one or combination of the prothrombin group factors except IX alone (isolated IX deficiency does not prolong prothrombin time). Lack of previous bleeding makes a severe hereditary deficiency of any of these factors unlikely.

■ **A child is bleeding excessively through a chest tube an hour after open heart correction of tetralogy of Fallot. Coagulation studies include platelet count 75,000/cu mm, clotting time (Lee-White) 25 minutes, prothrombin time 26 seconds, and partial thromboplastin time 135 seconds. What is the most likely cause of the bleeding, and which tests should be recommended to establish the cause?**

Heparin given at the time of operation possibly has not been sufficiently neutralized. This suspicion would be confirmed by prolongation of thrombin time not corrected by a 1:1 mix of the patient's plasma with normal plasma (proving presence of a circulating anticoagulant) and by in vitro correction of the thrombin time prolongation by addition of protamine. If protamine does not correct the prolongation, the problem probably is disseminated intravascular coagulation and fibrinolysis.

■ **A 20-year-old patient with acute leukemia has a platelet count of 5000/cu mm, petechiae, ecchymoses, and gastrointestinal bleeding. Four hours after the initial transfusion of platelets (6 units) the platelet count has risen only to 7000, and bleeding continues. What type of leukemia might this be?**

Promyelocytic leukemia is likely, for it typically produces the disseminated intravascular coagulation syndrome with consumption of platelets and plasmatic coagulation factors. Appropriate tests would include prothrombin and thrombin time determinations, fibrinogen assay, and tests for fibrin-split products.

■ **What is a likely type of coagulation defect in an infant who bleeds abnormally from the umbilicus in the first 2 weeks of life?**

This is characteristic of congenital factor XIII deficiency. Poor wound healing is a hallmark of this disorder.[2]

REFERENCES

1. Bennett, B., and Ratnoff, O. D.: Detection of the carrier state for classic hemophilia, N. Engl. J. Med. 288:342, 1973.
2. Duckert, F.: The fibrin stabilizing factor, factor XIII, Blut 26:177, 1973.
3. Estes, J. W.: The kinetics of heparin, Ann. N. Y. Acad. Sci. 179:187, 1971.
4. Feinstein, D. I., and Rapaport, S. I.: Acquired inhibitors of blood coagulation. In Spaet, T. H., editor: Progress in hemostasis and thrombosis, vol. 1, New York, 1972, Grune & Stratton, Inc.
5. Kidder, W. R., et al.: The plasma protamine paracoagulation test: clinical and laboratory evaluation, Am. J. Clin. Pathol. 58:675, 1972.
6. Marder, V. J., Matchett, M. O., and Sherry, S.: Detection of serum fibrinogen and fibrin degradation products: comparison of six technics using purified products and application in clinical studies, Am. J. Med. 51:71, 1971.
7. Mielke, C. H., Jr., et al.: The standardized normal Ivy bleeding time and its prolongation by aspirin, Blood 34:204, 1969.
8. Soloway, H. B., et al.: Differentiation of bleeding diatheses which occur following protamine correction of heparin anticoagulation, Am. J. Clin. Pathol. 60:188, 1973.
9. Weiss, J. H., and Hoyer, L. W.: Von Willebrand factor: dissociation from antihemophilic factor procoagulation activity, Science 182:1149, 1973.
10. Weiss, J. H., et al.: Defective Ristocetin-induced platelet aggregation in von Willebrand's disease and its correction by factor VIII, J. Clin. Invest. 52:2697, 1973.
11. Yin, E. T., and Wessler, S.: Rabbit plasma inhibitor of the activated species of blood coagulation factor X, J. Biol. Chem. 246:3594, 1971.

CHAPTER 7

Cytogenetics

Cytogenetics implies the study of genetic composition by microscopy. Only rather gross defects involving whole chromosomes or segments of chromosomes can be detected in this way, but a number of well-characterized conditions can be diagnosed by cytogenetic methods. Inborn errors of metabolism dependent on single enzymatic defects are not detectable by microscopic examination of chromosomes.

The requirements for an understanding of cytogenetics include familiarity with the concepts of the structure of deoxyribonucleic acid (DNA), genes, chromosomes, mitosis and meiosis. Any uncertainties about the mechanics of mitosis and meiosis should be dispelled by reviewing the subject before undertaking a study of cytogenetics. A good review can be found in the text by Lynch and associates.

Eggen, R. R.: Cytogenetics. In Davidsohn, I., and Henry, J. B., editors: Todd-Sanford clinical diagnosis by laboratory methods, ed. 15, Philadelphia, 1974, W. B. Saunders Co.

Lynch, M. J., et al., editors: Medical laboratory technology and clinical pathology, ed. 2, Philadelphia, 1969, W. B. Saunders Co.

■ **What is the normal chromosomal count in interphase diploid human cells?**

The count is 46, consisting of 23 pairs in the female and 22 pairs plus an X and a Y in the male.

■ **What comprises an interphase chromosome?**

The chromosome consists of two strands of deoxyribonucleic acid (DNA) in a helical coil.

■ **What are homologous chromosomes?**

Homologous chromosomes are morphologically identical and have identical genetic loci that bear allelic genes. Each of two homologous chromosomes originates from a different parent.

■ **What is a chromatid?**

It is one of two mirror image chromosomes joined by a centromere in a metaphase cell during mitosis and meiosis.

- **What is the number of chromatids in a normal human somatic cell in metaphase?**

There are ninety-two chromatids.

- **How many chromosomes are present in the nucleus of a human sperm or ovum?**

Twenty-three are present.

- **Which determines the male phenotype: the presence of only a single X chromosome or the presence of a Y chromosome in association with one or more X chromosomes?**

Presence of a Y chromosome determines male phenotype regardless of the number of X chromosomes present. XO (Turner's syndrome) has a female phenotype despite presence of only one X chromosome, and XXY (Klinefelter's syndrome) has a male phenotype despite presence of two X chromosomes.

- **How can the Y chromosome be selectively stained in interphase and metaphase nuclei?**

The Y chromosome can be selectively stained in either interphase or metaphase nuclei by quinacrine hydrochloride or quinacrine mustard. The preparation is examined by ultraviolet microscopy.

- **What is the Lyon hypothesis?**

It is the hypothesis advanced by Mary Lyon to correlate the incidence of Barr bodies (sex chromatin) with cytogenetic observations in various conditions. The hypothesis states that Barr bodies arise from the random heterochromatization of one X chromosome in each normal female cell. Recent evidence is more consistent with inactivation of only part of the X chromosome (the long arms) rather than of the whole chromosome.

- **Theoretically, what proportion of female somatic cells have Barr bodies?**

Theoretically, 100% have Barr bodies. However, with ordinary staining technics, they are recognizable only in nuclei that are oriented so that the Barr body can be recognized as being adjacent to the nuclear membrane.

- **Which routine stains are adequate for demonstrating of Barr bodies?**

Standard hematoxylin and eosin and Papanicolau stains as well as more specialized technics will demonstrate Barr bodies.

- **What kind of cells in buccal scrapings should be counted to determine incidence of Barr bodies?**

Epithelial cells with open nuclei should be counted. To obtain these cells, the first (superficial) scrapings should be discarded, and slides with the second (deeper) scrapings should be prepared.

■ **Approximately what proportion of buccal cells from normal females show Barr bodies when stained with hematoxylin and eosin?**

About 50% show Barr bodies. Approximately 33% of buccal cells show them in marginal position, and 17% show them in submarginal position.

■ **What is the incidence of Barr bodies in buccal mucosal cells from normal men?**

Barr bodies occur in 0% to 7% with a variety of stains.

■ **Buccal scrapings from a mother and her female infant show 5% chromatin-positive cells in each. Interpret this finding.**

A low Barr body incidence is usual in postpartum mothers and newborn infants. Ingestion of antibiotics can also lower the count.

■ **Identify the structures marked by arrows in Wright-stained blood films. Which of these structures should be counted as drumsticks?**

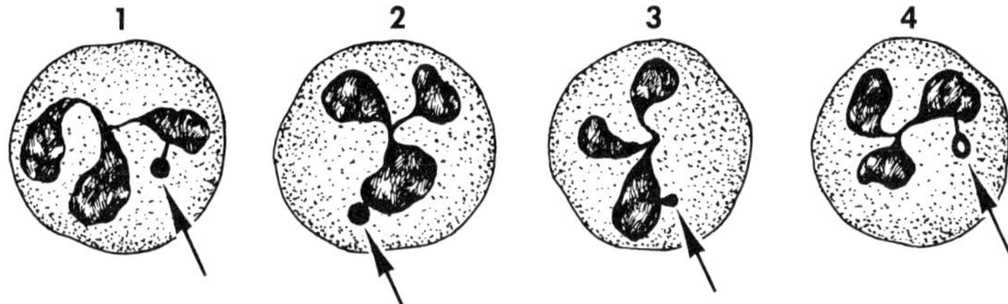

1. Drumstick
2. Sessile nodule (balloon; should also be counted as a drumstick)
3. Club (Clubs are found equally in both sexes.)
4. Racquets (They are of unclear significance. They resemble drumsticks but have pale centers.)

■ **What is the frequency of drumsticks in polymorphonuclear leukocytes in females?**

They occur in about 1.5% of the polymorphonuclear leukocytes, but the frequency occasionally is as low as 0.6%.

■ **What is the frequency of drumsticks in polymorphonuclear leukocytes in normal males?**

They are absent or present in a frequency of up to 0.4%.

■ **Describe briefly the technic of chromosome analysis (karyotyping).**

Cells (usually white blood cells or bone marrow cells) are cultured in vitro. After growth is established, a stathmokinetic agent (colchicine) is introduced to arrest mitosis at metaphase. The cells then are treated with a hypotonic solution to cause swelling and dispersal of chromosomes before preparing stained films on slides.

■ **Define a metaphase chromosome. At what stage of the cell cycle can chromosomes be visualized?**

A metaphase chromosome is composed of two chromatids joined by a centromere. Chromosomes are visualized during mitosis.

■ **How many metaphase figures should be counted in routine karyotyping?**

At least thirty should be counted to avoid missing mosaics.

■ **What proportion of cells are nonmodal (contain fewer or more than forty-six chromosomes) in young people (less than 30 years) and in older adults (more than 70 years)?**

1. Young people: less than 5%
2. Older adults: less than 10%

■ **In meiosis, is the reduction division the first or second division?**

Reduction occurs in the second division.

■ **Describe the characteristics of the sex chromosomes in metaphase.**

The X chromosome is indistinguishable on morphologic grounds from other chromosomes of group C. The Y chromosome resembles others of group G but may be slightly larger, and its long arms tend to be more nearly parallel.

■ **What is meant by "mitotic nondisjunction"?**

It is failure of homologous chromatids to separate during mitosis. This failure results in one daughter cell with an extra chromosome, whereas the other daughter cell lacks the chromosome.

■ **What is the difference between the first meiotic division and a mitotic division?**

In the first meiotic division, chromatids do not separate but remain attached by their centromeres. Instead, intact homologous metaphase chromosomes are segregated. This results in daughter cells with differing chromosomal and genetic complements. In mitotic division chromatids separate, and the daughter cells have identical chromosomal and genetic complements.

■ **Describe two types of nondisjunction that can occur during meiosis.**

Nondisjunction in the first meiotic division results in an extra chromosome in each of two identical gametes and a deficiency of the chromosome in another two identical gametes. Nondisjunction in the second meiotic divison yields a gamete with a double dose *of the same chromosome* and a gamete deficient in that chromosome.

■ **What is a chromosomal mosaic?**

It is an individual with two or more cell lines. Mosaicism results from an error in mitosis or another nonlethal chromosomal event occurring after fertilization.

■ **What is a translocation?**

It is the result of simultaneous breaks in two chromosomes with cross-reunion. Since the free (telomere) ends of chromosomes are inert, fracture of only one chromosome results in deletion rather than translocation.

■ **What is a chromosomal deletion?**

It is the loss of a portion of a chromosome.

■ **Compare homologous and nonhomologous translocations.**

In homologous translocations the event takes place between homologous chromosomes. In nonhomologous translocation the chromosomes involved are different members of the same group or members of different groups.

■ **What are isochromosomes, and what are their genetic compositions?**

They are formed by division of the centromere along the horizontal rather than the sagittal plane. Each isochromosome contains a double dose of the genetic material normally present in one arm of a chromosome.

■ **Name two human diseases with chromosomal deletions.**

Most examples of chronic granulocytic leukemia show deletion of the short arms of a group G chromosome (chromosome-22) in bone marrow cells (Philadelphia chromosome). Patients with the cat's cry syndrome (epiglottic hypoplasia, mewing cry, hypertelorism, and mental deficiency) show deletion of the short arm of a group B chromosome.

■ **What is the Christchurch chromosome (Gp—Ch[1]), and what is its significance?**

It is a group G chromosome having deletion of its short arms. It has been noted in association with a variety of congenital abnormalities and leukemias and in many clinically normal relatives of these patients. It may well be an incidental finding without phenotypic significance.

■ **What is the most common chromosomal abnormality in mongolism?**

It is trisomy of one of the group G chromosomes (chromosome-21). It accounts for more than 85% of all mongols.

■ **What other chromosomal abnormalities are present in some mongols?**

D/G or G/G translocations (familial translocation mongolism) are present. The genetic material on the short arms of the translocated chromosomes is lost, but individuals receiving the abnormal chromosome consisting of two long arms receive an extra dose of genetic material from the long arm of the group G chromosome. This abnormality is roughly equivalent to group G trisomy in phenotype. It accounts for less than 10% of mongols.

■ **What is the chromosomal number of the mother of a child with familial translocation mongolism?**

It is 45. A group G chromosome is absent, but most of its genetic material is present in the abnormal chromosome arising from translocation.

■ **What are the expectations for the offspring of female carriers of translocation mongolism?**

A third of the offspring will be normal; a third will be carriers, and a third will be mongols. Note that a fourth possible genotype is not represented by these three phenotypes. It is a complement of forty-five normal chromosomes with absence of a group G chromosome, and it is lethal. Consequently the offspring can be of only three types.

■ **Can the male be a carrier of translocation mongolism?**

The male can carry translocation mongolism, but only about 1 of 12 children sired will be mongols. About 5 of 12 will be carriers, and 5 of 12 will be normal.

■ **Describe the epidemiology of the common form of mongolism.**

It is sporadic and most often occurs in infants of mothers over 35 years of age. The incidence is 1 per 2000 births for mothers under age 30 and rises to 1 per 50 births for women over 45 years of age.

■ **What is the likelihood that the child born after a sporadic mongol will also be mongoloid?**

The probability is 1 in 40 to 1 in 80.

■ **What chromosomal abnormality would one suspect in an infant with microphthalmus, sloping forehead, mental deficiency, deafness, multiple hemangiomas, polydactyly, and ventricular septal defect with patent ductus arteriosus?**

One would suspect the D (chromosome-13) trisomy syndrome.

■ **What is the prognosis for subsequent pregnancies after birth of a child with a D trisomy syndrome?**

The prognosis is good, because translocations account for only a few examples of this syndrome.

■ **What is the probable chromosomal abnormality in an infant with pointed occiput, mental deficiency, micrognathia, overlapping of fingers, low-set and deformed ears, malformed kidney, and ventricular septal defect with patent ductus arteriosus?**

The abnormality probably is the E (chromosome-18) trisomy syndrome. Most examples are sporadic, although inheritable examples caused by translocation have been reported.

■ **What is the modal number of chromosomes in patients with trisomy syndromes?**

The modal number of chromosomes in patients with trisomy syndromes is 47.

■ **Describe the salient phenotypic and cytogenic features of Turner's syndrome.**

Individuals with Turner's syndrome are phenotypic females with short stature, webbed neck, and streak ovaries. Cytogenetically they are XO (lacking one X chromosome) or XO/XX mosaics.

■ **What is the approximate incidence of Turner's syndrome?**

It is about 4 per 1000 live births.

■ **What are the likely phenotypic features of a woman with three X chromosomes (trisomy X)?**

Usually the woman is normal, but the likelihood of mental impairment is increased.

■ **Is the trisomy X condition likely to be passed on to the woman's children?**

No. All children examined have had normal karyotypes, evidently because XX ova are infertile.

■ **Which syndrome is indicated by a phenotypically male patient with testes less than 2.5 cm in greatest dimension, aspermia, gynecomastia, long extremities, hyalinization of seminiferous tubules and hyperplasia of Leydig cells, and increased excretion of FSH?**

These criteria indicate Klinefelter's syndrome.

■ **What is the incidence of mental deficiency in patients with Klinefelter's syndrome?**

Mental deficiency occurs in 25% of patients.

■ **What findings would one expect on examination of buccal scrapings for Barr bodies from a patient with Klinefelter's syndrome?**

One would find a female pattern with or without multiple Barr bodies in some nuclei.

■ **Explain why patients with Klinefelter's syndrome have Barr bodies but are phenotypically male.**

They have multiple X chromosomes but at least one Y chromosome. The Y chromosome is the determinant of maleness.

■ **Describe the essential phenotypic and karyotypic features of the XYY syndrome.**

The features are aggressiveness, antisocial behavior, and occasionally mental deficiency in men who tend to reach more than 6 feet in height and have two or more Y chromosomes.

■ **What are the karyotypic features of the testicular feminization syndrome?**

Patients with the testicular feminization syndrome have normal karyotypes.

CHAPTER 8

Feces and intestinal absorption

Certain aspects of examination of the feces are covered in the sections on bacteriology, parasitology, and hematology.

Bauer, J. D., Ackermann, P. G., and Toro, G.: Clinical laboratory methods, ed. 8, St. Louis, 1974, The C. V. Mosby Co.

Beeler, M. F., and Kao, Y. S.: The examination of feces. In Davidsohn, I., and Henry, J. B., editors: Todd-Sanford clinical diagnosis by laboratory methods, ed. 15, Philadelphia, 1974, W. B. Saunders Co.

■ **Name a food and an injectable dye that will color the stool red.**

Beets and Bromsulphalein (BSP) will color the stool red.

■ **Name three extraneous substances that will color the stool black and two that will color it green.**

Bismuth, charcoal, and iron will color the stool black. Green vegetables and calomel will color the stool green.

■ **Name three conditions in which copious pus is passed with the stool.**

Copious pus indicates an abscess or a fistula communicating with the large intestine, chronic ulcerative colitis, or chronic bacillary dysentery. Copious pus is evidence against amebic dysentery.

■ **How much blood is normally lost from the alimentary tract daily?**

Less than 2.8 ml is lost.

■ **How much blood must be lost in a single upper gastrointestinal hemorrhage to color the stool dark?**

To color the stool dark, 50 to 75 ml of blood must be lost.

■ **List three peroxide-dependent reagents for detection of blood in the stool in order of decreasing sensitivity.**

The reagents are orthotolidine, benzidine, and guaiac.

■ **What is the principle of detection of blood by the above reagents?**

Peroxidase in red blood cells causes release of oxygen from hydrogen peroxide. The nascent oxygen changes the color of the reagent by oxidation.

■ **What happens to peroxidase activity of blood as it passes through the gastrointestinal tract?**

An 80- to 120-fold decrease in peroxidase activity occurs during passage through the gastrointestinal tract.

■ **Which of the above reagents for detection of fecal blood will give false positive reactions because of meat in the diet?**

The orthotolidine and benzidine tests will give false positive reactions.

■ **Is a patient who is receiving oral iron supplements likely to have false positive benzidine, orthotolidine, and guaiac test results for occult fecal blood?**

Ferrous sulfate and most other oral iron preparations will cause false positive guaiac test results, but not false positive benzidine and orthotolidine test results. However, certain medicinal iron preparations (ferrous fumarate and ferrous carbonate) will give false positive reactions with all three tests.

■ **What hazard is attached to working with benzidine?**

Benzidine is a carcinogen.

■ **To perform a reasonably accurate determination of fecal excretion of a given substance (for example, stercobilinogen) per 24 hours, for how long a time should feces be collected?**

Three days is usually sufficient for clinical purposes.

■ **Describe a microscopic screening test for excess neutral fecal fat.**

On a microscopic slide, mix a small amount of feces with two drops of 95% ethanol followed by two drops of saturated ethanolic Sudan III or oil red O. More than a few drops of stained neutral fat per high power field indicates pancreatic steatorrhea.

■ **Using the microscopic test for neutral fecal fat, how can mineral oil be distinguished from fat?**

Before performing the test, add several drops of 36% acetic acid to a small amount of the stool on a microscopic slide, and heat over a flame until slight boiling occurs. After this treatment, mineral oil can be stained but fat cannot because of conversion to soaps.

■ **Why does the microscopic method for detection of neutral fat in feces fail to detect most examples of steatorrhea?**

The method for neutral fat fails in most patients, other than some with pancreatic steatorrhea, because the excess fat is present as soaps and in other combined forms (split fat).

■ **How should feces be examined to detect excessive amounts of split fat microscopically?**

To detect split fat, add several drops of 36% acetic acid to a 5 mm. smear of feces on a slide, add two drops of alcoholic Sudan III solution, and place a cover slip over the slide. Heat the slide gently over a flame until boiling barely commences, and repeat the heating process twice. Examine while still warm.

■ **What microscopic findings indicate excessive fecal excretion of split fat?**

Split fat is present in excess when more than 100 sudanophilic globules 1 to 4 μm in diameter are present per high-power microscopic field (magnification $\times 430$).[2]

■ **Describe a titrimetric method for measurement of fecal fat.**

In the method of van de Kamer, feces are emulsified, an aliquot is refluxed with alcoholic KOH to hydrolyze triglycerides, and excess HCl is added to convert sodium soaps to fatty acids. The fatty acids are extracted with petroleum ether, and an aliquot of the petroleum ether is titrated with NaOH using a phenolphthalein end point.

■ **In the presence of normal intestinal mucosa and a normal length of intestine, what are the prerequisites for absorption of fat?**

Pancreatic lipase, conjugated bile salts, and alkaline intestinal pH are the prerequisites.

■ **What is the normal rate of fecal fat excretion?**

The normal rate is 3 gm plus 2% of the daily dietary fat intake, or usually less than 5 gm/24 hr.

■ **List ten causes of enterogenous (as differentiated from hepatogenous and pancreatic) steatorrhea.**

Celiac disease (gluten sensitive), tropical sprue, intestinal lymphoma, lymphangiectasis, Whipple's disease, amyloidosis, abetalipoproteinemia (acanthocytosis), surgical loss of intestine, blind loop syndrome (bacterial deconjugation of bile acids), and Zollinger-Ellison syndrome (low intestinal pH) all cause enterogenous steatorrhea.

■ **What is the significance of a low serum level of carotenoids?**

It is consistent with any malabsorption syndrome in which fat is poorly absorbed; but low levels are also seen in febrile illnesses, hepatic disease, and poor dietary intake.

■ **How is the D-xylose intestinal absorption test performed, and what are the normal ranges?**

Twenty-five grams of D-xylose is dissolved in water and administered orally. Urine collected for 5 hours afterward should contain more than 3 gm of D-xylose (mean 6.5 gm). If renal insufficiency is present, the blood level at

2 hours should be determined. It should be more than 19 mg/dl (mean 36 mg/dl). D-xylose concentration is measured by conversion to furfural followed by formation of a chromagen with *p*-bromoaniline. If the urine initially is negative for reducing substances, any quantitative reduction method that is suitable for glucose can be used for xylose.

■ **What is the significance of abnormal results of the xylose tolerance test?**

Abnormal results of the test indicate enterogenous malabsorption. The results of the test are normal in malabsorption syndromes secondary to hepatic or pancreatic disease.

■ **Describe the lactose tolerance test for detection of lactose deficiency.**

The procedure is similar to the glucose tolerance test, but 100 gm of lactose is substituted for 100 gm of glucose. The peak blood sugar rise should be 40 mg/dl or higher.

■ **What are the limitations of the x-ray film digestion test for fecal proteolytic enzymes?**

The test is valid only in children less than 5 years old. Adults may have little proteolytic activity in the stool because of bacterial inactivation of the enzymes.

■ **How great a decrease in pancreatic secretion of lipase must occur before onset of steatorrhea (fat greater than 7 gm/24 hr), and by how much must trypsin output be reduced to cause creatorrhea (stool nitrogen greater than 2.5 gm/24 hr)?**

The secretion of each enzyme must be less than 10% of normal before the abnormalities occur.[1]

■ **What is the normal fecal output of organic anion, and how is the output affected in pancreatic steatorrhea, adult celiac disease, disaccharidase deficiency, malabsorption after intestinal and gastric resections, and intestinal lymphoma?**

The normal output is 13.1 ± 1.2 mEq/24 hr for college students, and it is unaffected by changes in carbohydrate, cellulose, and organic acid content of diet. In all of the various types of malabsorption listed above, the fecal organic anion output is increased two to five times.[3]

REFERENCES

1. DiMagno, E. P., Go, V. L. W., and Summerskill, W. H., Jr.: Relations between pancreatic enzyme outputs and malabsorption in severe pancreatic insufficiency, N. Engl. J. Med. 288:813, 1973.

2. Drummey, G. D., Benson, J. A., Jr., and Jones, C. M.: Microscopical examination of the stool for steatorrhea, N. Engl. J. Med. 264:85, 1961.

3. Fernandez, L. B., et al.: Fecal acidorrhea, N. Engl. J. Med. 284:295, 1971.

CHAPTER 9

Fluids of serous cavities and joints

Fluids from serous cavities and joints are too often thoughtlessly discarded. Laboratory examination, particularly by microscopy and bacteriologic culture, is often rewarding and will sometimes reveal an unsuspected diagnosis.

Bauer, J. D., Ackermann, P. G., and Toro, G.: Clinical laboratory methods, ed. 8, St. Louis, 1974, The C. V. Mosby Co.

Jessar, R. A.: The synovial fluid. In Hollander, J. L., and McCarty, D., editors: Arthritis and allied conditions, ed. 8, Philadelphia, 1972, Lea & Febiger.

Krieg, A. F.: Cerebrospinal fluid and other body fluids and secretions. In Davidsohn, I., and Henry, J. B., editors: Todd-Sanford clinical diagnosis by laboratory methods, ed. 15, Philadelphia, 1974, W. B. Saunders Co.

■ **How are transudates distinguished from exudates?**

Transudates have protein concentrations of less than 3 mg/dl and specific gravities of less than 1.016, whereas exudates have protein levels of 3 gm/dl or more and specific gravities of 1.016 or more.

■ **What conditions are associated with transudates into the serous cavities?**

Congestive heart failure, cirrhosis of the liver, portal and hepatic venous thrombosis, hypoalbuminemia secondary to cirrhosis, starvation, malabsorption or protein-losing enteropathy, and renal failure are all associated with transudates into the serous cavities.

■ **What conditions are associated with exudates into the serous cavities?**

Infarcts, infections, irritations (acute pancreatitis), and neoplasms are associated with exudates into the serous cavities.

■ **Does a protein content of less than 3 gm/dl and a specific gravity of less than 1.016 in a serous effusion rule out an infection or neoplasm?**

No. Approximately 25% of all infections (tuberculosis, for example) or neoplasms will give rise to effusions fitting the criteria of transudates. Furthermore, a high protein content or high specific gravity does not rule out the conditions that more commonly are associated with transudates, particularly when they are chronic and when they occur after diuretic therapy.

■ **Can the lactic dehydrogenase (LDH) content of a fluid be used to distinguish infections and malignant effusions from transudative effusions?**

Yes. The LDH activity is at least as good a criterion as protein content or specific gravity in separating these types of effusions. Malignant and infective effusions have high LDH activity.

■ **What types of fluids from serous cavities contain fibrinogen and form a clot?**

Exudates contain fibrinogen and form a clot.

■ **What is a pseudochylous effusion, and what is its significance?**

It is a fluid with a milky appearance because of presence of cholesterol crystals. There is no specific significance. Cholesterol crystals sometimes form in long-standing effusions.

■ **What causes chylous effusions?**

Chylous effusions occur after traumatic rupture of the thoracic duct, during obstruction of the duct by neoplasm, in presence of lymphangiomas, and without identifiable cause (idiopathic).

■ **How can chylous effusions be distinguished from pseudochylous effusions?**

Chylous effusions have the consistency and appearance of milk, and the fluid clears and decreases in volume on alkalinization and extraction with ether. Orally administered lipophilic dye appears in chylous effusions.

■ **Cholesterol pericarditis is characterized by opaque milky pericardial fluid containing cholesterol crystals but without high triglyceride concentrations. The fluid does not separate into two layers on standing. What are the most commonly associated diseases?**

Cholesterol pericarditis is associated most often with hypothyroidism, and it also occurs in tuberculous pericarditis, carcinoma, rheumatoid arthritis, mitral stenosis, and other causes of chronic heart failure.[1]

■ **What is the diagnosis of a pericardial effusion that shows protein concentration 6.3 gm/dl, total lipid 1.45 gm/dl, cholesterol 230 mg/dl, and triglycerides 850 mg/dl?**

The diagnosis is chylopericardium.[1]

■ **What type of cell predominates in effusions caused by nontuberculous bacterial infections?**

Neutrophilic granulocytes predominate.

■ **What type of cell usually predominates in tuberculous effusions?**

Lymphocytes usually predominate.

■ **Can acid-fast organisms usually be recognized in stained sediments from tuberculous pleural effusion?**

They cannot usually be recognized. They must be sought by culture.

■ **What is Meigs' syndrome?**

It is ascites and pleural effusion associated with an ovarian fibroma.

■ **What is Dressler's syndrome?**

It is a postmyocardial infarct syndrome consisting of pericarditis with effusion, fever, and sometimes pneumonitis with pleural effusion. The effusions may be sanguineous.

■ **What other conditions may cause sanguineous effusions?**

Pulmonary infarcts, malignant neoplasms, bacterial infections including tuberculosis, and trauma may cause sanguineous effusions.

■ **Which of the following features help distinguish intestinal (mesenteric) infarction from acute pancreatitis: foul odor, presence of bacteria, prune juice color, markedly elevated amylase activity?**

The first three features indicate infarction of the intestine. Markedly elevated amylase activity occurs in both conditions. Bacteria may be present in ascitic fluid beginning 6 hours after onset of symptoms in intestinal infarction.

■ **How much fluid normally is present in a hip or knee joint?**

Normally, 0.1 to 4.0 ml is present.

■ **What is the appearance of normal joint fluid?**

It is clear and colorless or light yellow.

■ **Does synovial fluid normally clot?**

No. A clot indicates the abnormal presence of fibrinogen, which is usually an indication of inflammation.

■ **What substance gives synovial fluid its high viscosity?**

The substance is hyaluronic acid, which normally is present in a concentration of approximately 3.5 mg/ml of fluid.

■ **What is the principal protein present in normal synovial fluid, and what happens to the synovial fluid protein pattern in inflammatory conditions?**

Normally, 60% to 75% of the protein is albumin, and the total protein concentration is only 1.1 to 2.1 gm/dl. Inflammatory fluids show a protein pattern that approaches that of serum.

■ **What is the Ropes test?**

Add several drops of synovial fluid to 20 ml of 5% acetic acid. Normally, a mucin clot forms within 1 minute. Shake to determine friability. A poor, friable clot indicates inflammation.

■ **What substance in synovial fluid is responsible for a normal Ropes test and its ability to be drawn out into a string?**

The substance is hyaluronic acid. The degree of polymerization of the hyaluronic acid is more important than its concentration.

■ **What results of the Ropes test would one expect in synovial fluid from degenerative joint disease, effusions after trauma, rheumatic fever, lupus erythematosus, rheumatoid arthritis, and gout?**

A fair to good mucin clot is characteristic of the above conditions, except rheumatoid arthritis and gout, in which the clot usually is poor.

■ **What should be used as a diluent in performing cell counts on synovial fluid?**

Physiologic saline or 0.3% saline should be used if hemolysis of red blood cells with preservation of leukocytes is desired. Acetic acid cannot be used, because it precipitates hyaluronic acid.

■ **What are the normal total leukocyte and differential counts of synovial fluid?**

The total count should be between 13 and 300/cu mm, and the differential count should show no more than 25% granulocytes with the rest of the cells divided among lymphocytes, monocytes, histiocytes, and synovial lining cells.

■ **What is the typical cell count in synovial fluid from an osteoarthritic or Charcot's joint?**

The leukocyte count is fewer than 2000/cu mm with a predominance of lymphocytes.

■ **What level of the total cell count and what percentage of granulocytes in the differential count strongly favor a diagnosis of pyogenic bacterial arthritis over one of rheumatic fever, rheumatoid, gouty, or tuberculous arthritis?**

A total leukocyte count of at least 60,000/cu mm with 75% or more granulocytes probably indicates pyogenic bacterial arthritis.

■ **What are the average and maximum synovial fluid cell counts in rheumatic fever, rheumatoid arthritis, gout, pseudogout, and tuberculous arthritis?**

The average counts are approximately 15,000/cu mm with slightly higher counts in tuberculous arthritis than in the other arthritides. The counts can occasionally exceed 50,000/cu mm.

■ **What is the value of synovial fluid glucose determination?**

Large differences between blood and synovial fluid glucose concentrations favor a diagnosis of pyogenic bacterial or tuberculous arthritis (mean differences approximately 60 mg/dl for tuberculous arthritis and 80 mg/dl for bacterial arthritis). Differences in excess of 50 mg/dl can also occur in rheumatoid and gouty arthritis.

■ **With what other feature of synovial fluid does the glucose concentration correlate most closely?**

It correlates inversely with the cell count.

■ **What cell type usually predominates in the synovial fluid in rheumatoid and gouty arthritis?**

Polymorphonuclear leukocytes usually predominate.

■ **What are the typical features of synovial fluid in arthritis associated with lupus erythematosus?**

Clear to turbid fluid, a good mucin clot test, a leukocyte count of approximately 3000/cu mm, a small blood-synovial fluid glucose difference, and, in some instances, presence of lupus erythematosus cells are the typical features.

■ **What are RA cells (ragocytes)?**

They are polymorphonuclear leukocytes with cytoplasmic granules 0.5 to 2 μm in diameter. RA cells are present in 95% of synovial fluids from patients with rheumatoid arthritis. They may also occur in septic arthritis, gout, and other inflammatory conditions.

■ **How can RA cells be recognized?**

Their granules are dark when viewed unstained in wet preparation, and they are stainable supravitally with 0.2% brilliant cresyl blue or Sternheimer-Malbin stain (dark gray) or with oil red O (red) in fixed preparations.

■ **What do the granules of RA cells contain?**

They contain a complex of rheumatoid factor and IgG.

■ **What is the rheumatoid factor?**

It is an anti-**IgG** macroglobulin that is present in the synovial fluid and usually in the serum of patients with rheumatoid arthritis.

■ **How do complement levels of joint effusions associated with rheumatoid arthritis, gout, and Reiter's syndrome compare with each other?**

When corrected for protein content of the fluid, rheumatoid effusions have strikingly low levels of hemolytic complement and specific fractions C1, C2, C3, and C4. The levels in rheumatoid arthritis are less than half those of gouty arthritis and a third those of Reiter's syndrome.[2]

■ **How do immunologic events within the joint cavity explain the low complement level and the presence of neutrophilic polymorphonuclear leukocytes in the effusion?**

An IgG rheumatoid factor reacts with the autologous IgG, and the complex activates complement with resultant formation of chemotactic factors. The IgG-IgG$_{RF}$ complex may react with an IgM rheumatoid factor with resultant further activation of complement. Phagocytosis of the complexes by the neutrophils may lead to more inflammation by release of lysosomal enzymes.[2]

■ **How can the urate crystals of gouty arthritis be differentiated from the calcium pyrophosphate crystals of pseudogout by microscopy?**

Urate crystals are short rods with rounded or needlelike ends. Calcium pyrophosphate crystals are rodlike or rhomboid with sharp corners. Urate crystals have a strong negative birefringence, whereas calcium pyrophosphate crystals have a weak, positive birefringence in polarized light.

■ **When do cholesterol crystals occur in joint fluid, and how can they be recognized?**

They occur in old rheumatoid and other chronic effusions and may be recognized as strongly birefringent, notched rectangles.

REFERENCES

1. Csanády, M., and Kovács, G.: Isolated massive chylopericardium, Ann. Thorac. Surg. 15:427, 1973.

2. Ziff, M.: Pathophysiology of rheumatoid arthritis, Fed. Proc. 32:131, 1973.

CHAPTER 10

Fungi

The text by Conant and associates is a classic treatise covering basic concepts of fungal morphology, laboratory technics, and fungal diseases from clinical, pathologic, and mycologic viewpoints. The manual by Beneke and Rogers contains excellent gross and microscopic photographs in color. The work by Emmons, Binford, and Utz is also recommended. The chapter by Kaufman remains an authoritative discussion of serodiagnosis of fungal diseases.

Beneke, E. S., and Rogers, A. L.: Medical mycology manual, Minneapolis, 1971, Burgess Publishing Co.
Conant, N. F., et al.: Manual of clinical mycology, ed. 3, Philadelphia, 1971, W. B. Saunders Co.
Emmons, C. W., Binford, C. H., and Utz, J. P.: Medical mycology, ed. 2, Philadelphia, 1970, Lea and Febiger.
Kaufman, L.: Serodiagnosis of fungal diseases. In Blair, J. E., Lennette, E. H., and Truant, J. P., editors: Manual of clinical microbiology, Bethesda, Md., 1970, American Society for Microbiology.

■ **List the four classes of fungi.**

The four classes are Phycomycetes, Ascomycetes, Basidiomycetes, and Fungi Imperfecti.

■ **To which class do most of the pathogenic fungi belong?**

They belong to the Fungi Imperfecti.

■ **What distinguishes the Fungi Imperfecti?**

They show no sexual reproduction.

■ **What basic morphologic feature distinguishes fungi from bacteria?**

Fungi are eukaryotic (the nucleus is demarcated by a membrane).

■ **Why are most fungi periodic acid–Schiff (PAS) positive?**

Their cell walls are composed mainly of carbohydrates (chitin, glucan, and mannan).

■ **How do fungi stain with the Gram stain?**

They are all gram positive.

■ **Identify the class of fungi indicated by the fruiting bodies in the illustration below. Which of the drawings shows sexual spore formation?**

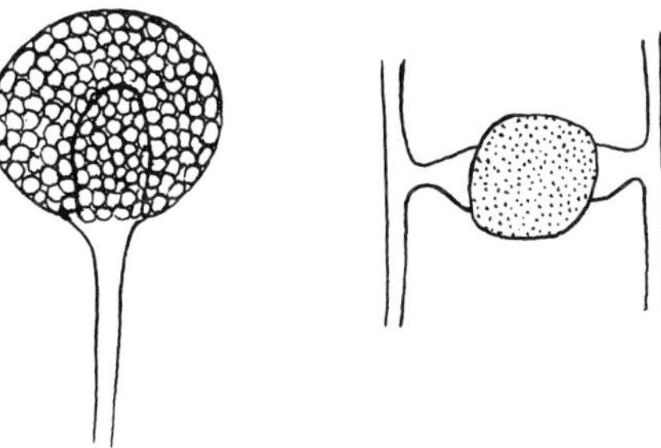

The fruiting bodies indicate class Phycomycetes. On the left is a sporangium, formed on the end of a specialized hypha called a sporangiophore, and containing asexual spores (sporangiospores). On the right is a zygospore that is formed by union of tips of two hyphae (sexual spores).

■ **Name the two types of spores shown below.**

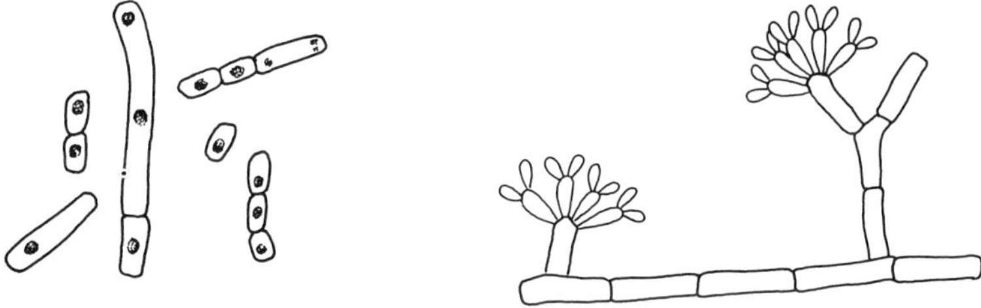

On the left are the arthrospores of *Geotrichum candidum,* and on the right, borne on specialized hypha called conidiophores, are the conidia (spores) of *Fonsecaeae pedrosoi.* The conidia are the terminal structures. Note the characteristic elongation of the *G. candidum* arthrospores.

■ **Describe the essential parts of a conidiophore. What are microconidia?**

A conidiophore consists of a swollen hypha (vesicle) or flask-shaped hypha (sterigma) on which the spores (conidia) are borne. A microconidium consists of only a single spore usually borne laterally on the hypha.

■ **Describe a simple method for microscopic examination of skin lesions in suspected dermatophytoses.**

Mount scrapings in a mixture of equal parts of 10% potassium hydroxide and fountain pen ink.

■ **Which of the dermatophytes fluoresce under Wood's light?**

Microsporum species (green), some *Trichophyton* species (gray-green), and *Malassezia furfur* (yellow-brown) fluoresce.

■ **How is a definitive diagnosis of *Malassezia furfur* infection (tinea vesicolor) made in the laboratory?**

It is made by demonstration of spores and fragments of hyphae in the stratum corneum of the epidermis. The organism has not been cultured.

■ **Which genera of dermatophytes most commonly infect hair of the scalp (tinea capitis), dry skin (tinea corporis), moist skin (tinea cruris, jockey itch, athlete's foot), and the nails (tinea unguium)?**

Tinea capitis is most often caused by *Microsporum* or *Trichophyton* species, tinea corporis by *Trichophyton* and *Microsporum* species, tinea cruris by *Epidermophyton floccosum* and *Trichophyton* species, and tinea unguium by *Trichophyton* species.

■ **What are microconidia and macroconidia?**

They are asexual spores. Microconidia are single spores, and macroconidia are septate structures containing multiple spores.

■ **Which of the dermatophytes produce numerous well-developed macroconidia when cultured?**

Well-developed macroconidia are produced by *Microsporum* species and *Epidermophyton floccosum*.

■ **Identify the macroconidia shown below.**

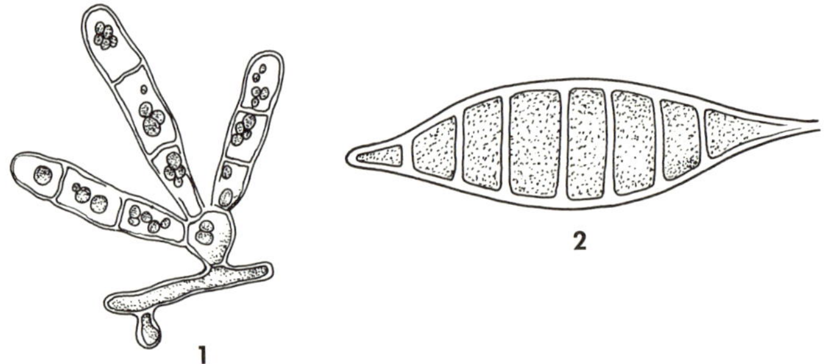

1. *Epidermophyton floccosum*
2. *Microsporum canis*

■ **Which genus of dermatophytes produces racquet-shaped and spiral hyphae, numerous microconidia, but only rare macroconidia?**

These characteristics indicate the genus *Trichophyton*.

■ **Which dermatophytes produce severe tinea capitis with shield-shaped ectothrix hyphal masses attached to the scalp and surrounding one or multiple hair shafts and complex, branched hyphae (favic chandeliers)?**

These characteristics indicate *Trichophyton schoenleini* or *T. violaceum,* which are the causes of favus.

■ **Which fungus produces the structures shown below when grown on corn-meal agar?**

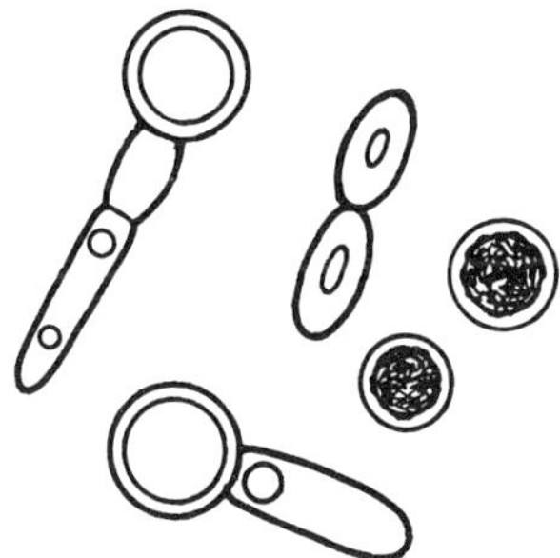

These structures are produced by *Candida albicans.* It is identified by the thick-walled chlamydospores.

■ **Describe a method for distinction of *C. albicans* from other species of *Candida* within 3 hours.**

C. albicans is distinguished by the appearance of germ tubes within 3 hours when incubated at 37° C in human serum, sheep serum, or trypticase soya broth.[3]

■ **Identify a *Candida* species that assimilates dextrose, maltose, and sucrose, produces gas from each, but fails to assimilate lactose.**

The organism is *C. albicans.*[1]

■ **What types of infections can *Candida albicans* produce?**

It can produce tinea cruris, vaginitis, thrush, esophagitis, and infections of internal organs including bacterial endocarditis and lung abscesses.

■ **The three fungi whose typical budding morphology is shown below grow in the yeast phase at 37° C and form mycelia when cultured at room temperature. Identify them.**

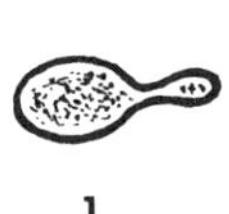
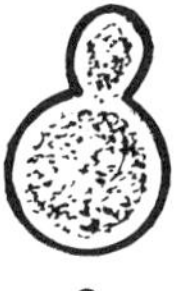
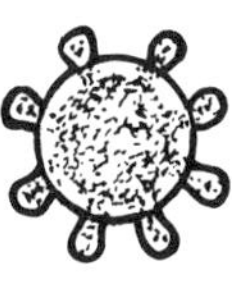

1. *Histoplasma capsulatum*
2. *Blastomyces dermatitidis*
3. *Paracoccidioides brasiliensis*

Note the slender, easily fractured attachment of the *H. capsulatum* bud, the thick attachment of the *B. dermatitidis* bud, and the multiple buds of *P. brasiliensis* (pilot wheel appearance).

■ **The illustration below depicts an organism grown from a tongue lesion on Sabouraud's glucose agar at room temperature for 3 weeks. What is it?**

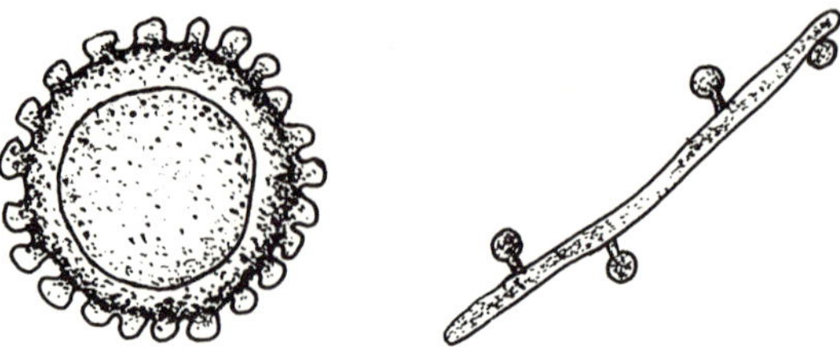

The illustration shows a mycelium with microconidia and a tuberculate chlamydospore of *Histoplasma capsulatum*.

■ **What immunologic tests are available for diagnosis of histoplasmosis?**

A skin test and tests for precipitating and complement-fixing antibodies are available.

■ **If histoplasmosis is suspected, what should be done before a skin test?**

Blood should be obtained for serologic studies. Intradermal injection of histoplasmin antigen may result in an anamnestic rise in precipitating and complement-fixing antibodies. However, the rise does not occur until 2 or 3 days after injection of the antigen.

■ **What is the typical response of the white blood cell count to disseminated histoplasmosis?**

Leukopenia is the typical response.

■ **A pathogenic fungus grows as a yeast at both room temperature and 37° C. Name the two most likely possibilities of its identity.**

It is probably *Cryptococcus neoformans* or *Torulopsis glabrata*.

■ **What biochemical reaction distinguishes *Cryptococcus neoformans* from *Torulopsis glabrata* and *Saccharomyces*?**

C. neoformans produces urease and gives a positive reaction on Christensen urea agar.[2]

■ **What is the characteristic structure of *C. neoformans*?**

It is a budding yeast with a broad, mucoid capsule.

■ **In the mouse virulence test for identification of *C. neoformans*, how long may the mouse live after inoculation?**

The mouse may live for 6 days to 3 weeks after inoculation with *C. neoformans*.[2]

■ **Are *C. neoformans* and *H. capsulatum* carried by pigeons and other birds?**

These fungi have not been isolated from the birds, but they do grow luxuriantly in their droppings.

■ **What is the identity of a nonencapsulated yeast that does not form hyphae at room temperature, produces no urease, and assimilates dextrose and sucrose but not lactose, maltose, or trehalose?**

The organism with these characteristics is *Torulopsis glabrata.*[1]

■ **The illustrations below pertain to a patient with cavitary pulmonary disease. Identify the fungus and state which form occurs in tissues and which occurs only in cultures.**

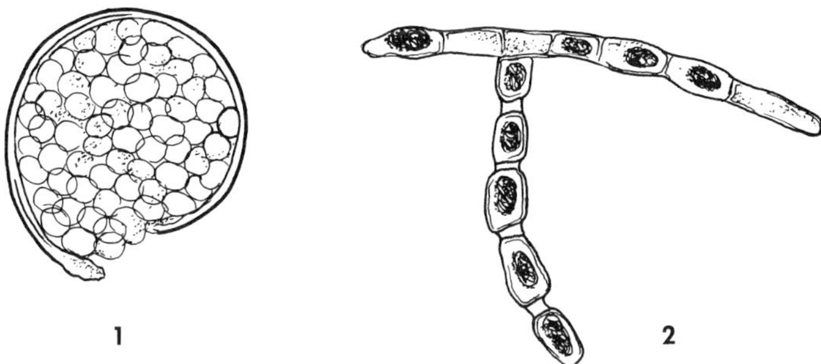

The fungus is *Coccidioides immitis.* Sporangia (1) occur only in tissues. In a culture at room temperature, hyphae break up into chains of arthrospores (2). Arthrospores occur only rarely in tissues.

■ **Which fungus has asteroid and cigar-shaped forms in pus and in culture at room temperature produces mycelia bearing single lateral conidia and conidiophores with clusters of pyriform conidia as in the illustration below?**

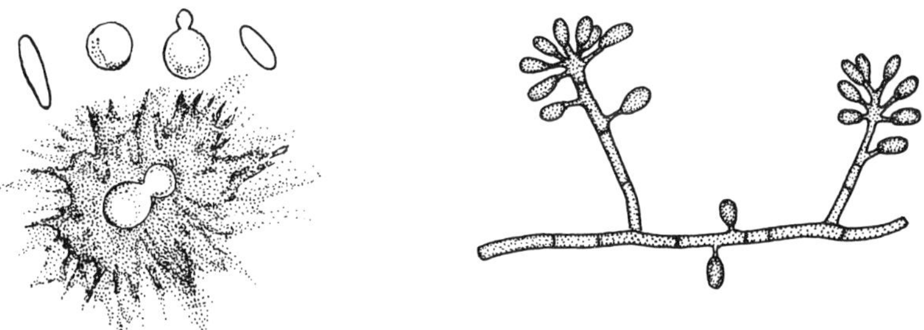

These criteria indicate *Sporothrix schenckii* (formerly called *Sporotrichum schenckii*). The asteroid form results from precipitation of immune globulins on the fungal cell. Recognition in tissue or in smears of pus usually requires special stains or direct immunofluorescence microscopy.

■ **What is the usual appearance of infection with *Sporothrix schenckii* in an early stage?**

The appearance is an ulcer of the skin at the site of inoculation and subcutaneous nodules along lymphatics.

■ **In what form does *S. schenckii* grow at 37° C?**

The yeast phase grows at 37° C.

■ **Why is a positive complement fixation test result in a titer of 1:8 with _Blastomyces dermatitidis_ not a firm basis for diagnosis?**

Patients with histoplasmosis frequently show complement-fixing antibodies to _Blastomyces_ organisms.

■ **What is the lowest significant titer of yeast phase _Histoplasma capsulatum_ complement-fixing antibody?**

It is 1:16 or 1:32.

■ **In what circumstances do patients with active histoplasmosis not have high titers of complement-fixing antibodies?**

For reasons that are not understood, some patients fail to develop titers higher than 1:8 against either yeast-form or mycelial antigen. Patients with progressive, disseminated disease and patients with malignant lymphomas, in particular, may be anergic.

■ **Is the latex agglutination test more reliable in the diagnosis of acute or chronic histoplasmosis? What titers are significant?**

It is a reliable test for diagnosis of acute histoplasmosis. Titers of 1:32 or higher are significant. The agglutinating antibodies may fall to low titer or become undetectable after several months.

■ **What is the significance of positive results of a complement fixation test in low titer (1:2 or 1:4) with coccidioidin?**

They are consistent with coccidioidomycosis but are not diagnostic.

■ **Name the genera represented in the illustration below. Which genus has species that cause mycosis of internal organs?**

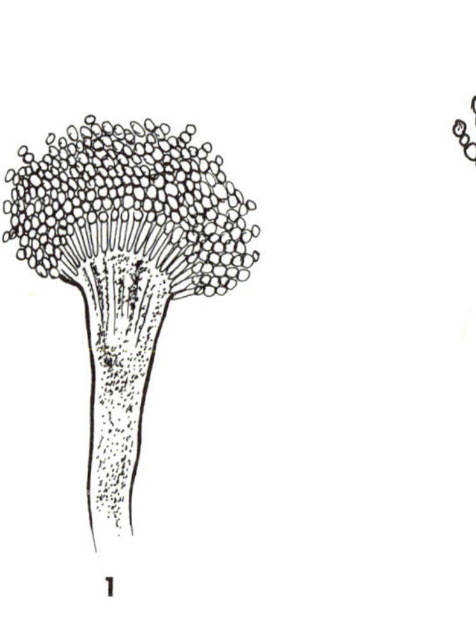
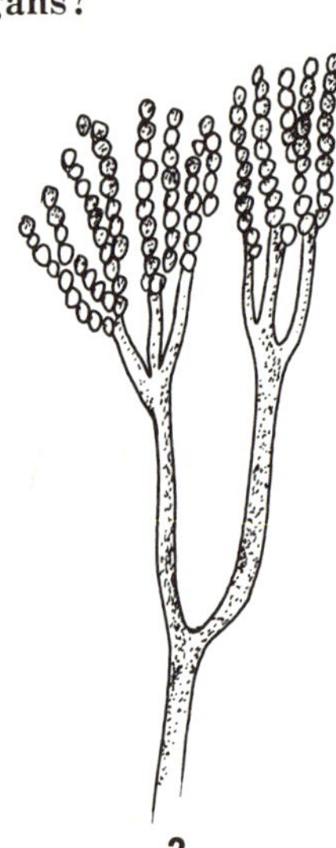

1

2

1. *Aspergillus*, conidiophore
2. *Penicillium*, conidiophore (*"Penicillium* brush")

Aspergillus fumigatus can produce progressive visceral infections.

■ **Which fungi are likely to produce a fulminating orbital cellulitis with cerebral invasion in uncontrolled diabetics?**

The likely fungi are those of class Phycomycetes. These include the genera *Absidia, Mucor, Rhizopus, Mortierella, Basidiobolus, Entomophthora*, and *Hyphomyces*.

■ **What morphologic characteristic distinguishes the Phycomycetes in tissues and in culture?**

Large (6 to 50 μm diameter) hyphae with few or no septa distinguish the Phycomycetes.

■ **Which fungi most commonly produce serious infections in patients with leukemia and malignant lymphoma?**

Serious infections are produced by *Candida albicans, Aspergillus fumigatus, Cryptococcus neoformans, Histoplasma capsulatum*, and Phycomycetes, but *C. albicans* and *A. fumigatus* account for most of the fungal infections in these patients.

■ **What is a mycetoma (maduromycosis)?**

A mycetoma is a localized swollen lesion, usually on a foot or hand, involving skin, subcutis, fascia, and bone, with draining sinuses. The purulent drainage contains granules formed of colonies of the causative organism.

■ **Which organisms cause mycetomas (maduromycosis)?**

Bacteria of genera *Streptomyces* and *Nocardia*, and fungi of genera *Madurella, Allescheria, Phialophora, Aspergillus*, and others cause mycetomas.

■ **What is chromoblastomycosis?**

It is a chronic mycosis of the skin and subcutis caused by species of *Cladosporium, Fonsecaea*, and *Phialophora*. These fungi have a brownish color in tissues, but do not form buds (blastospores). The disease produces warty cutaneous nodules, usually on the feet and legs. The nodules progress to papillomatous vegetations and may ulcerate.

■ **What are the dematiacious fungi?**

The demitiacious fungi are pigmented fungi that cause subcutaneous abscesses with a granulomatous component. They are soil and wood saprophytes that gain access to the body through injury. *Phialophora gougerotii, P. spinifera, P. richardsiae*, and *Cladosporium bantianum* comprise the dematiacious fungi.

■ **Brown hyphae found in a brain abscess are illustrated below. What is their identity?**

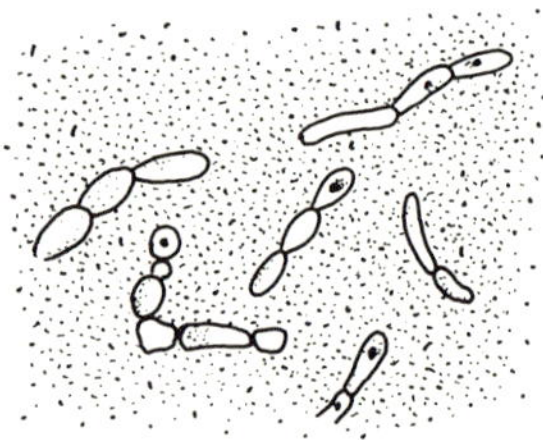

The brown hyphae are *Cladosporium bantianum*. This is the only one of the dematiacious fungi that is known to cause brain abscesses.

REFERENCES

1. Dolan, C. T.: A practical approach to identification of yeast-like organisms, Am. J. Clin. Pathol. 55:580, 1971.
2. Dolan, C. T., and Woodward, M. R.: Identification of *Cryptococcus* species in the diagnostic laboratory, Am. J. Clin. Pathol. 55:591, 1971.
3. Joshi, K. R., et al.: The formation of germ tubes by *Candida albicans* in sheep serum and trypticase soya broth, Am. J. Clin. Pathol. 60:839, 1973.

CHAPTER 11

Gastric analysis

A modern text should be consulted, since old terms and technics have given way to new ones.

Bauer, J. D., Ackermann, P. G., and Toro, G.: Clinical laboratory methods, ed. 8, St. Louis, 1974, The C. V. Mosby Co.
Cannon, D. C.: Examination of gastric and duodenal contents. In Davidsohn, I., and Henry, J. B., editors: Todd-Sanford clinical diagnosis by laboratory methods, ed. 15, Philadelphia, 1974, W. B. Saunders Co.

■ **What are the four major indications for the performance of a gastric analysis?**

The indications are (1) to determine the presence of anacidity, (2) to measure the amount of acid production in patients with the symptoms of peptic ulcer, (3) to reveal the hypersecretory state in the Zollinger-Ellison syndrome, and (4) to evaluate the completeness of vagotomy.

■ **What are the colors of Topfer's reagent in alkaline pH and acid pH, and what is its pH range?**

It is red in strongly acidic solutions and yellow in weakly acidic and in basic solutions. Its range of color change is pH 3.5 to 4.5.

■ **With maximal histamine stimulation, what pH level separates patients with pernicious anemia from normal subjects?**

The pH of the gastric fluid in pernicious anemia does not fall below pH 6.0.

■ **Describe the procedure for determination of basal HCl output.**

The basal HCl output in a fasted, medication-free patient is determined by withdrawing gastric fluid by continuous aspiration for 1 hour beginning 30 minutes after intubation to allow accommodation to the procedure.

■ **What is the normal basal gastric hydrochloric acid (HCl) output?**

The mean is 1.3 to 4.0 mEq/hr, and the normal range is up to 14 mEq/hr.

■ **What proportions of normal subjects and patients with duodenal ulcer have basal HCl secretions in excess of 10 mEq/hr?**

Only 4% of normal subjects and 15% of duodenal ulcer patients have basal HCl secretions that exceed 10 mEq/hr.

■ **What is the normal basal gastric secretory volume?**

It is 50 to 100 ml/hr.

■ **How is the augmented histamine test performed?**

Histamine 0.04 mg/kg of body weight is injected subcutaneously on completion of the 1-hour basal gastric secretion collection. At this dose of histamine, the response of parietal cells is maximal. An antihistamine may be given intramuscularly 30 minutes before histamine injection to decrease side effects, since antihistamine does not interfere with the gastric secretory effect of histamine. Gastric fluid is collected for 1 hour. The maximum response to histamine occurs 15 minutes after injection and continues for 30 minutes.

■ **What is the normal range of gastric HCl output during the augmented histamine test, and what proportion of duodenal ulcer patients exceed the upper limit of normal?**

The normal range is 5 to 39 mEq/hr of HCl. About 40% of ulcer patients exceed a gastric HCl output of 39 mEq/hr.

■ **Define anacidity in the augmented histamine test, and comment on its significance.**

Anacidity is failure of the pH to fall below 6.0. It is specific for pernicious anemia, although it occurs in a minority of gastric carcinoma patients, in some patients with rheumatoid arthritis, iron deficiency anemia, steatorrhea, myxedema, and nutritional megaloblastic anemia, and in relatives of patients with pernicious anemia.

■ **What is Histalog?**

It is a histamine analogue, 3-beta-aminoethyl pyrazole dihydrochloric acid (betazole), and it is a satisfactory substitute for histamine for gastric secretory studies.

■ **What gastric secretory features are typical of the Zollinger-Ellison syndrome?**

1. One-hour basal HCl secretion in excess of 14 mEq
2. Maximal HCl secretion in excess of 39 mEq/hr
3. Basal/maximal HCl secretion ratio in excess of 0.6 (doubtful range 0.4 to 0.6)
4. Twelve-hour overnight secretion exceeding 2 L. and 100 mEq HCl (The mean values for normal subjects are about 600 ml and 18 to 30 mEq HCl, and for ordinary duodenal ulcer patients they are 1000 ml and 60 mEq HCl.)

■ **What tests other than routine gastric analysis may be helpful in the diagnosis of the Zollinger-Ellison syndrome?**

Measurement of serum gastrin levels both fasting and after intravenous calcium infusion is helpful.[1,2]

■ **How may one differentiate between patients with the Zollinger-Ellison syndrome and pernicious anemia, both of which have elevated serum gastrin levels?**

Intragastric infusion of 0.1 N HCl produces a prompt decrease in the gastrin levels in patients with pernicious anemia.[1,2]

■ **What is the procedure for determination of titrable acidity in gastric secretion?**

Titrable acidity, expressed in milliequivalents per liter, is determined by titration of an aliquot of gastric fluid to pH 7.0 with 0.1 N NaOH. If a pH meter is not available, the end point can be approximated with phenol red indicator.

■ **A 12-hour overnight gastric secretion specimen from a patient with a duodenal ulcer has a volume of 800 ml, and 9.0 ml of 0.1 N NaOH is required for titration of a 10 ml aliquot to pH 7.0. How many milliequivalents of H^+ does the entire specimen contain?**

It contains 72 mEq H^+.

■ **What is the principle of tubeless gastric analysis?**

Azure A, a dye, is released from a cation exchange resin by H^+ ions in the stomach, absorbed in the intestine, and excreted in the urine. It is not absorbed by an achlorhydric subject and will not appear in his urine.

■ **What are the pitfalls of tubeless gastric analysis?**

The dye may be released by other cations (Na^+, Mg^{++}, K^+, Ca^{++}, Al^{+++}). It is unreliable in presence of renal failure, malabsorption, pyloric obstruction, severe urinary retention, and in patients who have had a subtotal gastrectomy or gastroenterostomy.

■ **Describe the Hollander test for completeness of vagotomy.**

1. Collect gastric secretions in 15-minute increments for 2 hours after a 12-hour overnight fast.
2. Inject intravenously 0.20 unit of insulin per kilogram of body weight. Collect gastric secretions in 15-minute increments for 2 hours, and draw blood for glucose determination at 30, 60, and 90 minutes.

■ **What are the criteria for incompleteness of vagotomy by the Hollander test?**

1. The Hollander test is valid only if acid is secreted basally or after histamine stimulation and if the blood sugar drops to 50 mg/dl or lower (usually 30 minutes after insulin injection).

2. Vagotomy is probably incomplete if the basal secretion of acid is in excess of 2 mEq/2 hr or if the secretion after insulin injection exceeds the baseline secretion by more than 0.5 mEq/2 hr.

- **Are fasting serum gastrin levels low, normal, or elevated in patients with ordinary duodenal ulcers?**

They are normal.[1,2]

- **Do patients with pernicious anemia and other patients with achlorhydria have high, low, or normal serum gastrin levels?**

Their serum gastrin levels are high. This apparently is because secretion of HCl inhibits secretion of gastrin.[1,2]

REFERENCES

1. Trudeau, W. L., and McGuigan, J. E.: Relations between serum gastrin levels and rates of gastric hydrochloric acid secretion, N. Engl. J. Med. 284:408, 1971.
2. Yalow, R. S., and Berson, S. A.: Radioimmunoassay of gastrin, Gastroenterology 58:1, 1970.
3. Zaterka, S., and Neves, D. P.: Maximal gastric secretion in human subjects after Histalog stimulation: comparison with augmented histamine test, Gastroenterology 47:251, 1964.

CHAPTER 12

Hematology

The sections on hematology in the recommended comprehensive textbooks are adequate for learning the fundamentals of hematology. More detailed information is found in the hematology textbooks by Williams, Wintrobe, and Miale. The illustrations and technical methodology in the section by Bauer in *Gradwohl's Clinical Laboratory Methods and Diagnosis* are excellent. The text by Harris and Kellermeyer is an inexpensive and superlative reference for study of anemias.

Bauer, J. D.: Hematology. In Frankel, S., Reitman, S., and Sonnenwirth, A. C., editors: Gradwohl's clinical laboratory methods and diagnosis, ed. 7, St. Louis, 1970, The C. V. Mosby Co.

Harris, J. W., and Kellermeyer, R. W.: The red cell, rev. ed., Cambridge, Mass., 1970, Harvard University Press.

Miale, J. B.: Laboratory medicine—hematology, ed. 4, St. Louis, 1972, The C. V. Mosby Co.

Williams, W. J., et al.: Hematology, ed. 1, New York, 1972, McGraw-Hill Book Co.

Wintrobe, M. M.: Clinical hematology, ed. 7, Philadelphia, 1974, Lea & Febiger.

HEMOGLOBIN AND GENERAL TOPICS

- **What is the best anticoagulant (1) for collecting blood for fragility testing and (2) for a complete blood count?**

  1. Heparin
  2. EDTA

- **Why is balanced oxalate unacceptable as an anticoagulant for determining blood urea nitrogen and electrolytes?**

  It contains a mixture of NH_4^+ and K^+.

- **How do EDTA, oxalate, and citrate prevent blood coagulation?**

  All three chelate calcium.

- **What is the principle of the cyanmethemoglobin method for measuring hemoglobin? Why is it the preferred method?**

  Drabkin's solution (ferricyanide-cyanide) oxidizes the iron present to

Fe^{+++}, which combines with cyanide to form cyanmethemoglobin. The absorption at 540 nm is then measured. This method measures all forms of hemoglobin except sulfmethemoglobin, can utilize a stable standard, and is reliable ($\pm$ 2% to 5%).

■ **What are the normal blood hemoglobin levels for adults, infants, and children?**

The normal range for men is 14 to 18 gm/dl, and for women it is 12 to 16 gm/dl. Newborn infants have high levels (average of 19 gm/dl in capillary blood on first day) that fall rapidly. The nadir occurs at 1 to 2 years with a mean of 12.5 gm/dl.

■ **How high are hemoglobin concentrations in the umbilical cord blood of newborn infants, and how do cord blood levels compare with levels in capillary and central venous blood?**

The cord blood hemoglobin levels are usually between 14 and 19 gm/dl in normal infants. Capillary and central venous blood hemoglobin levels are several gm/dl higher.

■ **What clinical feature does methemoglobinemia produce?**

It produces cyanosis by preventing hemoglobin combination with oxygen.

■ **How is methemoglobin normally reduced to hemoglobin by the body?**

The most important system is NADH-methemoglobin reductase. Other systems are ascorbic acid, reduced glutathione, and NADPH-methemoglobin reductase.

■ **Describe the three types of methemoglobinemia. Which is the most frequent?**

The most common is the acquired form caused by a myriad of drugs. The two hereditary forms include a deficiency of NADH-methemoglobin reductase (autosomal recessive) and certain hemoglobinopathies.

■ **List ten of the more common drugs that are capable of changing hemoglobin to methemoglobin.**

The drugs are acetanelid, antipyrine, chlorates, ferrous sulfate, iodine, nitrites, nitroglycerin, phenacetin, primaquine, and sulfonamides.

■ **What dye is valuable for the treatment of secondary methemoglobinemia, and why?**

Methylene blue is capable of greatly accelerating the normal cell reconversion mechanism for methemoglobin.

■ **How does sulfhemoglobin differ in its stability from the other abnormal hemoglobin pigments?**

Sulfhemoglobin cannot be converted back to normal hemoglobin and remains in the corpuscles until they break down.

■ **What drugs have been reported to produce sulfhemoglobinemia?**

Sulfonamides and aromatic amine drugs (phenacetin, acetanilid) produce sulfhemoglobinemia.

■ **Why is carboxyhemoglobin dangerous to the individual?**

Carboxyhemoglobin cannot bind oxygen and is therefore unavailable for oxygen transport.

■ **Are low levels of carbon monoxide in the air dangerous?**

Yes. Because the affinity of hemoglobin for carbon monoxide is 210 times greater than for oxygen, carboxyhemoglobin concentration can increase to dangerous levels with chronic exposure to low atmospheric concentrations (0.1% or less). Major sources are automobile exhausts and cigarette smoke.

■ **What is the blood half-life of carboxyhemoglobin after exposure?**

The half-life is approximately 5 hours.[9]

■ **What are the colors of oxyhemoglobin, carboxyhemoglobin, methemoglobin, and sulfhemoglobin?**

Oxyhemoglobin is bright red, carboxyhemoglobin is cherry red, methemoglobin is chocolate brown, and sulfhemoglobin is mauve lavender.

■ **Why must blood samples be obtained promptly when the presence of abnormal hemoglobin pigments is suspected?**

Except for sulfhemoglobin, the abnormal pigments disappear rapidly on cessation of exposure and the institution of therapy.

■ **What is the basis for the identification of the various hemoglobin pigments?**

They have characteristic absorption spectra.

■ **What is Katayama's test?**

It is a simple test for differentiating oxyhemoglobin and carboxyhemoglobin. The former turns greenish brown, and the latter turns rose red when mixed with ammonium sulfide in a slightly acid solution.

■ **Give the formulae for the mean corpuscular volume (MCV), mean corpuscular hemoglobin (MCH), and mean corpuscular hemoglobin concentration (MCHC).**

$$\text{MCV} = \frac{\text{Hematocrit (\%)} \times 10}{\text{Red cell count/cu mm in millions}}$$

$$\text{MCH} = \frac{\text{Hemoglobin (gm/dl)} \times 10}{\text{Red cell count/cu mm in millions}}$$

$$\text{MCHC} = \frac{\text{Hemoglobin (gm/dl)} \times 100}{\text{Hematocrit (\%)}}$$

■ **Which is greater, the venous hematocrit or the whole body hematocrit?**

The venous hematocrit is greater. Whole body hematocrit = 0.9 × venous hematocrit.

■ **What are the principles involved in electronic cell counting?**

Cells are detected by changes in electrical resistance (voltage pulse) as the cells pass through an aperture. In an alternative approach, cells deflect a constant light beam. When the voltage pulse system is employed, the quantitative amount of voltage charge is proportional to the cell volume and permits calculation of the MCV.

■ **What does the osmotic fragility test actually measure?**

It measures the degree of spherocytosis of the red blood cells. Spherocytosis may be inherited, or it may occur in acquired hemolytic anemia.

■ **What is the principle of the osmotic fragility test?**

Red blood cells suspended in a hypotonic solution of sodium chloride take up water, swell, and eventually burst. The greater the degree of spherocytosis, the less water the cell has to imbibe before it bursts.

■ **List those conditions with a decreased osmotic fragility of red blood cells.**

The conditions are iron deficiency anemia, thalassemia, sickle cell disease, jaundice, postsplenectomy, polycythemia, target cell anemias, and liver disease.

■ **Do mechanical and osmotic fragility parallel one another?**

They do not always parallel one another. Red cells with increased osmotic fragility also show increased mechanical fragility, but the reverse is not necessarily true.

■ **What sort of cells show an increased mechanical fragility without increased osmotic fragility?**

This condition indicates sickled and agglutinated cells.

■ **What plasma factors affect the erythrocyte sedimentation rate (ESR)?**

ESR is increased by increases in plasma levels of fibrinogen, alpha, beta, and gamma globulins, and cholesterol. ESR is decreased by increased plasma levels of albumin, and it is rarely decreased by cryogel formation.

■ **Which ESR method is most sensitive to mild elevation of the above reactive plasma proteins?**

The Wintrobe method is more sensitive than the Westergren method.[1]

■ **What effects do anemia and microcytosis have on ESR?**

Anemia increases and microcytosis decreases ESR.

■ **List various conditions or diseases in which an increase in the ESR is usually found.**

An increase is usually found in pregnancy (after the fourth month), acute and chronic infections, malignant diseases, most connective tissue diseases, dysproteinemias, and conditions involving tissue necrosis.

- **What are the normal ranges of the various white blood cells in a differential count on peripheral blood of adults?**

The ranges are lymphocytes, 25% to 33%; monocytes, 2% to 6%; polymorphonuclear leukocytes, 50% to 70%; eosinophils, 1% to 4%; and basophils, 0.25% to 0.50%.

- **How do the normal white blood cell differential counts of children differ from those of adults?**

Children have higher proportions of lymphocytes (averaging 60% in the first year and 36% in the tenth).

- **What proportion of the available granulocyte pool is present in the circulating blood?**

About half is present.

- **What are Dohle bodies, and when are they present?**

They are remnants of cytoplasmic RNA staining pale blue with Wright's stain. They are seen in polymorphonuclear neutrophils in patients with infectious diseases, burns, aplastic anemia, after administration of toxic agents, and in the May-Hegglin anomaly.

- **What is the Pelger-Huet anomaly, and what is its significance?**

It is a hereditary autosomal dominant condition in which there is a failure of segmentation of polymorphonuclear leukocyte nuclei. It is of little significance but should not be confused with a left shift of the differential count or the pseudo-Pelger anomaly seen in some patients with granulocytic leukemia.

- **What is the Chediak-Higashi syndrome?**

It is a lethal anomaly in which monocytes and granulocytes contain giant cytoplasmic peroxidase-positive granules. Associated abnormalities are photophobia, partial albinism, frequent pyogenic infections, malignant lymphoma, and leukemia.

- **What are the effects of ACTH administration (adrenals intact) on the neutrophil, lymphocyte, and eosinophil levels in the circulating blood?**

They are neutrophilia, lymphopenia, and eosinopenia, respectively.

- **Which of the bacterial infections are characterized by leukopenia?**

Typhoid fever, paratyphoid fever, sometimes tularemia and brucellosis, and others when infection is overwhelming, are characterized by leukopenia.

- **What changes in the platelet count would one expect in the following dis-**

eases or conditions: posthemorrhagic anemia, pernicious anemia, polycythemia vera, postsplenectomy, and posttrauma (including surgery)?

Platelet counts are usually increased in all the above conditions except pernicious anemia, in which they are almost always significantly diminished.

■ **Which of the leukemias are generally associated with a decreased platelet count, and which are generally associated with an increased platelet count?**

Decreased numbers of platelets are seen late in the course of chronic lymphocytic leukemia or in any of the acute leukemias. Increased numbers may be
seen in chronic granulocytic leukemia.

■ **Why are red blood cells eosinophilic?**

Hemoglobin has an affinity for acid dyes.

■ **Why do reticulocytes stain polychromatophilic with Wright's stain?**

They contain residual cytoplasmic RNA (which stains basophilic), in addition to hemoglobin.

■ **What is the significance of basophilic stippling of red blood cells?**

It may indicate exposure to lead (not necessarily lead poisoning). There
is no direct relationship between the degree of toxicity and the number of
stippled cells. In the absence of exposure to lead, it indicates accelerated regeneration of erythroid cells or impairment of hemoglobin synthesis.

■ **What are Heinz bodies?**

They are denatured hemoglobin within red cells seen in the acute phase of
certain hemolytic anemias, especially those associated with hypersensitivity to
certain chemicals (glucose-6-phosphate dehydrogenase deficiency).

■ **Are Heinz bodies visible in erythrocytes stained by the Wright method?**

Heinz bodies are not visible in routine Wright-stained blood films, but they
can be demonstrated by supravital staining with brilliant cresyl blue, crystal
violet, Nile blue sulfate, and a variety of other dyes.[4]

■ **Are normoblasts normally present in the peripheral blood?**

They are not present except in newborns and young infants.

■ **In adults, what is the significance of normoblasts in the peripheral blood?**

They indicate accelerated regeneration or disturbed release of red blood
cells, and their number roughly correlates with the extent of the bone marrow
reaction.

■ **What is a leukoerythroblastic reaction, and what is its significance?**

A leukoerythroblastic reaction denotes the presence of both normoblasts and
immature neutrophils in the peripheral blood. It most often indicates space-

occupying disturbances of the marrow (metastatic cancer, myelofibrosis, multiple myeloma).

■ **List those diseases or conditions associated with an absolute lymphocytosis.**

Lymphocytic leukemia, pertussis, infectious lymphocytosis, infectious mononucleosis, exposure to sunlight, exposure to high altitude, and tuberculosis are associated with an absolute lymphocytosis.

■ **List the diseases or conditions with which an absolute monocytosis is associated.**

Typhoid fever, infectious mononucleosis, subacute bacterial endocarditis, tuberculosis, brucellosis, certain parasitic infections (malaria, kala-azar, trypanosomiasis, amebic dysentery), Rocky Mountain spotted fever, and occasionally other infections are associated with an absolute monocytosis.

■ **What are the maximum and average numbers of lobes in the nuclei of polymorphonuclear leukocytes in the peripheral blood of normal individuals?**

The maximum number is 5, with an average of 3.5.

■ **List the diseases or conditions associated with eosinophilia.**

Allergic disorders (asthma, urticaria, etc.), certain skin diseases (pemphigus, dermatitis herpetiformis), parasitic infestations (especially tissue parasites such as roundworms), certain hematopoietic diseases (chronic granulocytic leukemia, pernicious anemia, etc.), Hodgkin's disease, postsplenectomy, postirradiation therapy, periarteritis nodosa, familial eosinophilia, and hypoadrenocorticism are associated with eosinophilia.

■ **List the diseases or conditions associated with basophilia.**

Chronic myelocytic leukemia, erythremia (polycythemia vera), and occasionally hemolytic anemia and postsplenectomy are associated with basophilia.

■ **How can myeloblasts be differentiated from lymphoblasts histochemically?**

Myeloblasts contain Sudan black B-positive and peroxidase-positive granules, whereas lymphoblasts do not.

■ **What are the normal ranges of the myeloid/erythroid ratio in adult and infant bone marrow?**

It is 3:1 to 4:1 in adults. At birth it is 1.85:1, rising to 11:1 by 2 weeks of age, after which it falls to adult levels by 1 year of age.

■ **Briefly describe the changes in cellularity of the sternal marrow with aging.**

It is 100% cellular up to 5 years of age, then it decreases to about 75% by

15 years of age. It then decreases more slowly to about 50% by 70 years of age.

■ **Under conditions of stress (hemolysis or blood loss with optimum nutrition), what is the maximum capacity to which the bone marrow can increase the output of red blood cells?**

It can increase the output six to eight times the normal rate.

■ **What proportion of an injected tracer dose of radioactive iron is used for red blood cell production?**

About 70% to 75% is used. The remaining 25% to 30% enters the liver.

■ **What is the normal ^{51}Cr-labeled red blood cell half-life?**

The half-life is 28 to 38 days. It is not 60 days, because about 1% of the isotope is eluted from the erythrocytes per day.

■ **What is the normal red blood cell survival?**

It is about 120 days.

■ **Describe the Ashby differential agglutination test for red cell survival.**

Red cells having a different antigen from the recipient's are transfused. Specimens are drawn shortly after transfusion and, at a later time, unagglutinated red blood cells are counted after adding a potent agglutinating serum for the recipient's cells.

■ **What is the corrected reticulocyte count in a patient who has a hematocrit of 30% and 6% reticulocytes?**

The corrected count is $6\% \times \dfrac{30}{45} = 4\%$.

■ **What are the effects of high-titer cold agglutinins on red blood cell measurements by automated counting methods?**

Formation of microaggregates results in erroneously low red blood cell counts and hematocrits, spurious macrocytosis, and poor reproducibility.[5]

■ **What is the most definitive method of confirming the diagnosis of hypersplenism?**

It is prompt and permanent restoration of the normal hematologic state after splenectomy. Increased spleen/liver ratio of radioactivity after injection of ^{51}Cr red cells is suggestive of hypersplenism, but it is not completely reliable as a predictive sign for response to splenectomy.

■ **Which of the following may result from hypersplenism: anemia, leukopenia, thrombocytopenia, lymphopenia?**

All but lymphopenia may result from hypersplenism.

■ **What changes in the peripheral blood are usual in patients whose spleens have recently been removed?**

Thrombocytosis, eosinophilia, lymphocytosis, circulating siderocytes, and Howell-Jolly bodies are common in such patients.

■ **What enzymatic change does the liver show in erythropoietic porphyria?**

An increase in δ-aminolevulinic acid synthetase has been observed in liver biopsies.[2]

■ **What proportion of erythrocytes in the peripheral blood show red fluorescence in patients with erythropoietic porphyria?**

Fluorescence is shown by 7% to 25%.[2]

ANEMIAS AND IRON METABOLISM

■ **Describe the major hematologic findings in the peripheral blood after acute blood loss.**

The platelet count rises within an hour, followed by leukocytosis with a peak at 2 to 5 hours. An increased number of reticulocytes appear at 24 to 48 hours. The hematocrit, hemoglobin concentration, and red cell count may increase briefly in presence of shock and then decrease during the next 48 hours, with 14% to 36% of the ultimate fall in hematocrit occurring within the first 2 hours after the hemorrhage.

■ **Which returns to the normal level first after an acute hemorrhage, the hemoglobin or the red cell count?**

The red cell count returns to normal about 2 weeks before the hemoglobin level.

■ **What is the most common cause of anemia?**

Iron deficiency is the most common cause.

■ **What is the normal total body iron store, and what is its distribution?**

The normal total body store is 4 to 5 gm, of which 60% is in red blood cells, 3% to 4% in myoglobin and enzymes, and the rest in ferritin and transferrin.

■ **What is the average daily iron intake in the diet, and what percentage of the daily intake is absorbed by the gastrointestinal tract?**

Twelve to 18 mg is taken in the diet, of which 10% to 12% is absorbed.

■ **About how much iron is needed by the average woman during pregnancy?**

Approximately 280 mg is needed for the fetus and placenta plus 200 mg for the iron lost in the blood at parturition, and 170 mg for normal losses.

■ **To what protein is iron bound in the blood?**

Iron is bound to transferrin.

■ **How does transferrin migrate electrophoretically?**

It migrates as a beta globulin.

■ **What is the normal range of serum iron and iron-binding capacity in the blood?**

The normal range of serum iron is 70 to 150 μg/dl, and that of total iron binding capacity is 250 to 400 μg/dl.

■ **List three conditions that lead to an elevation of the iron binding capacity.**

Iron deficiency, pregnancy, and oral-contraceptive therapy will lead to an elevation.

■ **List two causes of decreased iron-binding capacity.**

Chronic infection and decreased plasma proteins will decrease iron-binding capacity.

■ **List diseases or conditions in which there is an elevation of the serum iron level.**

Hemolytic anemia, hemochromatosis, transfusion siderosis, erythroid hypoplasia (as seen in lead poisoning, for example), and an increase in the release of iron stores (such as liver necrosis) will produce an elevation.

■ **List causes of a decrease in the serum iron concentration level.**

This decrease is caused by a decrease in the body's stores (such as iron deficiency anemia), decreased release from the body's stores (as is seen in chronic infection), rheumatoid arthritis, chronic renal disease, and cancer.

■ **What are the bone marrow findings in iron-deficiency anemia?**

They are absence of stainable iron and normoblastic hyperplasia with small normoblasts that have frayed margins and irregular shapes.

■ **Microcytosis is found in what anemias besides iron-deficiency anemia?**

It is found in thalassemia, sideroblastic anemias, and hereditary sex-linked anemia.

■ **What is a key feature distinguishing iron-deficiency anemia from other hypochromic anemias?**

Absence of stainable iron in the bone marrow is a key feature. Prussian blue stain is used for this purpose, and this will stain iron in hemosiderin and ferritin.

■ **List the causes of macrocytic anemias.**

The causes are vitamin B_{12} deficiency caused by decreased absorption (pernicious anemia, sprue, or after gastric or bowel resection), increased utilization of vitamin B_{12} (intestinal blind loop syndrome, *Diphyllobothrium latum* infestation, chronic hemolytic anemias, various malignancies), and folic acid deficiency (malabsorption, dietary deficiency as in alcoholism, pregnancy, and chemotherapy with methotrexate and certain other drugs).

■ **What congenital defects in absorption of vitamin B_{12} have been described?**

Absence of intrinsic factor, presence of an abnormal intrinsic factor, faulty transport of B_{12} across the ileal cell, and absence of transcobalamin II have been described.[7]

■ **What hematologic changes should be anticipated in patients receiving methotrexate, diphenylhydantoin (Dilantin), the diuretic triamterene (Dyrenium), or the antimalarial pyrimethamine (Daraprim)? What is the explanation for the changes?[8]**

Megaloblastic anemia secondary to deficiency in folinic acid may occur in patients who receive the drugs named. The deficiency results not from malabsorption of folic acid but from inhibition of its reduction to the active form, folinic acid.

■ **What are the bone marrow findings in megaloblastic anemias?**

Megaloblastic hyperplasia, basophilic stippling of red blood cells, multiple Howell-Jolly bodies, giant metamyelocytes, and large megakaryocytes are found in the bone marrow.

■ **What are the findings in the peripheral blood in patients with megaloblastic anemia?**

Pancytopenia with macrocytosis, anisocytosis, poikilocytosis, basophilic stippling, multiple Howell-Jolly bodies, occasional megaloblasts, and leukopenia with giant granulocytes showing excessive numbers of nuclear lobes are found in the peripheral blood.

■ **In addition to the bone marrow, what organ systems are affected in pernicious anemia?**

The gastrointestinal tract and central nervous system are affected.

■ **Do all patients with pernicious anemia have histamine-fast achlorhydria?**

Except for those patients with the juvenile form in which free acid is usually present, patients with pernicious anemia are achlorhydric.

■ **Describe the Schilling test. What are the normal ranges?**

One microgram of radioactive B_{12} given orally is followed 2 hours later by a large flushing dose of B_{12} given parenterally. Normally, 5% to 40% of the radioactive dose is excreted in the urine in 24 hours.

■ **What is FIGLU, and what is its significance?**

Folic acid is required for conversion of formiminoglutamic acid (FIGLU) to glutamic acid in catabolism of histidine. FIGLU appears in urine in increased amounts after oral histidine load in folic acid deficiency, but unfortunately for the diagnostic value of the tests, it also appears in some patients with pure vitamin B_{12} deficiency (pernicious anemia).

■ **What daily doses of folic acid and vitamin B_{12} will correct specific deficiencies without affecting megaloblastic anemia caused by deficiency of the other vitamin?**

Doses of 1 to 5 μg of B_{12} or 50 to 200 μg of folic acid given parenterally are required.

■ **What is the effect of vitamin B_{12} deficiency (pernicious anemia) on urinary excretion of methylmalonic acid?**

Methylmalonic acid excretion is increased in vitamin B_{12}–deficient subjects, because vitamin B_{12} is a coenzyme for methylmalonyl-CoA mutase, which converts methylmalonyl-CoA to succinyl-CoA.

■ **Name five hematologic effects of alcohol.**

Alcohol partly blocks the reticulocyte response to moderate doses of folate in folic acid deficiency, and in some patients it may cause thrombocytopenia, decreased megakaryocytes in the bone marrow, leukopenia secondary to maturation arrest in the marrow in alcoholic patients with pneumonia, and sideroblastic marrow in severe alcoholics. The latter effect may be secondary to interference with conversion of pyridoxine to pyridoxal phosphate, and it is reflected by rise in serum iron levels.[3]

■ **What is the effect of antibiotic therapy on measurement of serum folic acid concentration by the *Lactobacillus casei* bioassay?**

Antibiotic therapy results in falsely low assay values because the antibiotics inhibit growth of *L. casei*.

■ **What diseases or conditions may be associated with simple chronic anemia?**

Chronic infections, rheumatoid arthritis, and neoplastic and renal diseases may be associated with chronic simple anemia.

■ **Describe the peripheral blood picture in simple chronic anemia.**

The anemia is usually normocytic and normochromic but may be even microcytic as well (hypochromia precedes microcytosis).

■ **In those cases of simple chronic anemia with hypochromia, what is the status of the bone marrow iron?**

It is normal or increased in amount (the defect is in the movement of iron out of the reticuloendothelial system).

■ **What happens to the serum iron level and total iron-binding capacity (TIBC) in simple chronic anemia?**

The serum iron level is characteristically decreased, whereas the TIBC remains normal or is decreased.

■ **What is myelophthisic anemia?**

It is anemia secondary to replacement of bone marrow by abnormal tissue.

■ **What is the characteristic finding in the peripheral blood film in myelophthisic anemia?**

Leukoerythroblastosis (normoblasts and immature neutrophils) is found.

■ **What is the most sensitive indicator of metastatic carcinoma to bone marrow in the peripheral film?**

It is the presence of myelocytes.

■ **Describe the earliest changes in formed blood elements after 300 rads of total body irradiation.**

Lymphocytes are decreased in 24 hours, neutrophils are decreased in 5 days, red blood cells are slightly decreased in 24 hours, and platelets are decreased in about 4 days.

■ **What bone marrow abnormalities have been ascribed to chloramphenicol?**

Chloramphenicol apparently causes an irreversible aplastic anemia (in a small number of patients) and a reversible dose- and time-dependent pancytopenia (seen in about half of treated patients).

■ **Describe the characteristic laboratory findings in refractory sideroblastic anemia.**

Hypochromic, microcytic anemia with increased serum iron levels and saturation of iron binding protein, marked increase in iron stores in the bone marrow and other tissues, and large numbers of sideroblasts in the bone marrow are found.

■ **Pure red cell aplasia is often associated with what entity, and how often?**

Pure red cell aplasia is associated with thymoma in about half of the instances.

■ **What is the normal plasma hemoglobin concentration?**

It is 2 to 3 mg/dl.

■ **At what level of free hemoglobin does the plasma become pink?**

It becomes pink at 15 to 20 mg/dl.

■ **To what is free hemoglobin bound in the plasma?**

It is bound to haptoglobin.

■ **How high does the plasma hemoglobin level have to rise to produce hemoglobinuria?**

It must rise to 100 to 130 mg/dl. (At this level, the haptoglobin binding capacity is exceeded.)

■ **Which is the most sensitive detector of hemolysis: urine urobilinogen, fecal urobilinogen, or serum bilirubin?**

The level of fecal urobilinogen excretion is the most sensitive detector.

- **In obscure cases, how can the distinction between intracorpuscular and extracorpuscular causes for hemolysis be made?**

Normal compatible red cells injected into the blood of a patient with an intracorpuscular defect will survive normally, but they will have a shortened survival in a patient with an extracorpuscular abnormality. Defective red cells would show a shortened survival when injected into a compatible normal subject.

- **Describe the results of the following laboratory procedures in hereditary spherocytosis: MCV, MCH, MCHC, osmotic fragility, and the Coombs test.**

MCV and MCH are usually normal with a normal or increased MCHC. The osmotic fragility is usually increased, and the Coombs test result is negative.

- **How serious an illness is hereditary ovalocytosis?**

Ten to fifteen percent of those affected have mild anemia, but the others have no noticeable complication.

- **Why is glucose-6-phosphate dehydrogenase (G-6-PD) deficiency more often serious in male patients than in female patients?**

It is caused by an abnormality of a gene on the X chromosome so that both X chromosomes of a female would have to be involved, whereas only the one present in the male need be involved to cause a severe deficiency.

- **What drugs are known to increase the susceptibility to hemolysis in persons with G-6-PD deficiency?**

The drugs are primaquine, sulfonamides, nitrofurans, and aminoquinolones.

- **Next to G-6-PD deficiency, what is the most common enzyme deficiency producing a hemolytic anemia?**

Pyruvate kinase (PK) deficiency is the next most common enzyme deficiency.

- **List the three hemoglobin types found in normal people.**

They are hemoglobin A (Hb A), Hb F, and Hb A_2.

- **What are the polypeptide chains in Hb A, Hb F, and Hb A_2?**

They are Hb A ($\alpha_2\beta_2$), Hb F ($\alpha_2\gamma_2$), and Hb A_2 ($\alpha_2\delta_2$).

- **What are the normal concentrations of Hb F and Hb A at birth, at 4 months, and in adults?**

  1. Hb F: 80% at birth, 5% to 10% at 4 months, and less than 0.5% in adults
  2. Hb A: 15% to 40% at birth, 90% to 95% at 4 months, and greater than 95% in adults

- **What is the normal concentration of Hb A$_2$ in adults?**

It is less than 3.5%.

- **Which is the more serious, alpha or beta thalassemia?**

Alpha thalassemia is the more serious.

- **How do the homozygous differ from the heterozygous beta hemoglobinopathies?**

The former have no normal beta chains (i.e., no Hb A is produced).

- **What is the cause of the abnormal shape of sickle cells?**

The cause is orientation of the abnormal hemoglobin (Hb S) when oxygen is removed, to form fluid crystals (tactoids), which deform the cell.

- **What are the relative proportions of the hemoglobins present in sickle cell disease and heterozygous sickle cell trait?**

The proportions present in the homozygous condition are Hb S 60% to 90%, Hb F 1% to 40%, and Hb A$_2$ 3.5%; no Hb A is present. The proportions present in the heterozygous condition are Hb A 60% to 80% and Hb S 20% to 40%; Hb F is not increased.

- **What is the frequency of the sickle cell trait in American blacks? Is it a serious condition?**

It occurs in about 10% of all American blacks. Usually it causes complications only under conditions of hypoxia or acidosis.

- **Describe the changes in osmotic and mechanical fragility of red cells in Hb S and in Hb C diseases.**

Mechanical fragility is increased in both. The osmotic fragility is decreased in sickle cell disease and is biphasic in Hb C disease.

- **List the following hemoglobins in order of their mobility of pH 8.6 paper electrophoresis: A, C, D, E, F, S.**

The order (slowest first) is C, E, D and S, F, and A. Other hemoglobins such as A$_2$ require starch gel electrophoresis to be distinguished.

- **Which hemoglobinopathy characteristically shows the most target cells in the peripheral smear?**

Hb C disease, closely followed by Hb D disease, shows the most target cells.

- **A hemoglobinopathy associated with cyanosis from birth usually has what cause?**

It is usually caused by Hb M with alpha or beta chain abnormalities.

- **What are the functional defects in Hb M?**

Decreased O$_2$ binding in alpha chain disease, and decreased binding at high P_{O_2} but increased O_2 binding at low P_{O_2} in beta chain disease comprise the defects.

■ **How do the thalassemias differ from the hemoglobinopathies?**

Thalassemias show varying degrees of diminished synthesis of hemoglobin polypeptide chains rather than synthesis of abnormal hemoglobins.

■ **What are the features of the peripheral blood film in thalassemia major?**

The following characteristics are found: hypochromia, microcytosis, extreme poikilocytosis with bizarre shapes, target cells, siderocytes, reticulocytosis, normoblastosis, Cabot rings, and Howell-Jolly bodies.

■ **What changes in the serum iron level and bone marrow iron stores are characteristic of thalassemia major?**

Both are increased.

■ **What are the relative proportions of the hemoglobins in thalassemia major and in thalassemia minor?**

1. Thalassemia major: Hb F 40% to 60%, Hb A_2 normal or increased, Hb A always decreased considerably
2. Thalassemia minor: Hb F elevated up to 6% in half the cases, Hb A_2 elevated up to 7%, Hb A only slightly decreased making up the remainder

■ **How can Hb F be differentiated from Hb A?**

Hb F is more resistant to alkali denaturation than is Hb A, and Hb F also resists elution from red blood cells at pH 3.2 (Betke-Kleihauer test).

■ **Name three circumstances in which red blood cells of patients with paroxysmal nocturnal hemoglobinuria (PNH) show an abnormally sensitive lytic response.**

Exposure to antibodies, to acid pH (Ham test), and to hypertonic sucrose (sugar water test) will show an abnormally sensitive lytic response.

■ **What do all the laboratory tests for the membrane defect of paroxysmal nocturnal hemoglobinuria have in common?**

They all are tests for increased sensitivity to complement-mediated hemolysis.[6]

■ **Will PNH red cells be lysed by inactivated serum in acid pH?**

They will not be lysed, because complement (which is removed by inactivation) is required by lysis.

■ **What abnormalities are noted in the erythrocytes in peripheral blood films in microangiopathic hemolytic anemias?**

Burr cells, helmet-shaped cells, red cell fragments, and spherocytes are found.

■ **What diseases or conditions are associated with microangiopathic hemolytic anemia?**

Malignant hypertension, thrombotic thrombocytopenic purpura, cirrhosis, disseminated carcinoma, hemolytic-uremic syndrome, and disseminated intravascular coagulation are all associated with microangiopathic hemolytic anemia.

■ **What are incomplete warm autohemolytic antibodies?**

They are abnormal serum globulins that react with red cells predominantly at 37° C. They can produce acquired hemolytic anemia.

■ **What is a bithermal cold autohemolysin?**

It is an abnormal serum globulin that combines with red cells at low temperature (less than 20° C) and then produces hemolysis when the temperature rises above 25° C (optimum 40° C).

■ **What are monothermal cold autohemolysins?**

They are abnormal serum globulins that bind and hemolyze at temperatures between 15° to 30° C (best at slightly acid pH).

■ **Comment on the age distributions of warm- and cold-hemagglutinin autoimmune hemolytic anemias.**

The warm-hemagglutinin disease affects all age groups from infancy to old age without any striking preference. Cold-hemagglutinin disease occurs most often in old age, although rarely children are affected.

■ **In symptomatic cold-hemagglutinin autoimmune hemolytic anemias, what titers of cold agglutinins are usually found, and what is the usual upper thermal range of their activity?**

At 4° C the titer of cold agglutinin is usually in excess of 1:1000. The upper range of activity usually extends to 28° to 32° C.

■ **What conditions show increased autohemolysis?**

Spherocytosis, PNH, RBC enzyme deficiencies, autoimmune hemolytic anemias, and chemical hemolytic anemias (acetylphenylhydrazine) show increased autohemolysis.

■ **How do the antibodies of warm and cold autoimmune hemolytic anemias (AHAs) differ, and how can the difference be demonstrated, according to Dacie, by the Coombs test?**

In general, the warm AHAs show gamma globulin antibodies, whereas the cold AHAs will react with nongamma (complement) antibodies. One should mix antiglobulin reagent with serial dilutions of gamma globulin, and then test cells. If the gamma globulin prevents the antiglobulin reaction, warm antibodies are indicated. If it does not, complement is on the cells.

■ **What is the cause of symptomatic autoimmune hemolytic anemia?**

Why it occurs is unkown, but it is seen in patients with leukemia (mainly chronic lymphocytic), lymphomas, myeloproliferative disorders, macroglobulinemias, ovarian teratomas, various cancers, and the collagen diseases.

■ **How can one differentiate between acute and chronic cold agglutinin disease in the laboratory?**

The chronic type tends to show a negative reaction to the direct Coombs test. The acute type shows a positive reaction to both the direct and indirect Coombs tests. The antibody is an IgM antibody.

■ **Paroxysmal cold hemoglobinuria (PCH) is associated with what disease?**

PCH may be associated with syphilis (congenital or late). The antibody is an IgG antibody.

■ **Describe the Donath-Landsteiner test.**

It is a test for bithermal cold autohemolysin. Two tubes of blood are drawn. One is kept at 37° C. The other is placed in ice for 30 minutes then in a water bath at 37° C. After clotting, the serum from patients with PCH will show hemolysis only in the tube initially cooled.

■ **Is the result of the direct Coombs test positive in syphilitic chronic paroxysmal cold hemoglobinuria?**

No. The result is not positive, but the result of the indirect Coombs test is positive.

■ **Describe the peripheral blood in autoimmune hemolytic anemia.**

There is a normocytic, normochromic anemia with numerous reticulocytes, spherocytes, schistocytes, and often nucleated RBC.

■ **What abnormalities are noted in the blood of pregnant women?**

Decreased hemoglobin level, elevated ESR, slight leukocytosis in the third trimester increasing postpartum (up to 20,000/cu mm), mild increase in the iron-binding capacity in second semester increasing further during third trimester, slight thrombocytopenia, increased plasma volume (up to 140% in third trimester), increases in fibrinogen and a variety of transport proteins, and decreases in albumin and haptoglobin occur.

■ **Megaloblastic anemia of pregnancy is usually caused by what condition?**

It is caused by folic acid deficiency.

LEUKOCYTES AND PROLIFERATIVE DISORDERS

■ **Which of the cellular components of the blood have typically elevated counts in polycythemia vera?**

All three counts (red cells, leukocytes, and platelets) are elevated.

■ **Describe the leukocyte alkaline phosphatase (LAP) test.**

A peripheral blood film is fixed briefly in formol-ethanol and incubated with a suitable substrate (alpha-naphthyl acid phosphate) at pH 9.75. The degree of specific staining in each of 100 consecutively examined mature neutrophilic granulocytes is scored from 0 to 4. The total score for 100 neutrophils normally falls between 15 and 55.

■ **Is the alkaline phosphatase activity level of granulocytes altered in patients with polycythemia vera?**

Yes, it usually is significantly elevated.

■ **List the causes of secondary polycythemia.**

The causes are chronic hypoxia (high altitude, cyanotic heart disease, and chronic lung disease) and various benign and malignant tumors (renal carcinoma, ovarian carcinoma, and cerebellar hemangioblastoma).

■ **Describe the peripheral blood, bone marrow, lymph nodes, spleen, and liver in infectious lymphocytosis.**

The lymphocyte count is usually markedly increased (60% to 90% of WBC with WBC counts of 20,000 to 40,000); the bone marrow is unremarkable; lymph nodes are not enlarged but have prominent germinal centers; and the spleen and liver are rarely palpable.

■ **What are the salient features of infectious mononucleosis?**

Its characteristics are fever, lymphadenopathy, palpable spleen, absolute lymphocytosis (defined as more than 4500/cu mm in the adult and more than 8500/cu mm in the child, respectively), a typical lymphocytes, positive heterophile presumptive test result (titer 1:224) or differential test result (agglutinin absorbed by beef RBC, not by guinea pig kidney), or positive result of an infectious mononucleosis spot test.

■ **List the major complications of infectious mononucleosis.**

1. Central nervous system: Guillain-Barré syndrome
2. Heart: pericarditis
3. Liver: hepatitis
4. Spleen: rupture
5. Blood: thrombocytopenic purpura and hemolytic anemia

■ **Name five conditions other than infectious mononucleosis that may have atypical lymphocytes.**

Measles, chicken pox, mumps, infectious hepatitis, virus pneumonia, and other viral upper respiratory infections in children may have atypical lymphocytes.

■ **List some diseases and conditions associated with monocytosis.**

Tuberculosis (bad prognostic sign), subacute bacterial endocarditis, recovery from acute infections (good prognostic sign), Hodgkin's disease, agranulocytosis (good prognostic sign), fungus and rickettsial diseases, and Gaucher's and Niemann-Pick diseases are associated with monocytosis.

■ **What is meant by B and T lymphocytes?**

Lymphocytes are believed to have two sites of origin, the thymus (T) and the avian bursa (B) of Fabricius or its equivalent in mammals. B cells are the precursors of antibody-producing cells. The T cell line are the lymphocytes involved in cellular immunity.

■ **Define lymphopenia, and give four diseases with which it may be associated.**

Lymphopenia means fewer than 1000 lymphocytes per cubic millimeter of blood in adults or 1500/cu mm in children. Hereditary immune deficiency syndromes (Wiskott-Aldrich, ataxia-telangiectasia, Swiss-type agammaglobulinemia), Hodgkin's disease, some lymphosarcomas, radiotherapy, and cytotoxic and corticosteroid therapy are associated with lymphopenia.

■ **List the diseases or conditions in which an increased macroglobulin level may be found.**

An increased macroglobulin level may be found in Waldenstrom's macroglobulinemia, carcinomas, malignant lymphomas, chronic lymphocytic leukemia, collagen diseases, and chronic infections.

■ **Briefly describe the salient features of Waldenstrom's macroglobulinemia.**

Diffuse lymphoreticular proliferation associated with macroglobulinemia occurring in older people, adenopathy, chronic normochromic anemia, increased susceptibility to infection, visual defects, hemorrhagic states, and often hepatosplenomegaly are characteristic.

■ **How does macroglobulinemia affect the erythrocyte sedimentation rate?**

Macroglobulinemia markedly increases the ESR.

■ **What is the characteristic cell found in patients with Waldenstrom's macroglobulinemia, and where is it most often found?**

The lymphocytoid plasma cell (or plasmacytoid lymphocyte) containing PAS-positive intranuclear inclusions is found in the bone marrow, lymph nodes, spleen, and liver.

■ **How is the definitive diagnosis of Waldenstrom's macroglobulinemia made?**

It is made by immunoelectrophoresis (IgM globulin) or ultracentrifugation (19S).

■ **Are polycythemia, autoimmune hemolytic anemia, and thrombocytosis more common in chronic granulocytic or in chronic lymphocytic leukemia?**

Polycythemia and thrombocytosis occur often in chronic granulocytic leukemia, and autoimmune hemolytic anemia occurs in chronic lymphocytic leukemia.

■ **Which usually has the higher white blood cell count, chronic granulocytic leukemia or chronic lymphocytic leukemia?**

The counts are usually higher in chronic granulocytic leukemia with a characteristic range of 100,000 to 800,000/cu mm. In chronic lymphocytic leukemia, the counts usually are between 30,000 and 100,000/cu mm.

■ **What is the Philadelphia chromosome?**

It is a small acrocentric chromosome 22 with short arm deleted. It is seen in blood and marrow cells of some patients with chronic granulocytic leukemia during relapse.

■ **What is the half-life of granulocytes in the blood?**

The half-life of blood granulocytes is approximately 4 to 10 hours (range 4.4 to 15.3 hours).[11]

■ **During what age ranges are the various types of leukemia most often seen?**

1. Acute leukemia: less than 20 years of age
2. Chronic granulocytic leukemia: 20 to 50 years of age
3. Chronic lymphocytic leukemia: over 50 years of age
4. Monocytic leukemia: 30 to 60 years of age

■ **What is muramidase (lysozyme)?**

This low molecular weight enzyme is released from granulocytes and excreted in the urine. Large amounts are found with accelerated neutrophil and monocyte turnover, particularly monocytic leukemia.

■ **Are anemia and thrombocytopenia more often early or late manifestations of chronic leukemia?**

Both are usually not seen until the later stages.

■ **Which type of leukemia typically has a rapid course and a severe hemorrhagic diathesis with depressed levels of fibrinogen, prothrombin, factors V and XIII, and platelets, attributable to disseminated intravascular coagulation?**

Acute promyelocytic leukemia has these characteristics.

■ **What are the salient physical features and the peripheral blood appearances in myelofibrosis with myeloid metaplasia?**

They are massive hepatosplenomegaly and a blood film with marked anisocytosis, poikilocytosis, teardrop-shaped red blood cells, and a few nucleated red blood cells, myelocytes, and promyelocytes.

■ **List causes of granulocytic leukemoid reactions.**

Infections (pyogenic, *M. tuberculosis*), neoplastic replacement of bone marrow (with normoblasts present in blood), massive tissue necrosis (gangrene, bowel infarction), hemorrhage, hemolytic crisis, and Hodgkin's disease (the white blood cell count may be over 100,000 with many eosinophils) cause granulocytic leukemoïd reactions.

■ **List several causes of lymphocytic leukemoid reactions.**

Infectious lymphocytosis, infectious mononucleosis, varicella, and pertussis cause lymphocytic leukemoid reactions.

■ **Describe the nitroblue tetrazolium reduction test.**

The test is performed by incubating heparinized blood with nitroblue tetrazolium and examining stained films for blue-black formazan deposits in polymorphonuclear leukocytes. The test is reported as percent PMNs containing the deposits, which are formed by reduction of the dye by the leukocytes. A score of 10% or more has been taken as evidence for bacterial infection, but the test may be no more sensitive than the conventional white blood cell count and differential (with attention to vacuolization, toxic granulation, Dohle bodies and immaturity of granulocytes) in detecting infection.[10]

■ **Describe the leukocyte alkaline phosphatase index in chronic granulocytic leukemia, leukemoid reaction, polycythemia vera, and agnogenic myeloid metaplasia (myelofibrosis).**

It is zero or low in chronic granulocytic leukemia and high in the other conditions.

■ **Other than unknown causes, what is the most frequent cause of agranulocytosis?**

The most frequent cause is drug allergy or sensitivity with the production of antileukocytic autoantibodies.

■ **Briefly describe the various marrow pictures that may be seen in agranulocytosis.**

The marrow may appear normocellular except for a maturation arrest of the granulocytes at the promyelocyte level; it may show myeloid hyperplasia with a similar maturation arrest as above; it may show myeloid hypoplasia; it may show only an increase in reticulum and plasma cells; or it may appear similar to the marrow of patients with acute granulocytic leukemia.

■ **What is the significance of Auer rods in immature leukocytes?**

Auer rods (azurophilic, peroxidase-positive cytoplasmic inclusions) are virtually pathognomonic for leukemia (myeloblastic, myelomonocytic, and myeloerythroblastic forms).

■ **Which acid phosphatase isoenzymes are predominant in Gaucher cells,**

mature lymphocytes and lymphocytes of chronic lymphocytic leukemia, and the "hairy lymphocytes" of leukemic reticuloendotheliosis? Which of these isoenzymes is not inhibited by $L^{(+)}$ tartaric acid?

Isoenzyme O is specific for Gaucher cells, 3 is the only isoenzyme present in mature lymphocytes and lymphocytes of chronic lymphocytic leukemia, and 5 is the isoenzyme present in the hairy lymphocytes (reticulum cells) of leukemic reticuloendotheliosis. Only isoenzyme 5 is not inhibited by $L^{(+)}$ tartaric acid.[12]

REFERENCES

1. Bull, B. S., and Brecher, G.: An evaluation of the relative methods of the Wintrobe and Westergren sedimentation methods, including hematocrit correction, Am. J. Clin. Pathol. 62:502, 1974.
2. Cripps, D. J., and MacEachern, W. M.: Hepatic and erythropoietic protophyria, Arch. Pathol. 91:497, 1971.
3. Eichner, E. H.: The hematologic disorders of alcoholism, Am. J. Med. 54:621, 1973.
4. Gasser, C.: Heinz body anemia and related phenomena, J. Pediatr. 54: 673, 1959.
5. Hattersley, P. G., et al.: Erroneous values on the Model S Coulter Counter due to high titer cold autoagglutinins, Am. J. Clin. Pathol. 55:442, 1971.
6. Jenkins, D. E., Jr.: Diagnostic tests for paroxysmal nocturnal hemoglobinuria, Sem. Haemat. 3:24, 1972.
7. MacKenzie, I. L., et al.: Ileal mucosa in familial selective vitamin B_{12} malabsorption, N. Engl. J. Med. 286: 1021, 1972.
8. The Medical Letter 14:52, 1972.
9. Peterson, J. E., and Stewart, R. D.: Absorption and elimination of carbon monoxide by inactive young men, Arch. Environ. Health 21:165, 1970.
10. Steigbigel, R. I., et al.: The nitroblue tetrazolium reduction test versus conventional hematology in the diagnosis of bacterial infection, N. Engl. J. Med. 290:235, 1974.
11. Uchida, T., and Kariyone, S.: Intravascular granulocyte kinetics and spleen size in patients with neutropenia and chronic splenomegaly. J. Lab. Clin. Med. 82:9, 1973.
12. Yam, L. T., Li, C. Y., and Lam, K. W.: Tartrate-resistant acid phosphatase isoenzyme in the reticulum cells of leukemic reticuloendotheliosis, N. Engl. J. Med. 284:357, 1971.

CHAPTER 13

Immunology and serology

Because serologic technics are applied to a variety of clinical disorders, an understanding of basic immunology has become important for all areas of the clinical laboratory. The book by Eisen is an excellent introduction to immunology. The chapters in *Todd-Sanford Clinical Diagnosis by Laboratory Methods* cover basic principles and technics of serology. Gell and Coombs' book is a more detailed correlation of serology with clinical disease. A new edition is in press.

Ashcavai, M., and Peters, R. L.: Manual for hepatitis B antigen testing, Philadelphia, 1973, W. B. Saunders Co.
Davidsohn, I., and Nelson, D. A.: Infectious mononucleosis. In Davidsohn, I., and Henry, J. B., editors: Todd-Sanford clinical diagnosis by laboratory methods, ed. 15, Philadelphia, 1974, W. B. Saunders Co.
Eisen, H. N.: Immunology: an introduction to molecular and cellular principles of the immune responses, New York, 1974, Harper & Row, Publishers.
Fudenberg, H. H., et al.: Basic immunogenetics, New York, 1972, Oxford University Press, Inc.
Gell, P. G. H., and Coombs, R. R. A.: Clinical aspects of immunology, ed. 2, Oxford, 1968, Blackwell Scientific Publications, Ltd.
Pusch, A. L.: Serodiagnostic tests for syphilis and other diseases. In Davidsohn, I., and Henry, J. B., editors: Todd-Sanford clinical diagnosis by laboratory methods, ed. 15, Philadelphia, 1974, W. B. Saunders Co.
Smith, J. L.: Spirochetes in late seronegative syphilis, penicillin notwithstanding, Springfield, Ill., 1969, Charles C Thomas, Publisher.

■ **What are the four subunits of gamma globulins and their molecular weights?**

Gamma globulins have subunits of two light chains each with a molecular weight of 20,000, and subunits of two heavy chains, each with a molecular weight of 53,000. One such unit of two L and two H chains constitutes an IgG molecule. IgM has five units. IgA may have two or more.

■ **What is the F_c fragment?**

It is a fragment consisting of the constant portions of the two heavy chains joined by a disulfide bond. F_c fragment binds complement.

184

■ **What is the F_{ab} fragment?**

It is a fragment consisting of either of the two light chains joined by a disulfide bond to the variable portion of a heavy chain. The F_{ab} fragment retains antigen binding capability.

■ **What is the Bence Jones protein?**

It is a globulin composed of light chains, kappa or lambda type, found in multiple myeloma, which is heat precipitable at 50° to 70° C and soluble at 100° C.

■ **How may one distinguish between the immunoglobulin classes?**

Each class has a characteristic unique H chain, designated by a Greek letter: IgG (gamma, γ), IgA (alpha, α), IgM (mu, μ), IgD (delta, δ), and IgE (epsilon, ϵ).

■ **What are the L chain types?**

They are kappa (κ) and lambda (λ).

■ **What is the variable region and its significance?**

Near the terminal end of both L and H chains is an area of marked variation in amino acid content from one antibody to another. It is believed that this region conveys antibody specificity to the molecule.

■ **What is a "secretory piece"?**

A secretory piece is a polypeptide fragment (MW 60,000) found on exocrine IgA that gives resistance to proteolysis. IgA is the dominant immunoglobulin in secretions.

■ **How may one crudely distinguish between IgG and IgM as being the active antibody in a sera?**

Substances such as mercaptoethanol will break the disulfide bridges between the five units in the IgM molecule, rendering it inactive as an antibody. IgG will retain its activity.

■ **Match the following:**

Antibody class	*Characteristic*
1. IgG	a. Responsible for severe transfusion reactions when transfused into congenitally deficient persons
2. IgA	b. Believed important in hay fever and other allergic phenomena
3. IgM	c. Crosses the placenta and can cause erythroblastosis fetalis
4. IgE	d. Binds complement and is a "complete" antibody

1. c; 2. a; 3. d; 4. b.

■ **Distinguish between cellular and humeral immunity.**

Cellular immunity is mediated by sensitized lymphocytes (T cells) that have antibody bound to their surface. Humeral immunity results from synthesis of antibody and its release into the circulation (B cells).

■ **Which is the more sensitive method for detecting paraproteins, serum protein electrophoresis or immunoelectrophoresis?**

Immunoelectrophoresis is the more sensitive method. Small amounts of paraproteins may not be detectable as a "spike" on a routine electrophoresis, but they will show as an aberrant band on immunoelectrophoresis.

■ **What is the order of reaction of the components of complement?**

The order of reaction is 1, 4, 2, 3, 5, 6, 7, 8, 9.

■ **How many molecules of IgM and IgG, respectively, are required to bind complement?**

One IgM or two IgG molecules are required.

■ **What are the variables that influence an agglutination reaction?**

Antigen concentration, antibody concentration, composition of the reaction medium, and temperature will influence an agglutination reaction.

■ **What are the two major antigens of Enterobacteriaceae, and what are the appearances of their agglutination reactions?**

Flagellar (H) antigens produce floccular agglutination that can be easily broken up by shaking. Somatic (O) antigens produce fine granular clumps that are difficult to break up by shaking.

■ **What is the Widal reaction?**

It is an agglutination reaction using killed *Salmonella typhi* for the detection of antibodies in serum.

■ **What are Vi antigens? When are antibodies to Vi antigens present?**

They are surface antigens peculiar to *S. typhi* and a few other strains of *Salmonella*. Antibodies to the Vi antigen appear during the course of an infection but tend to disappear soon after recovery. They are usually present in asymptomatic carriers.

■ **What is an anamnestic reaction?**

It is the phenomenon whereby a patient who has had previous contact with an antigen shows a rapid increase in antibody titers after reexposure to the antigen.

■ **In what circumstances can a patient have a negative agglutination test result 4 weeks after infection with *S. typhi?***

In addition to those few people in whom no explanation can be found, patients with agammaglobulinemia, advanced carcinoma, leukemia, and those treated with antibiotics may fail to show an increase in agglutinin titer 4 weeks after infection.

■ **How can the prozone phenomenon be at least partly overcome?**

It can be partly overcome by increasing the dilutions or inactivating the serum by heating at 56° C for 30 minutes.

■ **Although a bacterial agglutinin titer of 1:160 is suggestive of an infection, what is more diagnostic?**

A rise in titer during convalescence is more diagnostic.

■ **How is the serologic diagnosis of brucellosis made?**

An agglutinin titer of 1:80 or more is suggestive. A definite diagnosis is made by demonstrating a rising titer of agglutinins during the course of infection.

■ **How specific are the brucellosis agglutination tests?**

They cross-react with tularemia and cholera antibodies.

■ **Is a titer of 1:80 or greater for tularemia agglutinins specific for tularemia?**

No. Cross reactions occur with antibodies to rickettsiae and brucellae.

■ *Proteus* **OX 19 antigen is most useful in the serodiagnosis of which of the rickettsial diseases?**

It is useful in the serodiagnosis of epidemic and murine typhus and Rocky Mountain spotted fever.

■ **What complicating factors should be kept in mind in the interpretation of a positive Weil-Felix reaction?**

Patients treated with antibiotics before obtaining the specimen may not show a high agglutinin titer; anamnestic cross reactions occur; patients with recent *Proteus* species infections may have misleadingly high titers; and, occasionally, patients fail to develop agglutinins even though they have a rickettsial infection.

■ **Describe the principle of the serologic tests for the rheumatoid factor (RF).**

Red blood cells or other particles (latex, bentonite) coated with IgG gamma globulin are agglutinated by inactivated serum containing the RF, a group of macroglobulins with anti-IgG specificity. The serum is inactivated at 56° C to destroy a labile nonspecific agglutinating factor and to prevent the prozone phenomenon.

■ **What is the advantage of using a euglobulin fraction of the patient's serum in testing for the RF (Ziff modification)?**

Sera of some patients contain an inhibitor of the agglutination reaction that is not present in the euglobulin fraction containing the RF.

■ **What titers of the RF are significant?**

With the Hyland latex-particle RA test, titers of 1:16 or more are considered significant. Titers of 1:256 to 1:2048 are observed in most adults with rheumatoid arthritis. With other agglutination tests, the lowest significant titers range up to 1:40.

■ **What is the accuracy of the various tests for the RF?**

About 70% to 90% (average 85%) of adult patients with rheumatoid arthritis have significant titers, and 5% to 10% of sera from patients with other diseases react positively.

■ **What diseases give false positive reactions to RF tests?**

Systemic lupus erythematosus (30% to 40%), most instances of Sjögren's syndrome with or without arthritis, a variety of infectious diseases, and sera from the aged sometimes give positive reactions.

■ **What infectious diseases are particularly likely to give positive agglutination results of tests for the RF?**

Syphilis, tuberculosis, subacute bacterial endocarditis, leprosy, and kala-azar will often give positive results.

■ **In what variants of rheumatoid arthritis are results of the test for RF usually negative?**

In rheumatoid arthritis of children (Still's disease), the RF often is absent, and it usually is absent in ankylosing spondylitis.

■ **Does the RF test usually have negative results in patients with dermatomyositis, palindromic rheumatism, psoriatic arthritis, Reiter's syndrome, arthritis of ulcerative colitis, osteoarthritis, and gout?**

Yes.

■ **What is antistreptolysin O (ASO), and how is it detected?**

It is an antibody to a streptococcal hemolysin, and it is detected in serum by inhibition of lysis of group O red blood cells by streptolysin O extracted from group A streptococci.

■ **What level of ASO is considered definitely elevated?**

A level of 166 Todd units or more is definitely elevated.

■ **What is the meaning of a rise in ASO titer to significant levels?**

Such a rise indicates recent or current streptococcal infection, usually with a group A strain. It does not indicate that the patient is suffering from a complication (rheumatic fever or glomerulonephritis).

■ **What is the significance of an elevation of the ESR?**

It is a nonspecific indicator of inflammation, tissue necrosis (infarction), or alterations in serum proteins caused by other conditions.

■ **What is C-reactive protein (CRP)?**

It is an alpha globulin that forms a precipitate with the somatic carbohydrate C substance of pneumococci.

■ **What is the significance of a positive test result for C-reactive protein?**

It indicates an inflammatory process of nonspecific type or tissue necrosis (infarction).

■ **What is a direct hemagglutination test?**

It is a test for antibodies capable of agglutinating red blood cells previously coated with antigen. The test is useful in detecting antibodies to bacteria and in diagnosing toxoplasmosis.

■ **What is a hemagglutination-inhibition test for viruses?**

It is a test of the ability of serum to inhibit agglutination of red blood cells (chicken cells are often used) by certain viruses. The test is performed by incubating a mixture of cells, serum, and viral antigen. It is useful in detecting antibodies to rubella, poxviruses, mumps, and various viruses that cause encephalitis and other diseases.

■ **Must serum be specially prepared before performing hemagglutination-inhibition tests?**

Yes. It usually must be treated with trypsin and periodate or absorption with kaolin to remove nonspecific inhibitors.

■ **What is the appearance of a negative reaction to a hemagglutination test?**

The red blood cells settle to the bottom of the tube to form a compact button.

■ **What is the appearance of a positive reaction to a hemagglutination test (cells agglutinated)?**

The agglutinated red blood cells settle to the bottom of the tube in a diffuse granular pattern.

■ **What are the appearances of positive and negative reactions to hemagglutination-inhibition tests?**

They are the opposite of positive and negative hemagglutination tests, because hemagglutination occurs in the *absence* of antibodies.

■ **What is the principle of the complement fixation test?**

The test detects antigen-antibody reactions by the binding of complement that occurs during the reaction.

- **What is the system for detecting complement in complement fixation tests?**

Red blood cells and antiserum hemolytic for the cells are used (for example, sheep red blood cells and hemolytic antiserum produced by injecting sheep red blood cells into rabbits). When the cells and antiserum are mixed, hemolysis occurs only when complement is present. The test antigen and test are initially mixed with complement. If antibody is present, the complement will be bound, and when the red cells and hemolytic antisera are added, no hemolysis will occur.

- **What is the source of complement in complement fixation tests?**

Complement of known titer is added to each tube. The serum to be tested has been inactivated (complement destroyed) by heating to 56° C for 30 minutes.

- **In the complement fixation reaction, does hemolysis indicate the presence or the absence of antibodies?**

It indicates the absence of antibodies.

- **Describe the controls that are necessary with the complement fixation test, using the cardiolipin complement fixation test for syphilis as an example.**
  1. With serum control and antigen (cardiolipin) omitted, hemolysis should occur. Absence of hemolysis indicates anticomplementary serum.
  2. With antigen control, test serum omitted, and antigen included, hemolysis should occur.
  3. With corpuscle control and both complement and hemolysin omitted, hemolysis should not occur.
  4. With hemolytic system control and antigen and serum omitted, hemolysis should occur.
  5. With positive serum control, hemolysis should not occur.

- **What are the appearances of complement fixation test tubes showing 2+ and 4+ reactions?**

A 2+ reaction shows hemolysis of half the red blood cells, and a 4+ reaction shows no hemolysis.

- **In the complement fixation test, how can anticomplementary serums be tested?**

Run the test with the serum control (antigen omitted) and the patient's serum in serially doubled solutions. The test result is positive if the first dilution showing complete hemolysis with the serum control has little or no hemolysis with the patient's serum.

- **What is the principle of slide flocculation tests for syphilis?**

A lipid-containing antigen empirically known to react with serums from syphilitic patients is used. For the Venereal Disease Research Laboratories (VDRL) tests, the antigen is an extract of beef heart (cardiolipin), and cholesterol is added to make the particles large enough to be seen without magnification. Agglutination of the antigen by inactivated serum indicates a positive result.

■ **What is the FTA-ABS test?**

It is a test to detect antibodies to *Treponema pallidum* by immunofluorescence. The antigen consists of *T. pallidum* organisms cultivated in rabbit testes. The sorbent is an extract of a nonpathogenic Reiter treponeme containing group treponemal antigens. After exposure of the antigen on glass slides to the patient's serum mixed with the sorbent, the slides are washed and reacted with fluorescein-labeled antihuman globulin. Fluorescence of the treponemes indicates a positive result of the test.

■ **What advantages does the FTA-ABS test have over flocculation and complement fixation tests for syphilis?**

The FTA-ABS test is highly specific and will have negative results in various conditions causing false positive results of nontreponemal antigen tests. Furthermore, the FTA-ABS test results are positive in most patients who have tertiary syphilis but have negative nontreponemal antigen test results.

■ **What is the TPI test?**

TPI stands for *Treponema pallidum* immobilization and refers to the capacity of sera from syphilitic patients to immobilize living *T. pallidum* organisms. In specificity and sensitivity the TPI test is similar to the FTA-ABS test. The TPI test is available in only a few laboratories because it is technically difficult to perform.

■ **How soon after appearance of a syphilitic chancre will positive serologic test results develop?**

They will develop usually within 1 to 4 weeks.

■ **If a patient is adequately treated with penicillin during the primary or secondary stage of syphilis, what will the effects on the serologic tests probably be?**

The flocculation and complement fixation test results usually become negative within a year if treated during the primary stage or within 1½ years if treated during the secondary stage, but the FTA-ABS test results will probably remain positive.

■ **In long-term followup, what proportion of patients with syphilis who are initially seropositive will develop negative flocculation test results if untreated?**

At least 25% will develop negative flocculation test results.

■ **Describe the course of serologic findings in the infants in the following three situations:**
  1. **Mother seropositive with late latent syphilis**
  2. **Mother infected with syphilis in sixth month of gestation, infant congenitally syphilitic**
  3. **Mother infected with syphilis shortly before delivery, seronegative at time of delivery, infant congenitally syphilitic**

  1. The infant's serum is positive by flocculation, complement fixation, and antitreponemal antibody tests (FTA-ABS, TPI) with falling titers during first 6 months and spontaneous conversion to seronegativity.
  2. The infant is seropositive (flocculation, complement fixation, FTA-ABS, TPI) and remains seropositive.
  3. The infant is initially seronegative but converts to seropositivity within 6 months.

■ **List the conditions other than allied spirochetal diseases (yaws, pinta) that are most likely to cause false positive nontreponemal antigen test results for syphilis.**

They are malaria, leprosy, diphtheria-pertussis-tetanus immunization in children, disseminated lupus erythematosus, lymphogranuloma venereum, vaccinia, infectious hepatitis, periarteritis nodosa, rheumatoid arthritis, rheumatic fever, and infectious mononucleosis.

■ **What precautions are necessary in collecting blood for nontreponemal antigen tests for syphilis?**

The blood should be drawn before a meal (excess chyle interferes with the reaction); the blood alcohol level should be low (alcohol decreases the intensity of the reaction); and hemolysis (which may cause anticomplementary reactions) should be avoided.

■ **How can a laboratory diagnosis of syphilis be made in some patients with clinical evidence of central nervous system involvement in whom all serologic test results are negative?**

A diagnosis can be made by demonstration of spirochetes in spinal fluid with fluorescent treponemal antiserum.

■ **Describe the principle of the lupus erythematosus (LE) cell test.**

The LE factor (an IgG globulin) reacts with the nucleoprotein of exposed white cell nuclei and causes them to lose the granular chromatin pattern and to stain homogeneously. LE cells are neutrophils or monocytes that have phagocytosed the altered nucleoprotein.

■ **What antibody is responsible for a positive LE cell test?**

The antibody responsible is antinucleoprotein antibody, which is found in lesser frequency in other diseases, particularly of the collagen-vascular group. Other antibodies such as anti-DNA are also found in systemic lupus erythematosus.

■ **What is a "tart cell"?**

It is a phagocyte that contains a relatively unaltered nucleus in which the granular chromatin pattern is still visible. Tart cells are not indicative of lupus erythematosus.

■ **What conditions are necessary for demonstration of the LE phenomenon?**

Incubation of unanticoagulated or heparinized blood at room temperature or at 37° C is necessary. Complement must be present, and anticomplementary anticoagulants (oxalate, citrate, EDTA) inhibit the reaction.

■ **What proportion of patients with active SLE have positive results of the LE cell test?**

Positive results occur in 60% to 80% of the patients.

■ **Under what circumstances is a patient with SLE likely to have a negative reaction to the LE cell test?**

A negative reaction may occur when complement is depleted (actively progressing lupus nephritis), during intensive corticosteroid therapy, and during spontaneous remission.

■ **What serologic test result, if negative, effectively excludes the diagnosis of SLE?**

A negative immunofluorescence test result for antinuclear factor (ANF) practically excludes the diagnosis of SLE.

■ **How often is ANF present in the sera of patients with rheumatoid arthritis?**

ANF is demonstrable in about 15% of sera from patients with rheumatoid arthritis.

■ **What differences exist between the ANF of patients with SLE and the ANF of patients with rheumatoid arthritis?**

In rheumatoid arthritis, the ANF may be IgM and, in such cases, it is activated by heating to 65° C or by mercaptoethanol. The ANF of patients with SLE is IgG and is not inactivated by either procedure.

■ **In what other conditions is the test result for ANF likely to be positive?**

It is likely to be positive in active chronic hepatitis (three fourths), primary biliary cirrhosis (half), cryptogenic cirrhosis (two fifths), dermatomyositis and scleroderma (a third), necrotizing vasculitis (a fourth), and acute drug hypersensitivity states (a fifth).

■ **What drugs are associated with a positive ANF?**

Several drugs have been noted to induce a "lupus diathesis" with positive ANF and sometimes joint symptoms. Among these are hydralazine (antihypertensive), procainamide (antiarrhythmic), and isoniazid (antibiotic).[6]

■ **What types of antinuclear immunofluorescent patterns are associated with rheumatoid arthritis, SLE, and scleroderma as demonstrated in the standard ANF test?**

In rheumatoid arthritis and SLE the pattern may be speckled, homogeneous, or rim. In scleroderma it is usually nucleolar or homogeneous.[3]

■ **Why are precipitin tests for antithyroid antibodies of limited value in the diagnosis of Hashimoto's thyroiditis?**

The results are positive in high titer in only little more than half of the patients, and they are occasionally positive in other thyroid diseases (lymphoid thyroiditis, thyroid carcinoma, Graves' disease, primary myxedema).

■ **When are antithyroid antibodies virtually diagnostic of Hashimoto's thyroiditis?**

They are virtually diagnostic when they are present in high titers (1:250,000 or more).

■ **What is the clinical value of tests for antibodies to striated muscle and thymus in patients with myasthenia gravis?**

Almost all patients with myasthenia gravis who also have a thymoma have these antibodies. Their absence in a patient with myasthenia gravis rules out thymoma with a high degree of certainty.

■ **What disease of the liver can be ruled out if antimitochondrial antibodies are not present in the serum early in the disease process?**

Primary biliary cirrhosis can be ruled out with 90% certainty.

■ **What is alpha fetoprotein?**

It is a serum protein made in the livers of embryos and which usually is not present after the neonatal period. It is found in the serum of patients with hepatic carcinoma and less frequently in gonadal tumors.

■ **What is carcinoembryonic antigen (CEA), and in what conditions is it present in serum in abnormally high concentrations?**

CEA is an antigen present in embryonic tissues, adenocarcinoma of the large intestine, and adenocarcinomas originating in the stomach, small intestine, lung, pancreas, and occasionally other organs. Serum concentrations may be elevated in presence of the neoplasms listed above and in some patients with inflammatory disease of the bowel, cirrhosis, renal disease, chronic cigarette smoking, or sometimes without evident cause.[5]

■ **How sensitive is the CEA test on serum for detection of carcinoma of the large intestine?**

The CEA is elevated (2.5 to 3 ng/ml or more) in two thirds to three fourths of patients with known large intestinal carcinoma. Rates of positivity are highest in patients with metastatic neoplasm.

■ **What currently is the most practical use of CEA testing?**

The most practical use of CEA testing is to follow patients with documented colon cancer postoperatively for signs of recurrent tumor.

■ **What proportions of patients with pernicious anemia, relatives of these patients, patients with Graves' disease, and healthy controls have parietal cell antibodies?**

Eighty-four percent of pernicious anemia patients, 30% of their healthy relatives, 30% of patients with Graves' disease, and 5% of healthy controls have antibodies against parietal cells.[2]

■ **What is the presumptive test for infectious mononucleosis?**

Serial dilutions of the patient's serum inactivated at 56° C are incubated with suspensions of sheep cells. Agglutination of the cells in a titer of 1:224 or more supports the clinical diagnosis of infectious mononucleosis.

■ **What conditions, other than infectious mononucleosis, cause elevations in the presumptive test titer?**

Serum sickness, various infections, and blood transfusion cause such elevations.

■ **Describe the Davidsohn differential serologic test for infectious mononucleosis.**

Forssman antibodies agglutinate sheep red cells but are not specific for infectious mononucleosis. The Forssman antibodies are removed by exposure of serum to a guinea pig or horse kidney that contains Forssman antigen. Beef red blood cell stroma removes the antisheep cell antibodies that are specific for infectious mononucleosis. A positive differential test result consists of agglutination of the sheep red blood cells in a titer of 1:28 or more after absorption with guinea pig or horse kidney and failure of agglutination after absorption with beef red cell stroma.

■ **How specific is the differential test for infectious mononucleosis?**

False positive test results are rare.

■ **Describe the Lee spot test for infectious mononucleosis.**

Serum (which need not be inactivated) is dropped on a card. One drop is mixed with a guinea pig kidney suspension, and another drop is mixed with a suspension of beef erythrocyte stroma. Then each mixture is mixed with a suspension of horse red blood cells. The spots are examined for agglutination of the red cells after 2 minutes. A greater degree of agglutination by the drop of serum absorbed with guinea pig kidney than by the drop absorbed with beef erythrocyte stroma indicates a positive result. Serum from patients with infectious mononucleosis usually agglutinates the cells within 5 seconds. This test compares favorably with the Davidsohn differential test in sensitivity and specificity.[4]

■ **What is the interpretation of a rubella hemagglutination-inhibition (HI) test in which the 1:10 dilution tube shows no inhibition of agglutination?**

HI titers of less than 1:10 indicate that the patient probably has no immunity to rubella.

■ **How is the rubella HI test used to confirm the diagnosis of a clinical case of rubella?**

Blood specimens are taken within 3 days after onset of the rash, and a second specimen is taken 3 weeks later. Both serum specimens are tested concurrently for **HI** antibody. A fourfold increase in antibody titer from the first to second serum indicates that the patient has rubella.

■ **What is the principle of most radioimmunoassays (RIA)?**

The principle is competition between the unknown amount of antigen in the sample and a known amount of radioactive antigen for antibody combining sites. Antibody-antigen complexes are then separated from free antigen.

■ **List several technics used to separate antigen-antibody (Ag-Ab) complexes from free antigen.**

1. Precipitation of Ag-Ab with a second antibody directed against the first antibody, or by high salt concentration
2. Prior absorption of the antibody to the inside of a plastic test tube
3. Removal of unbound antigen by dialysis or by absorption on charcoal
4. Gel chromatography

■ **What is the principle of the counterelectrophoresis test (CEP), and what are its advantages?**

Two wells are punched in alkaline agar. A test sample for antigen is placed in the well on the cathodal side, and an antibody is placed in the anodal well. In alkaline agar, gamma globulin will migrate towards the cathode and most antigens will go towards the anode, thus "driving" antibody and antigen together. The advantages over standard agar diffusion are speed (hours versus days) and increased sensitivity.

■ **In the Ausria RIA test for Hb_sAg, what reagent is labeled?**

Antibody is labeled. Hb_sAg in the sample binds to unlabeled antibody coated inside a test tube. Labeled antibody will then bind in a "sandwich" manner.

■ **What is the approximate relative sensitivity of solid phase RIA vs. CEP in testing for HB_sAg?**

Solid phase RIA is approximately a hundred times more sensitive than CEP.[1]

REFERENCES

1. Alter, H. J.: Radioimmunoassay tests for hepatitis B surface antigen: problems, practicalities, and promises in Seminar on Current Technical

Topics. Washington, D. C., 1974, American Association of Blood Banks.

2. Chararin, I.: Pernicious anemia as an autoimmune disease, Br. J. Haematol. 23 (supp.) :101, 1973.

3. Husain, M., et al.: Antinuclear antibodies: clinical significance of titers and fluorescence patterns, Am. J. Clin. Pathol. 61:59, 1974.

4. Lee, C. L., Davidsohn, I., and Panczyszyn, O.: Horse agglutinins in infectious mononucleosis. II. The spot test, Am. J. Clin. Pathol. 49:12, 1968.

5. McCartney, W. H., and Hoffer, P. B.: The value of carcinoembryonic antigen (CEA) as an adjunct to the radiological colonic examination in the diagnosis of malignancy, Radiology 110:325, 1974.

6. Peltier, A. P., and Estes, D.: Antinuclear antibodies. In Iaachim, H. L., editor: Pathobiology annual, New York, 1972, Appleton-Century-Crofts.

CHAPTER 14

Instrumentation

The explosion in the area of instrumentation in the laboratory in recent years precludes any but the barest review of principles in this area. The incorporation of computers, television, and other electronic methods into laboratory measurement has only partly superseded the older instruments. Spectrophotometry and fluorometry still play an important role in the laboratory. Descriptions of these methods in *Todd-Sanford Clinical Diagnosis by Laboratory Methods* and in the book by Lee are helpful in understanding their principles.

Davidsohn, I., and Henry, J. B., editors: Todd-Sanford clinical diagnosis by laboratory methods, ed. 15, Philadelphia, 1974, W. B. Saunders Co.

Henry, R. J., Cannon, D. C., and Winkelman, J. W.: Clinical chemistry: principles and technics, ed. 2, New York, 1974, Harper & Row, Publishers.

Lee, L. W.: Elementary principles of laboratory instruments, ed. 3, St. Louis, 1974, The C. V. Mosby Co.

■ **Define absorbance (optical density, extinction).**

Absorbance is $\log_{10} 1/T$ or $2 - \log_{10} \% T$. T is transmitted energy per incident energy.

■ **Define absorptivity (extinction coefficient, specific extinction).**

Absorptivity is absorbance per unit length of energy path per unit concentration.

■ **What are the wavelength definitions of the following types of radiant energy: visible, near ultraviolet (uv), far uv?**

1. Visible: 380 to 780 nm
2. Near uv: 200 to 380 nm
3. Far uv: 10 to 200 nm

■ **State Beer's law.**

$P = P_o 10^{-abc}$ where P_o is incident power, P is transmitted power, a is absorptivity, b is length of light path, and c is concentration of the solute. Essentially this law states that the optical density is linearly proportional to solute concentration and is zero when the solute concentration is zero.

■ **Give three causes for deviation from Beer's law.**

   1. Interaction between solute and solvent
   2. Change in refractive index of solvent with added solute
   3. Interaction between molecules of solute or between the solute being measured and another (extraneous) solute

■ **State a formula for calculating centrifugal force in terms of gravities (g) when radius (R) in centimeters and revolutions per minute (N) are known.**

$$g = 1.118 \times 10^{-5} \times R \times N^2$$

■ **What is fluorescence?**

Fluorescence is the energy emitted as visible light shortly after the absorption of radiant energy by certain substances.

■ **What is the most efficient exciting energy utilized in fluorometric photometers?**

It is ultraviolet radiation.

■ **How does the sensitivity of fluorometry compare with spectrophotometry?**

It is 1000 to 10,000 times as sensitive as spectrophotometry.

■ **How does the concentration of the test substance within solution affect fluorescence?**

At low concentrations, the intensity of fluorescence is proportional to the concentration, but at higher concentrations the linear relationship is destroyed by absorption of the exciting energy by the solvent molecules and by the variation in solvation, disassociation, and association of the solute molecules.

■ **List the factors, in addition to solute concentration, that affect fluorescence.**

Dielectric constant of the solvent, pH, temperature, the presence of certain ions in solution (iodide, bromide, chloride, etc.) and the presence of other contaminants affect fluorescence.

■ **What is the function of the primary filter in a fluorimeter?**

It restricts the wavelength of the exciting energy.

■ **What is the function of the secondary filter in the fluorimeter?**

It limits the range of emitted fluorescence.

■ **Why is it necessary to use Pyrex or quartz cuvettes in the fluorimeter?**

Soft glass cuvettes have their own fluorescence.

■ **Briefly describe the general principal of the flame photometry.**

Certain electrons of atoms or molecules are raised to an increased energy state by heat or electricity. In dropping back to their initial energy level, the excited atoms or molecules emit the extra energy as light, which is measured by spectrophotometry.

■ **What is band width interference in flame photometry?**

It occurs when the spectrophometric band width is sufficient to include an emission line from an element other than the one being measured.

■ **What is background interference in a flame photometer?**

It occurs when a substance in the sample produces emission over a wide spectrum. Background intereference varies with the square of the band width.

■ **What is radiation interference?**

Radiation interference is produced by another element or an ion that causes the desired metal to emit more or less light. Increasing the dilution of the solution decreases the radiation interference.

■ **Describe the use of the internal standard in the flame photometry of sodium and potassium.**

The internal standard utilized is lithium, which is present in equal concentrations in the standard and test solutions. The energies emitted simultaneously from the lithium and the sodium or potassium are compared by a potentiometer.

■ **In flame photometry, certain cations and anions may interfere with accurate determination of sodium and potassium. Cation interference usually is positive at high flame temperatures but may be negative at low temperatures. Is anion interference (1) almost always positive, (2) almost always negative, or (3) also dependent on temperature of flame?**

Anion interference is almost always negative.

■ **Describe briefly the principle of the Coulter counter. How precise is the Coulter counter?**

The Coulter counter counts individual blood cells passing through a minute orifice. The blood cells are poor electrical conductors and modulate the electric current flowing through an electrical gate. The modulations are amplified and counted. The precision of this instrument is about $\pm 2\%$.

■ **What effect does the white cell count have on the red cell count performed on the Coulter counter?**

Both red and white cells are counted, but the latter are insignificant unless there is a leukocytosis of at least 30,000 cu mm.

■ **Explain why the leukocyte count may be falsely low in patients with chronic lymphocytic leukemia.**

The lymphocytes in these patients may be fragile and may be broken up in preparing the specimen, and hence may not be counted.

■ **Atomic absorption spectrophotometry is best suited for the measurement in serum of which of the following: calcium, sodium, potassium, magnesium, iron?**

Those that are present in trace amounts in serum, (i.e., calcium, magnesium, and iron) are best measured by atomic absorption spectrophotometry.

CHAPTER 15

Kidney

The review of renal function tests by Relman and Levinsky is brief and concise. The book by Wesson covers renal physiology in detail. Applications of measurement of renin activity have been developing rapidly in the recent literature.

Berman, L. B., and Vertes, V.: The pathophysiology of renin, CIBA Clinical Symposia, vol. 25, no. 5, 1973.
Relman, A. S., and Levinsky, N. G.: Clinical examination of renal function. In Strauss, M. B., and Welt, L. G., editors: Diseases of the kidney, ed. 2, Boston, 1971, Little, Brown & Co.
Wesson, L. G.: Physiology of the human kidney, New York, 1969, Grune & Stratton, Inc.

- **What is the average glomerular filtration rate in normal adults?**

  The rate is approximately 125 ml/min.

- **In the normal person, about what percentage of the water present in the glomerular filtrate is reabsorbed in the proximal tubule?**

  Approximately 85% is reabsorbed.

- **Is water absorption in the proximal tubule passive or active, that is, does the absorption of water require the expenditure of energy?**

  It is passive (does not require the expenditure of energy).

- **Is water selectively absorbed in the loop of Henle?**

  No. The loop of Henle is impermeable to water, but sodium is reabsorbed to render the luminal contents dilute.

- **Is water absorption in the proximal tubule, distal tubule, or both dependent on antidiuretic hormone secretion?**

  Water absorption is dependent on antidiuretic hormone secretion in the distal tubule only.

■ **Can water be absorbed by the collecting duct?**

It can be absorbed with antidiuretic hormone (ADH) stimulation.

■ **What percent of the sodium in the glomerular filtrate is reabsorbed in the proximal tubule?**

In the proximal tubule, 85% is reabsorbed.

■ **Is sodium reabsorption in the proximal tubule active or passive?**

It is active, requiring the expenditure of energy.

■ **What effect, if any, does aldosterone have on sodium reabsorption by the kidney?**

It increases sodium reabsorption in the distal tubule.

■ **Is potassium excreted or absorbed by the renal tubule?**

It is both excreted and absorbed.

■ **Briefly explain the mechanism of urinary excretion of uric acid.**

Uric acid is present in the glomerular filtrate, is reabsorbed actively by the tubules, and then reexcreted by the tubules.

■ **What is the minimum amount of urine excreted by a normal individual from whom fluids and food have been withheld for an extended period?**

The minimum amount is 300 ml per square meter of body surface or approximately 500 ml/24 hr.

■ **What are the extreme upper and lower limits of urine specific gravity?**

The limits are 1.001 to 1.040.

■ **What are the extreme limits of the urine pH?**

The limits are 4.8 to 8.0.

■ **Which of the buffers present in urine largely determines the urine pH?**

The urine pH is largely determined by $H_2PO_4^-:HPO_4^=$.

■ **Which of the major serum proteins is most readily and which is least readily filtered by the glomeruli?**

Albumin is most readily, fibrinogen least readily filtered.

■ **Is the albumin/globulin ratio in the glomerular filtrate the same as, increased, or decreased as compared with the albumin/globulin ratio in the blood?**

It is increased to about 10:1.

■ **Why is the measurement of serum creatinine a more accurate indicator of renal function than measurement of urea and nonprotein nitrogen?**

The rate of formation of creatinine is relatively independent of nutritional status and hepatic function, and it is not affected by gastrointestinal hemorrhage.

■ **What is the normal range of serum creatinine levels?**

The normal range is 0.5 to 1.2 mg/dl.

■ **How does one measure glomerular filtration rate?**

This rate is measured by determining the rate of excretion in the urine relative to its concentration in the plasma of some substance that is freely filtered by the glomerulus but is neither secreted nor reabsorbed to a significant degree by the renal tubules.

■ **Why are urea clearances less than creatinine clearances?**

A significant proportion of the filtered urea is reabsorbed by the renal tubules.

■ **Why are creatinine clearances usually greater than inulin clearances?**

The renal tubules secrete small amounts of creatinine.

■ **How is creatinine clearance measured?**

Creatinine clearance is the volume of plasma that can be cleared of creatinine by the kidney per minute. It is calculated by multiplying the urine volume by the urine creatinine concentration and dividing the product by the plasma creatinine concentration.

■ **What are the normal creatinine clearances for adults?**

The normal clearances are 70 to 140 ml/min. The average for women is about 100 ml/min, and for men it is about 120 ml/min.

■ **How is the maximum urea clearance calculated, and what is its normal range?**

The maximum urea clearance is calculated by the ordinary clearance formula when the rate of urine flow exceeds 2 ml/min. Its normal range is 64 to 99 ml/min.

■ **Does the rate of urine flow have any effect on the measured urea clearance?**

Yes. The apparent clearance decreases with decreasing urine flow.

■ **How is the standard urea clearance defined, and what are the normal limits?**

When the rate of urine flow is less than 2 ml/min, the square root of the urine volume replaces the urine volume in the clearance formula, and the result is the standard urea clearance. The normal range is 41 to 65 ml/min.

■ A patient has a plasma urea nitrogen concentration of 15 mg/dl and excretes 150 ml urine with a urea nitrogen concentration of 450 mg/dl during a 1-hour collection. What is his maximum urea clearance?

It is 75 ml/min.

■ What parameter of renal function does the phenolsulphonphthalein (PSP) test using an intravenous injection of 6 mg of the dye measure?

The test measures renal blood flow.

■ PSP excretion is dependent on renal blood flow and tubular function. Why is it possible to ignore the latter when interpreting PSP excretion?

The standard PSP dose produces plasma levels far below the tubular maximum for PSP excretion, and tubular function is seldom selectively compromised sufficiently to alter the PSP excretion.

■ What constitutes a normal result of the PSP test?

A normal result is excretion of at least 25% of the injected dye in 15 minutes.

■ What effect would one expect hypoalbuminemia (nephrotic syndrome) to have on the PSP test?

The PSP excretion during the first 15 minutes may be increased because of less albumin available to bind the dye.

■ Describe a more accurate measure of renal plasma flow than the PSP test.

Para-aminohippurate (PAH) or iodopyracet (Diodrast) clearance is a more accurate measure. Both substances are excreted by the renal tubules and are removed nearly completely from the plasma in one passage through the kidney.

■ What is the normal range of renal plasma flow?

The normal range is 600 to 700 ml/min, with males having somewhat higher flow than females.

■ Describe the urine dilution test.

The subject drinks 1200 ml of water within 30 minutes, and then the urine is collected over the next 4 hours. A normal individual will void the 1200 ml within the next 4 hours with a specific gravity as low as 1.003.

■ Describe the urine concentration test.

The patient has nothing to drink or eat after 6 P.M. The urine is then collected the following morning at 8 A.M., 9 A.M., and 10 A.M. A normal individual will have a urine specific gravity greater than 1.025 in one of the specimens.

■ What is the significance of a decrease in the ability to concentrate urine?

It indicates an abnormality of the distal tubule, a lack of antidiuretic hormone (ADH), or a significantly decreased number of functioning nephrons.

■ **What is the effect on the urine specific gravity of albumin and glucose?**

One gm/dl of albumin or glucose will raise the specific gravity of urine by approximately 0.003 unit.

■ **How does a patient with significant renal damage secondary to chronic glomerulonephritis maintain a low blood urea nitrogen level?**

He maintains a low blood urea nitrogen level by excreting large quantities of water (and therefore urea).

■ **Is the elevation of the blood urea nitrogen level an early indication of arteriolar nephrosclerosis?**

No. Elevation in the blood urea nitrogen occurs relatively late. Renal blood flow and glomerular filtration are usually decreased before the elevation of the BUN level.

■ **What is the extreme range of urine osmolality in a normal individual?**

It is 38 to 1400 mOsm/L.

■ **If red cells present in urine are crenated, is the urine osmolality high or low?**

It is high. Water leaves the red cells (leading to crenation) and enters the urine.

■ **What are the biochemical hallmarks of the nephrotic syndrome?**

They are massive proteinuria (3.5 gm/24 hr or more), decreased serum proteins, increased serum cholesterol, and increased serum lipids.

■ **Name several causes of the nephrotic syndrome.**

The nephrotic syndrome is caused by membranous glomerulonephritis, so-called "minimal change disease" (lipoid nephrosis), certain types of proliferative glomerulonephritis, diabetic glomerulosclerosis, amyloidosis, renal vein thrombosis, and occasionally drug reactions.

■ **Is the PSP excretion in patients with nephrotic syndrome usually increased, decreased, or normal?**

It is usually normal.

■ **What usually happens to the levels of total serum calcium and ionized serum calcium in patients with the nephrotic syndrome?**

The total serum calcium level is usually decreased, while the ionized calcium level is usually normal. These reactions are a reflection of the decrease in serum albumin to which calcium is bound.

■ **What diseases or conditions are generally associated with "postrenal" proteinuria?**

Inflammatory and degenerative disease of the renal pelves, ureter, bladder, prostate, and urethra is associated with "postrenal" proteinuria.

■ **List those diseases and conditions that have been associated with "pre-renal" proteinuria.**

Cardiac failure with passive congestion, ascites, fever, epilepsy after cerebral vascular accidents, hematologic diseases (anemia, leukemia, purpura), hyperthyroidism, intestinal obstruction, liver disease, and certain drugs are associated with "prerenal" proteinuria.

■ **List common renal diseases associated with proteinuria.**

Glomerulonephritis (acute and chronic), nephrotic syndrome, acute and chronic pyelonephritis, arteriolar nephrosclerosis, diabetic glomerulosclerosis, preeclampsia and eclampsia, and focal destructive lesions (carcinoma, tuberculosis, infarcts) are associated with proteinuria.

■ **Does the degree of proteinuria in renal diseases correlate with the severity of the disease?**

No. Frequently the degree of proteinuria decreases with increasing severity of the disease, especially when the glomeruli are damaged to the point of nonfunction.

■ **What is renin, where is it produced, and what is the most important physiologic stimulus for its release into the circulation?**

Renin is a highly specific proteolytic enzyme, it is produced by the juxtaglomerular cells of the kidney, and the most important physiologic stimulus for its release is decreased pressure in the afferent glomerular arteriole.[3,6]

■ **Describe the nature and electrophoretic mobility of the substrate on which renin acts, and cite the chemical changes that lead to production of a potent vasoconstrictor.**

Renin acts on an alpha-2 globulin to release a decapeptide, angiotensin I. A converting enzyme present in lung, plasma, and other organs splits two amino acids (His-Leu) from the carboxy terminus of the decapeptide to produce angiotensin II, an octapeptide with potent vasoconstrictor properties.[6]

■ **Apart from vasoconstriction, what important property does angiotensin II have?**

Angiotensin II is a potent stimulus for release of aldosterone from the adrenal cortex.[6]

■ **Describe the proper method for collecting and preserving blood for renin assay.**

The blood is collected into EDTA anticoagulant, immediately iced, centrifuged in the cold, and the plasma is frozen at $-20°$ C, at which temperature renin activity remains unchanged for many months.[6]

■ **How is renin activity measured?**

The patient's plasma is incubated with angiotensin substrate for a number of hours, and the angiotensin generated is measured by radioimmunoassay.

pH, temperature, and presence of substances to inhibit breakdown of angiotensin are critical to the analysis.[7]

- **At what time of day does the plasma level of aldosterone correlate closely with total daily aldosterone secretion, and when is plasma renin activity highest?**

The plasma level of aldosterone measured at noon correlates closely with total daily aldosterone secretion,[2] and plasma renin activity is highest in the morning.[6]

- **What effects do upright posture for 4 hr and low sodium intake (10 mEq/24 hr) have on plasma renin activity?**

Upright posture for 4 hours in a young subject on normal sodium intake doubles the plasma renin activity over recumbent levels. Three days of low sodium intake triples supine renin levels and increase upright renin levels sixfold.[6]

- **Is measurement of plasma renin level useful in the clinical study of patients with benign essential hypertension?**

Patients with benign essential hypertension have been divided into a group with subnormal plasma renin (20% to 30% of all patients), a group with elevated plasma renin (10% to 15%), and a residual group with normal plasma renin. The prognosis of the first group (subnormal plasma renin) is better than for the other two groups, and therapeutic approaches to the three groups are different.[1,5,8]

- **What levels of plasma renin and aldosterone characterize malignant hypertension?**

Most patients with malignant hypertension have elevated plasma renin levels, and plasma aldosterone levels are also elevated secondary to the effect of renin on the zona glomerulosa. In the rare patient with malignant hypertension complicating an aldosterone-secreting adrenal tumor, plasma renin level is decreased.[6]

- **Differential sodium excretion and angiographic studies suggest that partial obstruction of the left renal artery is the cause of a patient's hypertension. Which of the following conditions indicate a high probability that the hypertension will be cured by resection of the suspected kidney: (1) abnormally high peripheral plasma renin activity in relation to level of daily sodium excretion, (2) complete suppression of renin secretion from contralateral (assumedly normal) kidney, or (3) abnormally increased renal vein/renal artery renin level (V-A/A > 0.48) from suspect kidney?**

Each of the three conditions suggests that surgical therapy will be successful, because they are consistent with increased renin production only by the suspect kidney.[9]

■ **Does a ratio of renin activities in blood from the right and left renal arteries of 1.5 indicate that hypertension is caused by a renal vascular lesion?**

Since about 13% of patients with essential hypertension have a ratio of 1.5 or more, this can not be taken as conclusive evidence for a renal vascular causation of the hypertension.[8]

REFERENCES

1. Brunner, H. R., Sealey, J. E., and Laragh, J. H.: Renin as a risk factor in essential hypertension: more evidence, Am. J. Med. 55:295, 1973.
2. Bühler, F. R., et al.: Plasma aldosterone-renin interrelationships in various forms of essential hypertension; studies using a rapid assay of plasma aldosterone, Am. J. Cardiol. 32:554, 1973.
3. Davis, J. O.: The control of renin release, Am. J. Med. 55:333, 1973.
4. Koch-Weser, J.: Correlation of pathophysiology and pharmacotherapy in primary hypertension, Am. J. Cardiol. 32:499, 1973.
5. Laragh, J. H.: Vasoconstriction-volume analysis for understanding and treating hypertension: the use of renin and aldosterone profiles, Am. J. Med. 55:261, 1973.
6. Oparil, S., and Haber, E.: The renin-angiotensin system, N. Engl. J. Med. 291:389, 401, 1974.
7. Sealey, J. E., and Laragh, J. H.: Searching out low renin patients: limitations of some commonly used methods, Am. J. Med. 55:303, 1973.
8. Sealey, J. E., et al.: The physiology of renin secretion in essential hypertension, Am. J. Med. 55:391, 1973.
9. Vaughan, E. D., et al.: Renovascular hypertension: renin measurements to indicate hypersecretion and contralateral suppression, estimate renal plasma flow, and score for surgical curability, Am. J. Med. 55:402, 1973.

CHAPTER 16

Liver

Tests of hepatic function are discussed in various textbooks of laboratory medicine and diseases of the liver. Immunologic abnormalities in liver disease are particularly well covered in the text by Gell and Coombs.

Batsakis, J. G., Briere, R. O., and Markel, S. F.: Diagnostic enzymology, Chicago, 1970, American Society of Clinical Pathologists.
Combes, B., and Schenker, S.: Laboratory tests. In Schiff, L., editor: Diseases of the liver, Philadelphia, 1969, J. B. Lippincott Co.
Gell, P. G. H., and Coombs, R. R. A., editors: Clinical aspects of immunology, ed. 2, Oxford, 1968, Blackwell Scientific Publications, Ltd.

■ **In what organ system does the breakdown of hemoglobin into globin, iron, and biliverdin take place?**

It takes place in the reticuloendothelial system.

■ **In normal subjects, how is most of the bilirubin carried in the plasma?**

It is unconjugated and is bound loosely to albumin.

■ **Most of the bilirubin present in the bile of normal subjects is in what form?**

It is conjugated with glucuronic acid (mostly as the diglucuronide).

■ **Where does conjugation of bilirubin with glucuronic acid take place, and what enzyme is involved?**

The conjugation takes place in the hepatic parenchymal cells, and the responsible enzyme is glucuronyl transferase.

■ **What is the source of bilirubin?**

It is a reduction product of biliverdin produced in the reticuloendothelial system.

■ **What portion of the bilirubin excreted by the normal individual is derived from degradation of circulating red blood cells?**

The portion derived is 80% to 90%. The remainder is derived from other heme proteins, the bone marrow, and other sources.

- **What is the source of urobilinogen?**

It is produced in the intestine by bacterial reduction of bilirubin.

- **What is the fate of urobilinogen in the intestine?**

Some is excreted unchanged; some is oxidized in the intestine to sterocobilin; and some is reabsorbed from the intestine and is reexcreted in the bile by the liver.

- **Low levels of fecal urobilinogen are found under what circumstances?**

Low levels are found in the presence of obstructive jaundice or in patients receiving broad-spectrum antibiotics that suppress the bacteria that convert bilirubin to urobilinogen.

- **What is the principle of the van den Bergh reaction?**

Bilirubin couples with Ehrlich's diazo reagent (diazotized sulfanilic acid) to form a red-violet azopigment.

- **What are the direct and indirect van den Bergh reactions?**

Conjugated bilirubin is soluble in acidic aqueous solution and can react directly with the diazo reagent. Unconjugated bilirubin, however, is only slightly soluble in water at low pH and requires the addition of a solvent (alcohol) or an alkali (caffeine, sodium benzoate) in which both bilirubin and the diazo reagent are soluble for the two to react indirectly. Effective separation of direct-reacting and indirect-reacting fractions can be achieved only at low pH, because both fractions react rapidly at higher pH.

- **How are the concentrations of bilirubin pigments, total, direct-reacting, and indirect-reacting, determined in the clinical laboratory?**

Methods vary. In the widely used Malloy-Evelyn procedure, direct-reacting bilirubin is measured 5 minutes after addition of the low pH diazo reagent to serum. The total bilirubin is measured 30 minutes after the addition of an equal volume of methanol to the serum-diazo reagent mixture. Note that a dilution factor of 2 is introduced by adding the methanol. Indirect-reacting bilirubin is obtained by subtraction.

- **What is the range of serum bilirubin concentrations in adults? Is the bilirubin predominantly conjugated or unconjugated?**

The normal range of serum bilirubin is 0.1 to 1.0 mg/dl (occasionally a normal adult will have a level as high as 1.5 mg/dl). It is predominantly unconjugated.

- **What is the normal range of serum bilirubin levels of full-term infants during the first week of life?**

At birth, umbilical cord blood bilirubin concentration is less than 2.8 mg/dl (average 1.8 mg/dl), and it rises to a peak of 2 to 12 mg/dl (average 7.0 mg/dl) at 2 to 4 days of age. It falls to less than 2.0 mg/dl by the end of the first week.

■ **How do premature infants differ from full-term infants in regard to their normal serum bilirubin concentrations?**

Premature infants have a more prolonged rise to a higher level, reaching a peak of up to 20 mg/dl at 5 to 7 days. The fall is also delayed corresponding to the degree of prematurity.

■ **What is the explanation for the hyperbilirubinemia often seen in premature infants?**

It is the inability of liver cells to excrete conjugated bilirubin caused by immaturity of the glucuronyl transferase system.

■ **What are the criteria for abnormal neonatal hyperbilirubinemia?**

The criteria are jaundice appearing within 24 hours of birth in full-term infants or by 36 hours in premature infants, serum bilirubin 12 mg/dl or more in full-term infants or 20 mg/dl or more in premature infants, or bilirubin levels exceeding 2 mg/dl after 1 week in full-term infants, increase in serum bilirubin concentration exceeding 5 mg/dl in 24 hours, or direct-reacting bilirubin exceeding 15% of the total.

■ **What is kernicterus?**

It is pigmentation of the basal ganglia by unconjugated bilirubin, a condition that frequently leads to death. It usually develops during the first 5 days of life in the presence of severe hyperbilirubinemia, especially in premature infants and in the presence of hypoalbuminemia or acidosis.

■ **What is "breast milk" jaundice?**

Some breast-fed infants develop jaundice ascribed to the presence of pregnane-3(α)20(β)-diol in breast milk. This hormone inhibits glucuronyl transferase. The jaundice subsides when the infant is removed from the breast.

■ **Classify the causes of predominantly unconjugated hyperbilirubinemia. Give examples of each.**

1. Hemolytic jaundice: sickle cell anemia, malaria, erythroblastosis fetalis, congenital spherocytosis
2. Nonhemolytic overproduction jaundice: pernicious anemia and allied conditions
3. Familial and hereditary nonhemolytic, nonobstructive jaundice: Crigler-Najjar syndrome, Lucey-Driscoll syndrome, Gilbert's syndrome

■ **Classify the causes of predominantly conjugated hyperbilirubinemia. Give examples of each.**

1. Obstructive jaundice: pancreatic carcinoma, common duct stone, sclerosing cholangitis
2. Hepatocellular jaundice: viral hepatitis, toxic hepatic damage
3. Cholestatic jaundice: Dubin-Johnson syndrome, Rotor's syndrome, chlorpromazine-induced jaundice

■ **What is the maximum serum bilirubin concentration that can be reached on the basis of hemolysis alone? Why?**

It is approximately 3.5 mg/dl, because the rate of bilirubin excretion increases proportionately to the square of its concentration in the serum.

■ **In patients with hemolytic jaundice, what is the significance of a serum bilirubin concentration greater than 5 mg/dl, or conjugated bilirubin greater than 15% of the total?**

It indicates associated biliary obstruction or hepatocellular dysfunction.

■ **What is the Dubin-Johnson syndrome?**

It is a benign familial disease with fluctuating, predominantly direct-reacting, hyperbilirubinemia of moderate degree (in 90% of all patients it is less than 10 mg/dl) with onset frequently in childhood. The defect appears to be the impaired ability of liver cells to excrete conjugated bilirubin. Hepatic cells contain a coarse, granular, brown pigment.

■ **Briefly describe Gilbert's syndrome.**

It is a hereditary condition of chronic fluctuating, predominantly indirect-reacting hyperbilirubinemia (usually less than 6 mg/dl). It is associated with a normal life span and is usually asymptomatic. The defect is thought to be an inability to transport bilirubin from sinusoidal blood into the liver cells.

■ **What is the icterus index?**

It is an outmoded method of estimating the serum bilirubin concentration by comparing the color of the serum with a potassium bichromate standard.

■ **Why does a patient with hyperbilirubinemia consisting predominantly of conjugated bilirubin show icterus at a lower level than when unconjugated bilirubin predominates?**

Conjugated bilirubin diffuses into tissues more readily than unconjugated bilirubin.

■ **Describe the following in obstructive jaundice: conjugated/unconjugated serum bilirubin ratio, fecal urobilinogen, urine urobilinogen, and serum alkaline phosphatase.**

The conjugated/unconjugated bilirubin ratio is greater than 0.5; both urinary and fecal urobilinogen levels are decreased; and the serum alkaline phosphatase level is elevated.

■ **Describe the above parameters in hepatocellular jaundice.**

The conjugated/unconjugated bilirubin ratio is 0.2 to 0.7; the urine urobilinogen level may be increased; the fecal urobilinogen level may be decreased; and the serum alkaline phosphatase level is normal or slightly elevated.

■ **Describe the above parameters in drug-induced cholestatic jaundice.**

The conjugated/unconjugated bilirubin ratio is greater than 0.5; the urine urobilinogen level may be increased or decreased; the fecal urobilinogen level is decreased; and the serum alkaline phosphatase level is increased.

■ **Describe the sulfobromophthalein (Bromsulphalein) (BSP) excretion test.**

A dose of 5 mg/kg of body weight of BSP is injected intravenously. A serum sample is withdrawn at 45 minutes, and the amount of retained BSP is determined by spectrophotometer after alkalinization of the sample. Normal individuals retain less than 5% of the injected dose.

■ **Is BSP retention usually increased in obstructive jaundice, hepatocellular jaundice, and hemolytic jaundice?**

It is increased in obstructive jaundice and in hepatocellular jaundice, but is usually normal in hemolytic jaundice.

■ **What are the indications for requesting a BSP excretion test in patients with nonhemolytic jaundice?**

It is not indicated for diagnostic purposes, but only to follow the course of the disease. BSP and bilirubin hepatic excretory mechanisms are similar, and there is no additional information to be gained from a BSP test if the patient is jaundiced. The BSP excretion test is, of course, useful in detecting hepatic dysfunction in the presence of normal serum bilirubin levels.

■ **List the causes of increased BSP retention in addition to hepatocellular damage and bile duct obstruction.**

The causes are drug-induced cholestasis, decreased hepatic blood flow (congestive heart failure, shock), focal intrahepatic duct obstruction (tumor), fever, drugs (iopanoic acid [Telepaque]), and gross obesity and fluid retention (which make calculation of an appropriate dose difficult).

■ **How high can the urinary excretion of unconjugated bilirubin be in cases of severe hemolytic anemia?**

Unconjugated bilirubin does not appear in the urine.

■ **What are the characteristic laboratory findings in uncomplicated hemolytic anemia?**

An elevated serum bilirubin level (more than 80% unconjugated), absence of bilirubin from the urine, increased fecal and urinary urobilinogen levels, normal serum alkaline phosphatase level, normal BSP excretion, and normal serum transaminases are found. Other routine tests of liver function also show normal results.

■ **What are the laboratory findings most often associated with obstructive jaundice?**

Elevation of the serum bilirubin (predominantly conjugated) level, elevated serum cholesterol and alkaline phosphatase levels, slight to moderate increase in serum transaminases, decreased fecal and urinary urobilinogen levels, increased urine bilirubin excretion, and increased prothrombin time that responds to vitamin K given parenterally are found.

■ **Serum transaminase levels generally reach their highest point in which type of liver disease?**

Acute hepatic necrosis as seen in severe viral hepatitis or with liver toxins (carbon tetrachloride) is associated with the highest transaminase levels.[1,2]

■ **What are the laboratory findings most often associated with hepatocellular jaundice?**

Elevation of the serum bilirubin level, elevated serum globulin and decreased albumin levels, increased prothrombin time that fails to respond to vitamin K given parenterally, elevated serum transaminase levels, a normal or only slightly elevated serum alkaline phosphatase level, and an elevated urine urobilinogen (decreased hepatic clearing) level are found.

■ **Which of the following serum enzymes are elevated more in obstructive jaundice than hepatocellular disease: alkaline phosphatase, SGOT, SGPT, 5′-nucleotidase, γ-glutamyl transpeptidase, leucine aminopeptidase, ornithine carbamyl transferase, sorbitol dehydrogenase?**

Those more elevated in obstructive jaundice than hepatocellular disease are alkaline phosphatase, 5′-nucleotidase, leucine aminopeptidase, and γ-glutamyl transpeptidase.[1,2]

■ **What lesions are most likely to be associated with relatively high alkaline phosphatase levels and little or no jaundice?**

Space-occupying lesions (abscess, tumor, etc.) and partial occlusion of the biliary ductal system are the lesions.

■ **Under what conditions might there be an elevation of the serum hepatic alkaline phosphatase level with normal bilirubin levels and BSP excretion?**

These characteristics may be seen in patients with sarcoidosis, liver abscess, echinococcal cyst of the liver, primary or metastatic liver cancer, or with partial obstruction of the common bile duct.

■ **How can administration of vitamin K parenterally help to distinguish between hepatocellular and obstructive jaundice?**

Patients who have long prothrombin times because of vitamin K deficiency (obstructive jaundice) respond to vitamin K with a return of the prothrombin time toward normal. Patients with hepatocellular jaundice do not respond.

■ **What abnormalities of the serum cholesterol levels occur in severe hepatitis or cirrhosis and in obstructive jaundice?**

The serum cholesterol level is decreased in the former and is increased in the latter.

■ **Can serum levels of CPK, LDH, and lipase aid in the differential diagnosis of jaundice?**

They are of little if any help, since they are usually normal or only slightly elevated in patients with jaundice.

■ **What changes in the serum albumin and globulin levels ordinarily are found in patients with cirrhosis?**

Usually the albumin level is decreased, and the globulin level is increased.

■ **In patients with normal renal function, does the blood urea nitrogen level usually fall, rise, or remain unchanged with the advent of massive liver necrosis?**

It falls, because urea is being formed in lesser quantity.

■ **How may serum mucoprotein and haptoglobin levels help differentiate between the various forms of liver disease?**

They tend to be increased in patients with obstructive jaundice and low in patients with hepatocellular disease.[3]

■ **List four causes of increased blood ammonia levels.**

The causes are decreased urea synthesis (hepatocellular damage), portal hypertension with spontaneous or surgical portacaval shunts, increased amount of nitrogenous material within the intestine (gastrointestinal bleeding), and increased production of ammonia by the kidney (hypokalemia with metabolic alkalosis).

■ **Why should alkalosis be avoided in the patient with elevated blood ammonia levels?**

At 37° C, the pK_a of NH_4^+ is close enough to the pH of blood so that small changes of blood pH affect the NH_4^+/NH_3 ratio. Alkalosis favors the formation of NH_3, which enters tissues more readily than NH_4^+.

■ **Which of the following seems, at the present time, to be the most reliable diagnostic indication of hepatic coma: blood ammonia, CSF ammonia, CSF glutamine, CSF alpha-ketoglutaramate?**

Alpha-ketoglutaramate (α-kGM) is a neurotoxin formed from glutamine by transamination. CSF α-kGM levels in hepatic coma are elevated approximately tenfold above the normal mean of 3.6 μmol/L. Elevation of α-kGM in CSF appears to be the most reliable chemical indicator of hepatic coma.[7]

■ **High levels of serum cholesterol are most often seen in what type of liver disease?**

Intrahepatic cholestasis, especially primary biliary cirrhosis is associated with the highest cholesterol levels.

- **What are the usual significant laboratory findings, other than the liver function tests, in active chronic hepatitis?**

Patients with active chronic hepatitis typically have elevated gamma globulin levels with beta-gamma bridging on serum electrophoresis. They have an increased incidence of positive systemic lupus erythematosus (LE) test results, rheumatoid factor, antinuclear antibodies, and autoimmune complement fixation (AICF) test results. Most patients with active chronic hepatitis have serum antibodies against smooth muscle, and some lack smooth-muscle antibodies but are serologically positive for the Australia antigen.

- **What are the usual significant laboratory findings in primary biliary cirrhosis?**

The serum gamma globulin level usually is not elevated. Antibodies to mitochondria are almost invariably present, and consequently the AICF test result is usually positive in a high (1:64 or more) titer. Antibodies to nuclei and smooth muscle occur less frequently than in active chronic hepatitis. Serum bilirubin, alkaline phosphatase, cholesterol, and total lipid levels are markedly elevated, and transaminases and the results of flocculation tests are normal or only silghtly elevated.

- **When, in relationship to exposure, appearance of hepatitis-associated antigen (HB_sAg), and rise of serum glutamic oxaloacetic transaminase (SGOT), does anti-HB_sAg appear in the serum of patients with type B (MS-2) hepatitis? In which patients with type B hepatitis is anti-HB_sAg unlikely to be detectable?**

Anti-HB_sAg appears approximately 40 to 100 days after exposure, probably when the HB_sAg titer is at or just beyond its peak, and during the period of serum GOT elevation. It is undetectable in some patients with persistently high titers of HB_sAg, even by the sensitive radioimmunoprecipitation technic.[5]

- **How long does HB_sAg persist in ordinary cases of HB_sAg-positive acute viral hepatitis, and what is the significance of unusually long persistence of HB_sAg in these patients?**

HB_sAg usually persists for 1 to 13 weeks when studied by immunoelectro-osmophoresis. One study showed that it persisted longer than 13 weeks in 11 of 88 patients with HB_sAg-positive acute viral hepatitis, and that all of the eleven patients with persisting HB_sAg developed signs of chronic hepatitis. Biopsies showed chronic aggressive hepatitis in eight patients and chronic persistent hepatitis in two patients.[6]

- **Which of the following, measured in serum, is the most sensitive indicator of activity in chronic or slowly resolving hepatitis: conjugated cholic acid, alkaline phosphatase, transaminase, bilirubin, prothrombin time, sulfobromophthalein (Bromsulphalein) retention, albumin/globulin ratio?**

The conjugated cholic acid level is the most sensitive. More than 50% of patients with persisting histologic abnormality may have elevated conjugated cholic acid when other liver function tests have returned to normal.[4,7]

REFERENCES

1. Batsakis, J. G., Sodeman, T. A., and Deegan, M. J.: Enzymatic evaluation of hepatobiliary disease, Lab. Med. 5:33, 1974.
2. Burke, M. D.: Liver function, Human Pathol. 6:273, 1975.
3. Hartwell, R. M., and Hew, A. Y., Jr.: Non-enzyme hepatic function tests, Lab. Med. 5:24, 1974.
4. Korman, M. G., Hofmann, A. F., and Summerskill, W. H. J.: Assessment of activity in chronic active liver disease: serum bile acids compared with conventional tests and histology, N. Engl. J. Med. 290:1399, 1974.
5. Lander, J. J., et al.: Viral hepatitis, type B (MS-2 strain): detection of antibody after primary infection, N. Engl. J. Med. 285:303, 1971.
6. Nielsen, J. O., et al.: Incidence and meaning of persistence of Australia antigen in patients with acute viral hepatitis: development of chronic hepatitis, N. Engl. J. Med. 285:1157, 1971.
7. Soloway, R. D., et al.: Clinical, biochemical, and histological remission of severe chronic active liver disease: a controlled study of treatments and early prognosis, Gastroenterology 63:820, 1972.
8. Vergara, F., Plum, F., and Duffy, T. E.: Alpha-ketoglutaramate: increased concentrations in the cerebrospinal fluid of patients in hepatic coma, Science 183:81, 1974.

CHAPTER 17

Parasitology and medical entomology

Amebiasis, ascariasis, enterobiasis, hookworm, strongyloidiasis, and toxoplasmosis are among the parasitic diseases that are endemic in the United
States, and potential intermediate hosts are available for others that could become problems in the future (malaria, schistosomiasis). *Pneumocystis carinii*
has become a significant problem in immunosuppressed patients. Worldwide
jet travel makes possible exposure to parasites endemic in other parts of the
world. Consequently, we should be alert to the existence of parasites and
should be prepared to recognize them. A simplified approach to the study of
medical parasitology is best for the inexperienced, and for that purpose we
recommend the U. S. Naval Medical School publication, which is inexpensive
and yet is adequately illustrated. The section on parasitology by McQuay in
Todd-Sanford Clinical Diagnosis by Laboratory Methods is also adequate. Beck
and Barrett-Connor's text is concise. The texts by Brown and by Markell and
Voge are also sufficiently comprehensive and yet brief and practically oriented.
Belding's text remains the most comprehensive reference. Spencer and Monroe's atlas contains excellent color photographs.

Beck, J. W., and Barrett-Connor, E.: Medical parasitology, St. Louis, 1971, The
    C. V. Mosby Co.
Belding, D. L.: Textbook of parasitology, ed. 3, New York, 1965, Appleton-Century-
    Crofts.
Brown, H. W.: Basic clinical parasitology, ed. 3, New York, 1969, Appleton-Century-
    Crofts.
Markell, E. K., and Voge, M.: Medical parasitology, ed. 2, Philadelphia, 1965, W. B.
    Saunders Co.
McQuay, R. M., and Shaffer, J. G.: Medical protozoology, helminthology, and ento-
    mology. In Davidsohn, I., and Henry, J. B., editors: Todd-Sanford clinical diag-
    nosis by laboratory methods, ed. 15, Philadelphia, 1974, W. B. Saunders Co.
Spencer, F. M., and Monroe, L. S.: The color atlas of intestinal parasites, Spring-
    field, Ill., 1973, Charles C Thomas, Publisher.
U. S. Naval Medical School: Medical protozoology and helminthology, Washington,
    D. C., 1965, U. S. Government Printing Office.

PARASITOLOGY

■ **Name the four classes of protozoa.**

The four classes are Sarcodina (amebae), Mastigophora (flagellates), Ciliata (ciliates), and Sporozoa (plasmodia, coccidia, *Toxoplasma* species).

■ **What is a karyosome?**

It is the nucleolus of a protozoan.

■ **What is a kinetoplast?**

It is the structure at the root of a flagellum that consists of the blepharoplast together with the parabasal body.

■ **Describe the merthiolate-iodine-formalin (MIF) method for fixation and sedimentation of cysts and ova in stool.**

Prepare a stock solution of MIF by mixing 250 ml of distilled water, 200 ml of tincture of merthiolate, 25 ml of formaldehyde USP, and 5 ml of glycerine. Immediately before use, prepare the MIF solution by adding 0.3 ml of fresh Lugol's solution to 4.7 ml of MIF solution. Add 1 ml of feces to the MIF solution in vial and emulsify with a stick. Allow it to stand and examine a drop from the surface of the sediment.

■ **Which of the following technics is the most sensitive for detection of antibody to parasites: indirect hemagglutination (IHA), complement fixation (CF), bentonite flocculation, or latex agglutination?**

IHA is the most sensitive.[5]

■ **What is the length of the sexual cycle of malaria parasites in the mosquito?**

The sexual cycle is 8 to 21 days long. (*Plasmodium malariae* has the longest sexual cycle.)

■ **How often does fever recur in various forms of malaria?**

In vivax malaria (caused by *Plasmodium vivax*), ovale malaria (caused by *P. ovale*), and falciparum malaria (caused by *P. falciparum*) it recurs every other day, or daily in falciparum malaria. In quartan malaria (caused by *P. malariae*) it recurs every third day.

■ **Approximately how long are the initial attacks and periods of risk of recurrences of untreated malaria?**

1. Falciparum malaria: 11 days; 6 months
2. Vivax malaria: 3 weeks; 3 years
3. Ovale malaria: 14 days; 4 years
4. Quartan malaria: 6 months; 40 years

■ **Which mosquitoes transmit malaria?**

Only mosquitoes of the genus *Anopheles* transmit malaria.

■ **What are the incubation periods of various types of malaria in man?**

The incubation periods range from 8 to 37 days, with the following means: falciparum malaria, 12 days; vivax malaria, 14 days; ovale malaria, 18 days; quartan malaria, 28 days.

■ **Describe cytoplasmic inclusions in various types of malaria.**

Schüffner dots occur in vivax and ovale malaria, and Maurer dots occur in falciparum malaria. Inconspicuous inclusions may occur in quartan malaria.

■ **Which gametocytes and trophozoites are the most heavily pigmented?**

Trophozoites of *P. malariae* (in quartan malaria) are the most heavily pigmented.

■ **How many merozoites are there in the schizonts of the four types of malaria?**

P. malariae has six to twelve in rosette. *P. ovale* also has six to twelve. *P. falciparum* has eight to thirty-two, and *P. vivax* has twelve to twenty-four. In relapse, *P. ovale* may have twelve to sixteen merozoites.

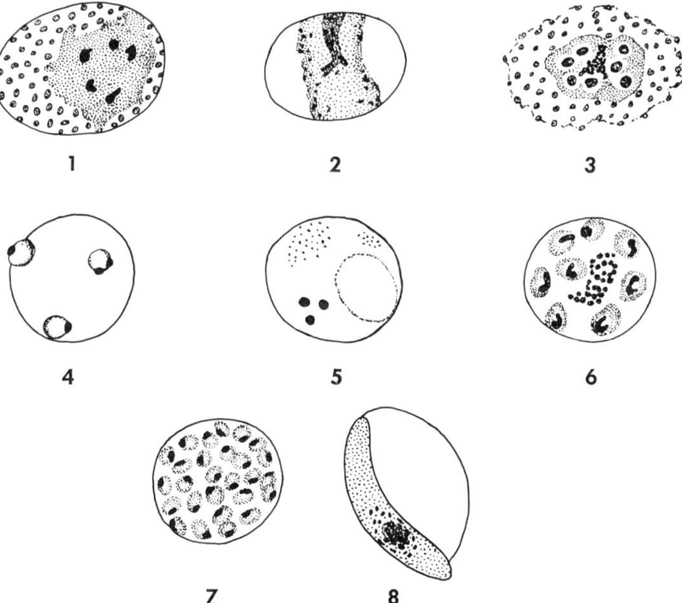

■ **Select the red blood cell in the above illustration that fits each of these descriptions: (1) *P. falciparum*, ring form, (2) *P. vivax*, early schizont, (3) *P. malariae*, trophozoite, (4) *P. malariae*, schizont, (5), *P. ovale*, schizont, (6) *P. falciparum*, macrogametocyte, (7) form not ordinarily seen in circulating blood, and (8) nonparasitized red cell.**

   1. No. 4 is the ring form of *P. falciparum*. Multiple rings occur in either vivax or falciparum malaria, but the young *P. falciparum* trophozoites

are smaller (a fifth of the diameter of the red cell) than those of *P. vivax* and are more often adherent to or protruding from the cell surface.

2. No. 1 is the early schizont of *P. vivax*. Note the enlargement of the red cell and Schüffner's dots. Cytoplasmic division lags behind nuclear division.

3. No. 2 is the trophozoite of *P. malariae,* showing the distinctive band shape.

4. No. 6 is the schizont of *P. malariae*. The arrangement of merozoites in rosette around pigment is typical.

5. No. 3 is the schizont of *P. ovale*. The enlarged, fimbriated red cell with Schüffner's granules identifies *P. ovale*.

6. No. 8 is the macrogametocyte of *P. falciparum.*

7. No. 7 is the schizont of *P. falciparum,* recognized by the large number of merozoites and lack of Schüffner's dots. It is seen in peripheral blood only rarely because the parasitized cells stick to vascular endothelium.

8. No. 5 shows a red cell with a Cabot ring, three Howell-Jolly bodies, and punctate basophilic stippling. No parasites are present.

■ **If a thin film shows one malarial parasite per fifty fields, how many will be seen in a thick film?**

Five to ten parasites per microscopic field will be seen.

■ **Comment on the applicability of serologic tests for malaria.**

Indirect fluorescent antibody (IFA) and indirect hemagglutination (IHA) tests are excellent screening tests in nonendemic areas, but are not satisfactory for speciation. In endemic areas the high prevalence of antibodies in the population renders serologic tests useless for diagnosis.[3]

■ **Name the four forms illustrated below that occur during the life cycles of various members of genera *Leishmania* and *Trypanosoma*.**

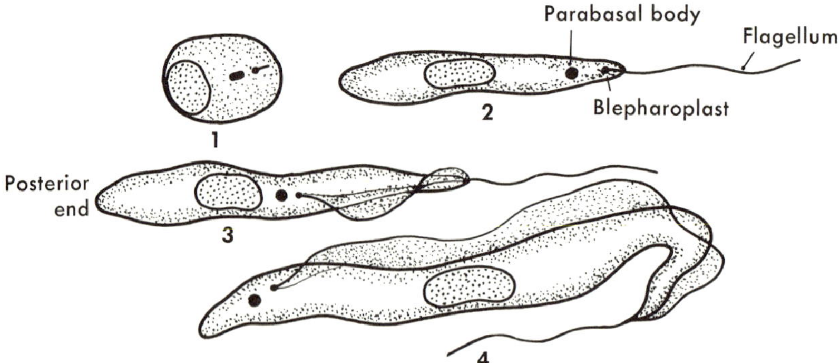

1. Leishmanial (intracellular only)
2. Leptomonad
3. Crithidial
4. Trypanosomal

■ **Describe the life cycle of *T. rhodesiense* and *T. gambiense*.**

The reservoir is wild and domestic animals. Trypanosomal forms multiply in human blood and lymph. The tsetse fly (*Glossina* species) transmits the infection. Crithidial forms multiply in the tsetse fly and become metacyclic in the salivary glands to infect humans when bitten.

■ **What are the laboratory approaches to diagnosis of African sleeping sickness?**

Aspirate a lymph node early in the disease, or use blood later. Movement of trypanosomes jiggles RBC in a tiny wet drop of blood. Stain thick and thin smears as for malarial parasites. Inoculate mice or guinea pigs. Their blood will be positive after a week or more.

■ **Which trypanosome exists in tissues of man?**

T. cruzi exists, often in heart muscle, in leishmanial form.

■ **What is the life cycle of *T. cruzi?***

Trypanosomal forms in blood do not multiply, but they penetrate cells and are transformed to leishmanial forms that multiply by fission. Then transformation to leptomonad and crithidial forms occurs. Crithidial forms become trypanosomes and circulate in blood. Crithidial forms multiply in the reduviid bug (*Triatoma* species), and metacyclic forms are passed in its feces, which are rubbed into puncture wounds. The metacyclic parasites enter the blood stream and penetrate tissue cells.

■ **How are *T. cruzi* infections diagnosed?**

Blood rarely is visually positive for trypanosomes except during febrile periods. Spinal fluid is also rarely positive. One method used is xenodiagnosis, in which reduviid bugs (laboratory-bred) are allowed to feed on the patient. Ingested trypanosomes can be recovered in 2 weeks. In another method, a dose of 5 to 10 ml of blood is injected into a guinea pig or puppy. Its blood may be positive in 2 weeks. At autopsy, one should search for leishmanial forms in the heart.

■ **What is the geographic distribution of kala-azar?**

Kala-azar is found in the Mediterranean countries, Asia Minor, China, India, South America, and the southern USSR.

■ **What organism causes kala-azar?**

Leishmania donovani causes kala-azar.

■ **What is the vector of leishmaniasis?**

It is the sand fly of genus *Phlebotomus*.

■ **Describe the life cycle of *L. donovani*.**

The reservoir is in dogs and other animals. Infected white blood cells

(WBC) are ingested by various species of *Phlebotomus,* in which leptomonad forms develop and proliferate and pass into the buccal cavity to be transmitted by bite. Leishmanial forms develop in macrophages of the viscera.

■ **How is leishmaniasis diagnosed?**

Giemsa-stained blood smears, and especially buffy coat smears, should be examined. Splenic, liver, and bone marow aspirations are useful. Bone marrow examination is becoming the standard diagnostic approach. Various presumptive tests (Sia test, Chopra's antimony test, Napier's serum test) depend on the presence of increased levels of macroglobulin in the plasma.

■ **What is the organism that causes cutaneous leishmaniasis (Bagdad boil), and what is its life cycle?**

The organism is *L. tropica.* It is indistinguishable from *L. donovani* (except serologically), and it has the same life cycle and insect vector. It occurs in the same general geographic area of the Mediterranean as *L. donovani,* but not in the same localities. The organism infects reticuloendothelial cells of the skin.

■ **To which class of phylum Protozoa does *Toxoplasma gondii* belong?**

It belongs to Sporozoa.

■ **What is the life cycle of *T. gondii?***

A mouse eats oocysts from a cat's stool. Sporozoites develop in the mouse and infect the muscle and brain. Schizogony occurs intracellularly in the mouse, and the organisms are ingested by the cat. Excystment and fertilization occur in the intestine of the cat, and oocysts are passed in the stool.[6,13]

■ **Which cells in the human being are immune to infection by *T. gondii?***

Red blood cells are immune.

■ **What proportion of the general population of the United States is immunoreactive against *T. gondii* by the indirect hemagglutination (IHA) or indirect fluorescent antibody (IFA) tests?**

About 20% to 30% are reactive by either method.[8]

■ **What IHA and IFA titers indicate recent infection with *T. gondii?***

IHA titers above 256 and IFA titers above 64 usually indicate recent infection.[8]

■ **What proportion of asymptomatic individuals have significant serum antibody titers against *T. gondii?* How long do titers remain elevated after an acute infection with *T. gondii?***

About 10% of asymptomatic individuals tested have "significant" titers. They remain elevated for 20 to 30 years except for the complement fixation test, which returns to normal within 2 to 4 years.[9]

■ **In tissue sections, how can *Toxoplasma* organisms be distinguished from *Leishmania* species or *Trypanosoma cruzi?***

Toxoplasma organisms lack a parabasal body and blepharoplast (kinetoplast), but they may have a tiny red-staining body between the nucleus and the attenuated end.

■ **Describe the life cycle of *Entamoeba histolytica*.**

Cysts are ingested and undergo excystation in the ileum. The metacystic form grows; each of the four nuclei divides once, and it splits into eight amebulae. Encystment occurs in the colon and begins with loss of motility and rounding up, then accumulation of glycogen, formation of chromatoid bodies, and formation of a cyst wall. Two nuclear divisions occur, giving rise to a total of four nuclei.

■ **Which intestinal ameba does not form cysts?**

Dientamoeba fragilis does not form cysts.

■ **Which of the cysts of intestinal amebae and flagellates have one nucleus?**

Chilomastix mesnili, Retortamonas intestinalis, and *Iodamoeba buetschlii* have one nucleus.

■ **Which cysts have four nuclei?**

Entamoeba histolytica, E. nana, Giardia lamblia, and *Enteromonas hominis* have four nuclei.

■ **What are the indications for examination of a fresh stool specimen for ova and parasites?**

The chief indications are to search for trophozoites of *Entamoeba histolytica* in suspected amebic dysentery or to identify *Dientamoeba fragilis* and *Trypanosoma hominis*. Since cysts of *E. histolytica* lose their morphologic characteristics on standing, when stool cannot be examined with minimum delay, it should be emulsified in 10% formol saline, MIF (merthiolate-iodine-formalin) solution, or Schaudinn's fluid. The latter preservative permits subsequent preparation of stained smears for trophozoites and cysts.[11,12]

■ **Which intestinal trophozoites are (1) less than 10 μm in diameter, (2) 10 to 12 μm in diameter, (3) 12 to 14 μm in diameter, and (4) 18 μm or more in diameter?**

1. Less than 10 μm in diameter: *Entamoeba nana* and small strains of *E. histolytica*
2. 10 to 12 μm in diameter: *Iodamoeba buetschlii* and *Dientamoeba fragilis*
3. 12 to 14 μm in diameter: *Entamoeba histolytica* from nondysenteric cases
4. 18 μm or more in diameter: *Entamoeba histolytica* from cases of amebic dysentery and *E. coli*.

■ **Which trophozoites show progressive unidirectional crawl?**

Entamoeba histolytica (small and large strains) typically and *E. coli* rarely show progressive unidirectional crawl.

■ **Which amebae have spherical trophozoites that resemble cysts?**

This description indicates *D. fragilis*.

■ **How do chromatoid bars of *E. histolytica* and *E. coli* differ?**

In *E. histolytica*, they are abundant, present in about 50% or more of cysts, and have rounded or cigar-shaped ends. In *E. coli*, they are scanty, are spicules or blocks with sharp points, and seldom are seen in more than 10% of cysts.

■ **Which of the intestinal amebae have no chromatin granules on the nuclear membrane?**

This characteristic indicates *D. fragilis*, *I. buetschlii*, and *E. nana*.

■ **Which intestinal ameba has a karyosome made up of four to six granules, usually in a circular pattern?**

This description indicates *D. fragilis*.

■ **Identify these intestinal amebae by the appearance of their nuclei in stained films.**

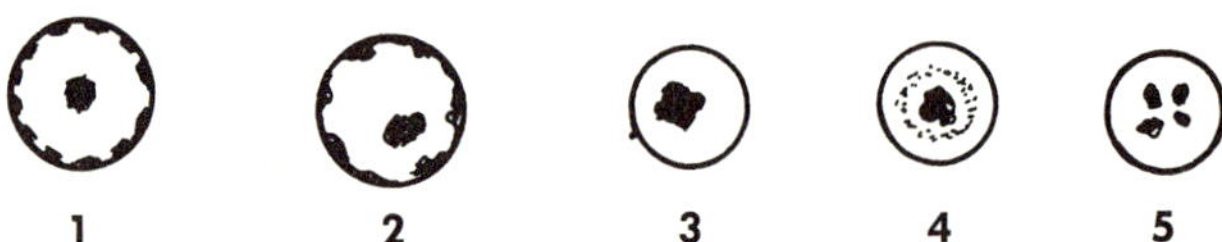

1. *E. histolytica*   4. *I. buetschlii*
2. *E. coli*   5. *D. fragilis*
3. *E. nana*

■ **After a barium meal, how much time must elapse before stool samples will be satisfactory for parasitologic examination?**

In individuals with ordinary intestinal transit times, at least 3 days must elapse.[14]

■ **For diagnosis of *E. histolytica* infection, are three stool specimens obtained at weekly intervals better than three specimens on consecutive days?**

The three specimens at weekly intervals are better because *E. histolytica* tends to appear in showers.[14]

■ **What proportion of asymptomatic carriers of *E. histolytica* will be revealed by microscopic examination of three stool unconcentrated specimens by an expert fecal microscopist?**

About 50% will be revealed. Examination of one formol-ether concentrated specimen will also reveal about 50%.[14]

■ **Do most patients with amebiasis show blood eosinophilia?**

Eosinophilia is not characteristic of amebiasis and suggests that the patient is also infected with helminths.[14]

■ **The serologic tests of choice for amebiasis are indirect hemagglutination (IHA), gel diffusion, and fluorescent antibody (FA). What are the sensitivities of these tests in detecting intestinal and hepatic amebiasis?**

Each test detects about 96% of hepatic infestations with *E. histolytica*, but IHA and gel diffusion detect only about 86% of cases of symptomatic amebiasis confined to the intestine, and the FA test detects only 50% of intestinal cases.[1,7,8]

■ **Describe the identifying characteristics of *Naegleria gruberi*. What disease does it cause, how is it contracted, and what is its prognosis?**

N. gruberi is a free-living ameba that exists as a trophozoite or cyst. The trophozoite in tissue resembles *E. histolytica* and ingests RBC, but it has a large, central karyosome surrounded by a halo. When culture fluid is diluted with water, it assumes an oval or pyriform shape with flagellae at one end. The disease is acquired by diving in freshwater ponds and has been reported from the southeastern United States and Australia. It causes a meningoencephalitis that has invariably been fatal.

■ **Identify the flagellates illustrated at approximately ×2000 magnification.**

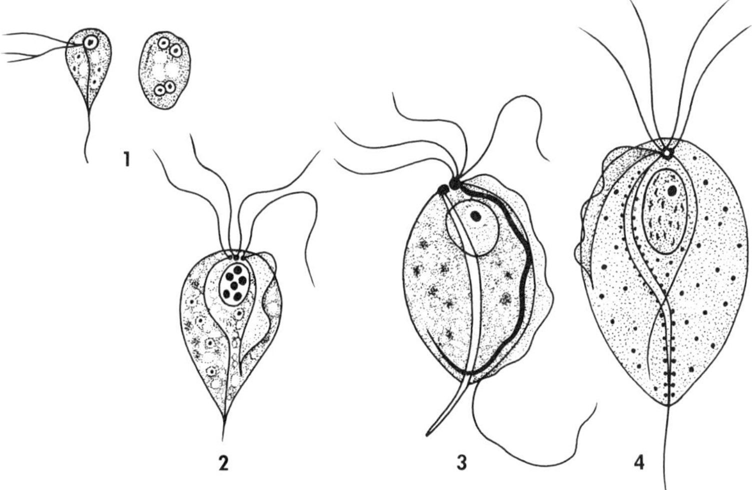

1. *Enteromonas hominis* trophozoite and cyst
2. *Trichomonas tenax* (oral cavity)
3. *T. hominis* (intestine)
4. *T. vaginalis* (vagina)

■ **Which of the intestinal flagellates shown in the illustrations below is pathogenic, particularly in patients with "acquired" hypogammaglobulinemia?**

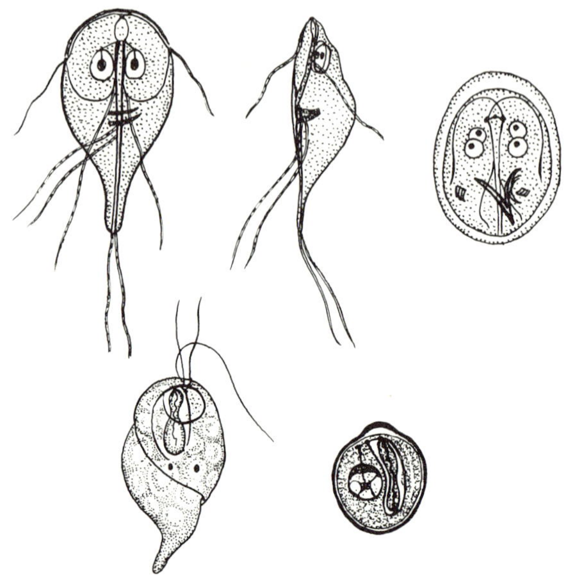

Giardia lamblia, shown in the top three drawings, is pathogenic.[2] On the left the parasite is seen from the front, in the center is the lateral view, and the cyst is shown on the right. The flagellate shown in the bottom of the figure is *Chilomastix mesnili.* Note the spiral groove in the vegetative form and the protuberance of the wall of the lemon-shaped cyst. *C. mesnili* is considered nonpathogenic.

■ **In patients with hypogammaglobulinemia and intestinal malabsorption, what is the appropriate method for diagnosis of *G. lamblia* infection?**

The parasite should be sought by examination of Giemsa-stained smears of duodenal aspirates. It often cannot be found in the stool of patients with symptomatic giardiasis.[2]

■ **Define the two larval forms of roundworms.**

Rhabditiform, the first larval form, is feeding and noninfective. Filariform, the second form, is infective but nonfeeding.

■ **How does *Trichinella spiralis* differ in its life cycle from the other parasitic roundworms?**

It is the only roundworm in which the same animal is both intermediate and definitive host. The entire life cycle is completed in cannibalistic rats, which furnish a reservoir for the parasite.

■ **Describe the life cycle of *T. spiralis.***

Encysted larvae in meat are ingested. They excyst in the small intestine and mature within 3 to 4 days. After copulation, females live 6 weeks and discharge 1500 larvae into the intestinal mucosa, and from there they enter the circulation. They encyst in skeletal muscle, beginning about 9 days after infection. Calcification of cysts begins at 6 to 12 months, but the larvae may live in the cysts for 10 years.

■ **During what period of the infection do *T. spiralis* organisms occur in the blood, and what is the efficacy of examining blood for diagnosis?**

They occur in the blood from about 9 days to 3½ weeks after infection. A search for the parasites in blood succeeds only occasionally.

■ **Describe three immunologic tests for trichinosis.**

1. A skin test is performed by intradermal injection of 1:10,000 diluted saline extract of powdered *Trichinella* larvae. Immediate (within 20 minutes) reaction indicates infection. Occasionally the response may be a delayed, tuberculoid one.
2. A precipitin test is performed by layering increasing dilutions of antigen, beginning with 1:100, over serum at room temperature. Formation of precipitate at the interface is a positive response.
3. Complement fixation, bentonite flocculation, IHA, latex agglutination, and FA tests are also available.

■ **When do immunologic tests become positive for trichinosis, and for how long do they remain positive?**

Positive results usually are not obtained until the end of the third week of infection, with results of the complement fixation test becoming positive first (about 16 days at the earliest). Results of the skin test remain positive up to 7 years, results of the precipitin test remain positive for 2 years, and results of the complement fixation test remain positive for 9 months.

■ **What causes false positive results of tests for trichinosis?**

Cross-reactions with other roundworms (*Trichuris* roundworms, for one) account for some, but the cause of most is unknown.

■ **Describe the use of muscle biopsy in diagnosis of trichinosis.**

Diagnosis may be made by biopsy of deltoid or gastrocnemius muscle 10 days or more after infection. One should spread fresh muscle between glass plates, compress it with screw clamps, and examine the muscle under low power with the microscope. Ordinary histologic sections of muscle often do not show the parasites.

■ **Which of the intestinal roundworms has the ability to propagate in the free-living state?**

This characteristic indicates *Strongyloides stercoralis*.

■ **Which of the intestinal roundworms develop free-living rhabditiform and filariform larvae, and which are infective only by ingestion of eggs?**

Strongyloides, Ancyclostoma, and *Necator* roundworms are free-living rhabditiform and filariform larvae. *Ascaris, Trichuris,* and *Enterobias* roundworms are infective by egg only.

■ **Which of the intestinal roundworms can carry out repeated reproductive cycles in man, resulting in superinfection?**

S. stercoralis has this capability.

■ **Describe *S. stercoralis,* and indicate how to differentiate free-living from parasitic and male from female.**

A free-living adult is about 1 mm long; a parasitic adult is 2 mm long. The former has an esophageal bulb; the latter does not. Males have posterior spicules and a gubernaculum.

■ **Is the diagnosis of *S. stercoralis* made by finding ova in the stool?**

No, these ova are rarely seen in the stool. They usually hatch in the intestine.

■ **Differentiate the rhabditiform larva of *Strongyloides* roundworms from that of hookworm. When would the need to do so arise?**

Both are about 0.25 to 0.5 mm long. Hookworm has a clearly visible buccal cavity, whereas that of *Strongyloides* roundworms is short and broad. Both have esophageal bulbs. Constipated patients with hookworm may pass rhabditiform larvae in the stool, and they could then be confused with *S. stercoralis* larvae, which normally hatch in the intestine.

■ **How large are adult hookworms?**

They are 8 to 12 mm long. The female is 2 mm longer than the male.

■ **How do the mouth parts of *Ancylostoma duodenale* differ from those of *Necator americanus?***

A. duodenale has two pairs of ventral, clawlike teeth and one pair of dorsal, knoblike teeth. *N. americanus* has two ventral cutting plates and two rudimentary dorsal plates.

■ **Describe the life cycle of the hookworm.**

The adult lives 3 to 8 years and produces 10,000 to 20,000 eggs per day. The rhabditiform larva feeds on organic debris for 3 days and molts; on the eighth day it stops feeding, the mouth closes, the esophagus elongates, and after the second molting it becomes a filariform larva. Once in the host, migration occurs through the lungs to the pharynx, and the adult fixed to the intestine begins to lay eggs in about 5 weeks.

■ **How much blood does an adult hookworm consume daily?**

It consumes 0.4 ml.

■ **What type of anemia results from infestation with hookworms?**

Iron-deficiency anemia results from infestation with hookworms.

■ **What is *Ancylostoma braziliense*, what diseases does it cause, and how does it cause them?**

Three strains of these hookworms exist, and dogs, cats, and man (geographically limited) are their definitive hosts. Dog and cat strains cause creeping eruption in man, for they are unable to penetrate the subdermal layer of skin. The human strain causes intestinal hookworm infection.

■ **What clinical condition is caused by *Ancylostoma braziliense* in North America?**

Creeping eruption (cutaneous larva migrans) is caused.

■ **Visceral larva migrans is caused by what parasites, and how are individuals infected?**

It is caused by *Toxocara canis* and *T. cati*. Infection is acquired by eating embryonated eggs in dirt. Freshly passed ova are not infective.

■ **What is the range of the size of adult *Ascaris lumbricoides*?**

The range is 20 to 45 cm long and 3 to 6 mm in diameter. The male is two thirds as long as the female and is more slender.

■ **With what might decorticate *Ascaris lumbricoides* ova be confused, and how may they be distinguished?**

They may be confused with hookworm ova. A thicker shell and undivided cell mass distinguish *Ascaris lumbricoides* ova.

■ **Describe the life history of *Ascaris lumbricoides* after ova are ingested by a human being.**

The ova hatch in the small intestine, and larvae enter the lymphatics and sojourn for 10 days in the lungs. They are 2 mm long when they leave the lungs via the trachea to enter the digestive tract, where they mature in the small intestine.

■ **Identify these three forms of *A. lumbricoides* ova.**

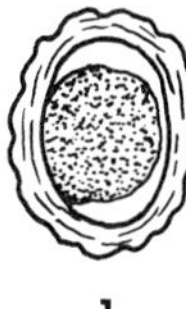
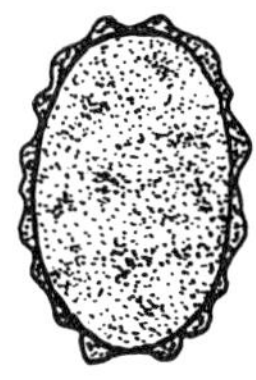
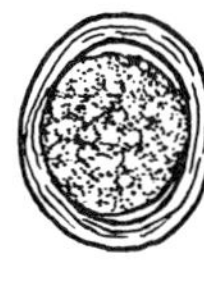

1. Fertilized
2. Infertile
3. Fertile and decorticate

■ **Are *Ascaris lumbricoides* ova resistant to drying?**

Yes, they survive for years when dried.

■ ***Trichuris trichiura* (formerly *Trichocephalus*) is known as the (1) guinea worm, (2) eyeworm, (3) whipworm, (4) ropeworm, (5) hookworm, (6) mouse hookworm, or (7) gooseworm?**

It is known as the whipworm.

■ **Describe the life cycle of *Trichuris trichiura*.**

Adults live attached to the cecum. Ova require at least 10 days in soil for embryonation. The larva attaches first in the small intestine and then passes to the site of adult attachment, the cecum (less commonly to the appendix or colon).

■ **Identify the forms illustrated below.**

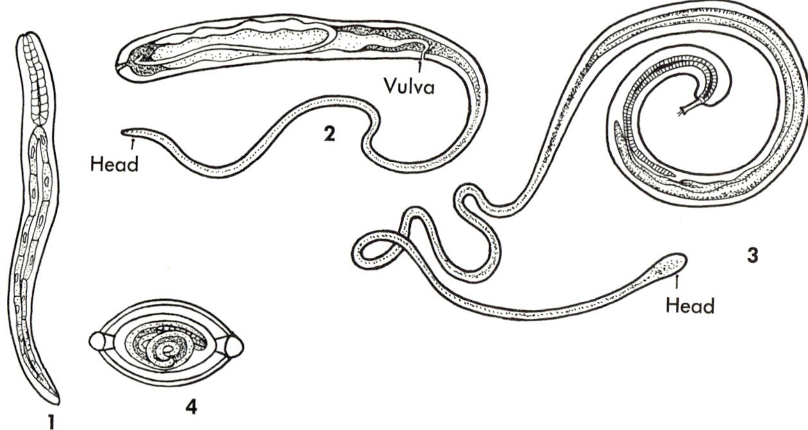

1. A larva
2. An adult female
3. An adult male
4. An embryonated ovum of *Trichuris trichiura*

■ **How large is the adult *Enterobius vermicularis?***

The male is 2 to 5 mm long, and the female is 8 to 13 mm long; the male is 0.1 to 0.2 mm in diameter, and the female is 0.3 to 0.5 mm in diameter.

■ **Where do adult *E. vermicularis* live?**

They live in the cecum and appendix.

■ **Describe the life cycle of *E. vermicularis*.**

Pressure of the gravid uterus on the esophagus of the female forces her detachment from the cecum. She migrates to perianal or perineal skin, deposits her eggs, and dies. Eggs are ingested by the same or another person, or they may be wafted in air currents and inhaled. They hatch in the duodenum, and the larva develops to maturity in the small intestine. It then attaches to the cecum where it grows to maturity.

■ **Identify the forms illustrated below.**

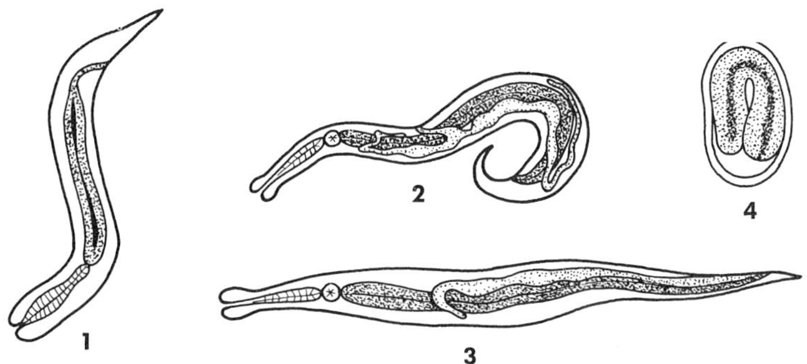

They are stages in the life cycle of *E. vermicularis.*
1. A larva
2. An adult female
3. An adult male
4. An embryonated ovum

■ **If only their ova are available, how can hookworm species be identified?**

They can be identified by culture. Filariform larvae of *Ancylostoma duodenale* have a slightly flattened head and narrow esophagus without constriction at the esophageal-intestinal junction and with inconspicuous, unequal esophageal spears. *Necator americanus* has a smaller, more cylindrical head, a broader esophagus with marked constriction, and conspicuous, equal esophageal spears. *A. braziliense* has a more slender tail than the other two species.

■ **What is the effectiveness of the scotch tape method for detection of ova on perianal skin?**

It is most effective for *E. vermicularis.* It will detect half of *Ascaris* infestations and a sixth of *Trichuris* infestations.

■ **What is the significance of serologic tests for intestinal nematode infestations?**

There is little significance, because the tests are not reliable.

■ **Name seven tissue roundworms.**

Wuchereria bancrofti, Brugia malayi, Loa loa, Onchocerca volvulus, Dracunculus medinensis, Acanthocheilonema perstans, and *Mansonella ozzardi* are tissue roundworms.

■ **What reproductive characteristic do these roundworms have in common?**

They all give birth to live young (microfilariae).

■ **What is the intermediate host for all tissue roundworms except *D. medinensis?***

The intermediate host is a dipterous insect.

■ **What happens to the microfilaria after it is ingested by the dipterous insect?**

If sheathed, it sheds its sheath, migrates through the gut wall to the thoracic muscles, molts twice, emerges as infective form, and enters the proboscis of the insect.

■ **How large are adult *Wuchereria bancrofti* roundworms? Where do they live?**

The male is 4 cm long, and the female is 8 cm long. They occupy the lymph nodes and release microfilariae periodically into the blood.

■ **What insects serve as intermediate hosts for *W. bancrofti?***

Mosquitoes of *Culex quinquefasciatus* (night-biting), *Aedes pseudocutellaris* (day-biting), and various anopheline species are the intermediate hosts.

■ **What are the dimensions of microfilariae of *W. bancrofti?***

The dimensions are 7×300 μm.

■ **Which of the other tissue roundworms does *Brugia malayi* resemble?**

B. malayi is similar to *W. bancrofti*. Its microfilariae are slightly smaller.

■ **What is the intermediate host for *Loa loa,* and what is its geographical distribution?**

The intermediate host is the deer fly (*Chrysops* species). *Loa loa* is found in central west Africa (Congo River area).

■ **What is the principal complication of onchocerciasis?**

It is blindness caused by a reaction to microfilariae trapped in the anterior chamber of the eye.

■ **Describe *O. volvulus* microfilariae.**

Unsheathed microfilariae occur in two sizes, one 0.25 mm and the other 0.35 mm long (one probably male, the other probably female). Both the anterior end and tail are free of nuclei.

■ **Describe lesions of onchocerciasis.**

Lesions of onchocerciasis are subcutaneous fibrous tumors containing male and female parasites. Microfilariae are released into a cyst within the tumor by the female.

■ **What is the intermediate host of *O. volvulus?***

It is the *Simulium* gnat (black gnat) of Africa and Central and South America.

■ **The female of which tissue roundworm is forty times as long as the male?**

The female of *Dracunculus medinensis* is forty times as long as the male.

■ **Describe the life cycle of *Dracunculus medinensis*.**

Microfilariae are discharged when the anterior end of the female comes in contact with water. Infective forms develop in the body of *Cyclops* organisms within about 10 days. The adults mature in body cavities after the definitive host ingests *Cyclops* organisms, and they migrate to subcutaneous tissue. Males are rarely seen. This roundworm infects man, dogs, cattle, and monkeys in Africa and occurs in foxes, raccoons, and minks in North America.

■ **Outline the methods of laboratory diagnosis of microfilariasis.**

Aspirate a lymph node for *Wuchereria* and *Brugia* species infestation, or a subcutaneous fibrous nodule for *Onchocerca* species infestation. *Wuchereria* and *Brugia* microfilariae are demonstrable in blood in heavy infections. Use Giemsa or hematoxylin stain on thick smears.

■ **Which of the tissue roundworms causes solitary pulmonary nodules?**

Dirofilaria immitis causes solitary pulmonary nodules. The organism is transmitted from dogs or other animals to man by mosquitoes. Infection is incidental to the life cycle, for man is not a definitive host.

■ **Which of the microfilariae found in human blood have no sheath?**

Onchocerca volvulus, *Acanthocheilonema perstans*, and *Mansonella ozzardi* have no sheath.

■ **Differentiate the various sheathed microfilariae found in human blood.**

W. bancrofti has no nuclei in the tip of the tail, while *B. malayi* does. *Loa loa* resembles *B. malayi* in distribution of nuclei, but it has ungraceful angular curves unlike those of *B. malayi*, and the terminal two nuclei of *B. malayi* are more distinctly separated than those of *Loa loa*.

■ **The illustrations below show the distal ends of three sheathed and three unsheathed microfilariae. Identify each.**

1. *W. bancrofti*
2. *B. malayi*
3. *Loa loa*
4. *O. volvulus*
5. *M. ozzardi*
6. *A. perstans*

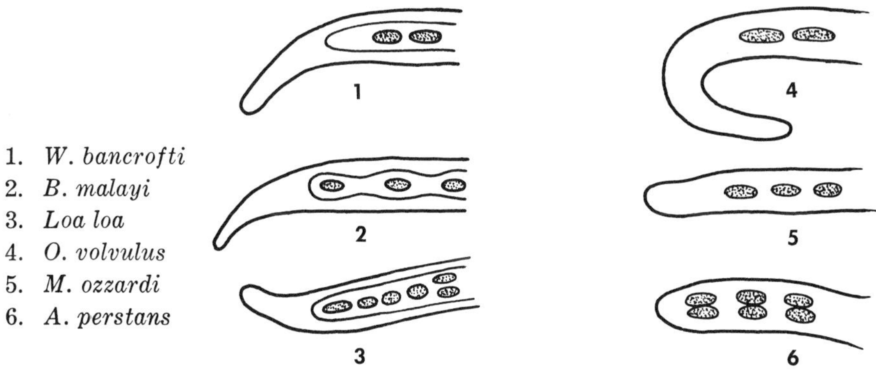

■ **Name the three classes of phylum Platyhelminthes.**

1. Turbellaria: free-living flukes
2. Trematoda: parasitic flukes
3. Cestoidea: tapeworms

■ **Operculate ova occur in which two classes?**

They occur in Trematoda and Cestoidea.

■ **Spined ova occur in which class?**

They occur in Trematoda (genus *Schistosoma*).

■ **In general, what is the first intermediate host of trematodes?**

It is generally a snail.

■ **Describe the typical life cycle of trematodes.**

The miracidium hatches from the ovum, swims about, and is eaten by or penetrates the epithelium of the snail. It becomes a sporocyst in the snail, forming within it germ balls that are immature rediae. Daughter sporocysts may arise from sporocysts. Immature cercariae form from germ balls that bud off the body wall of the redia. After maturation, they pass through the birth pore. The cercaria emerges from the snail's body. Depending on the species, it enters the definitive host, encysts on vegetation (metacercaria), penetrates the next intermediate host (fish, crayfish, crag, or second mollusk) or dies.

■ **Name one genus of flukes inhabiting blood vessels, three genera inhabiting the liver, four genera inhabiting the intestine, and one genus inhabiting the lung.**

1. Blood vessels: *Schistosoma*
2. Liver: *Fasciola, Opisthorchis, Clonorchis*
3. Intestine: *Heterophyes, Metagonimus, Fasciolopsis, Echinostoma*
4. Lung: *Paragonimus*

■ **Name the genera whose metacercariae encysts (1) on vegetation, (2) in fish, (3) in crayfish and crabs, and (4) in second mollusks.**

1. *Fasciola* and *Fasciolopsis* on vegetation
2. *Opisthorchis, Heterophyes, Metagonimus,* and *Clonorchis* in fish
3. *Paragonimus* in crayfish and crabs
4. *Echinostoma* in second mollusks (snails, fresh-water clams)

■ **Which flukes, parasitic for man, do not encyst after emerging from their first and only intermediate host?**

The schistosomes do not. They are also distinguished among pathogenic flatworms by forked tails of their cercariae and by unisexual reproduction.

■ **Which of the flukes cause cercarial dermatitis?**

Schistosomes cause cercarial dermatitis.

■ **When do symptoms of cercarial dermatitis appear, and when are they most intense?**

They appear within a few hours after the host bathes in contaminated water and reach a peak in 3 to 4 days.

■ **In which geographic regions does schistosomal dermatitis occur?**

It occurs in the north-central lakes region of the United States and Canada, Europe, Africa, parts of the Orient, and other regions in which lower mammal, bird, and human schistosomes occur.

■ **Which of the schistosomes that parasitize man is prevalent in the New World?**

Schistosoma mansoni is prevalent.

■ **Identify the ova.**

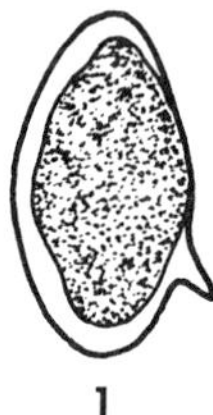 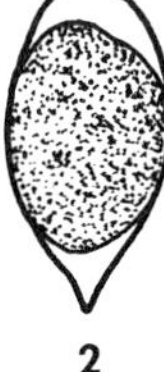 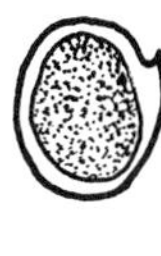

1. *S. mansoni*
2. *S. haematobium*
3. *S. japonicum*

■ **In what parts of the human body do the adults of the three schistosomes live?**

S. japonicum lives in veins of the small intestine, *S. mansoni* in veins of the large intestine, and *S. hematobium* in veins of the urinary bladder.

■ **Describe the adult schistosomes.**

Males are 9 to 22 mm long and females are 12 to 26 mm long, with *S. mansoni* being the smallest and *S. japonicum* being the largest. The body of the male is broad and folded to form the gynecophoral canal in which the narrow female is held.

■ **Describe the life cycle of human schistosomes.**

Ova are ready to hatch when passed. The miracidium enters the snail within 30 hours. Two generations of sporocysts occur so that 100,000 to 200,000 cercariae result from a single successful miracidium. The work-tailed cercariae enter the human host and mature into adults within veins.

■ **What are the disadvantages of current serologic tests for schistosomiasis and filariasis?**

The current serologic tests lack both good sensitivity and specificity. Only about 70% of lightly infected cases are serologically positive.[8]

■ **What is the geographic distribution of *Clonorchis sinensis?***

It is found in Japan, Korea, China, and southeastern Asia.

■ **Describe the life cycle of *C. sinensis*.**

The ovum is ingested by a snail where is hatches and becomes a sporocyst. The sporocyst gives rise to rediae, which in turn produce cercariae that leave the snail and encyst on freshwater carp or minnows and are ingested when the fish are eaten raw. The cercaria excysts in the duodenum and enters the common bile duct. It matures in the liver. The ova enter the intestine in bile and are passed in feces.

■ **In what geographic localities does *Fasciola hepatica* occur?**

It occurs in sheep-raising countries throughout the world.

■ **How does *F. hepatica* differ from *C. sinensis* in its journey through the human body?**

The metacercaria of *F. hepatica* penetrates the duodenum and migrates to the liver through the portal circulation rather than by entering the common bile duct from the intestine.

■ **In what form is *F. hepatica* ingested by man?**

It is ingested as the metacercaria encysted on aquatic vegetation that is eaten raw.

■ **Name two minute (1 to 2 mm) intestinal flukes that utilize snails as the intermediate host and encyst on fish.**

Two such intestinal flukes are *Metagonimus yokogawai* and *Heterophyes heterophyes.*

■ **Name the largest trematode parasite of man.**

The largest is *Fasciolopsis buski,* which lives in the duodenum and jejunum. It is 5 cm long.

■ **Describe the life cycle of *Fasciolopsis buski.***

The ovum matures over 3 to 6 weeks in water before the miracidium emerges. It enters a snail and reproduces through sporocysts and rediae. The metacercaria occurs on water chestnuts, and it excysts in the intestine after raw water chestnuts are eaten.

■ **The ova of *Fasciolopsis buski* are virtually indistinguishable from those of what organisms?**

They are indistinguishable from *F. hepatica* ova.

■ **What is the intermediate host for *Paragonimus westermani,* and on what does the cercaria encyst?**

The intermediate host is a snail of genera *Melanoides, Hua,* and others, and the encystation of the cercaria occurs on a crayfish or crab.

■ **How does *P. westermani* reach the lung?**

It excysts in the intestine and migrates over a 30-day period through the peritoneal cavity, diaphragm, and pleural cavity to reach the lung.

■ **What are the principal anatomic regions of tapeworms?**

The principal regions are the scolex, for attachment to the intestine; the neck, or germinative tissue from which proglottids are formed; and the strobila, the chain of proglottids that form fertile ova.

■ **Name the two orders of tapeworms, and describe their distinguishing characteristics. Give examples.**

1. Pseudophyllidea: scolex equipped with suctorial grooves (bothria) (example: *Diphyllobothrium latum*)
2. Cyclophyllidea: scolex equipped with round suckers (example: *Taenia* species)

■ **Are the tapeworms unisexual or hermaphroditic?**

They are hermaphroditic.

■ **Which genus of tapeworms has two gonopores in each proglottid?**

Dipylidium species have two gonopores in each proglottid. (The name derives from this fact.)

■ **Which of the tapeworms lay operculate ova?**

Pseudophyllidea (*Diphyllobothrium* species) lay operculate ova.

■ **Name and describe the six illustrated larval forms occurring in various tapeworms.**

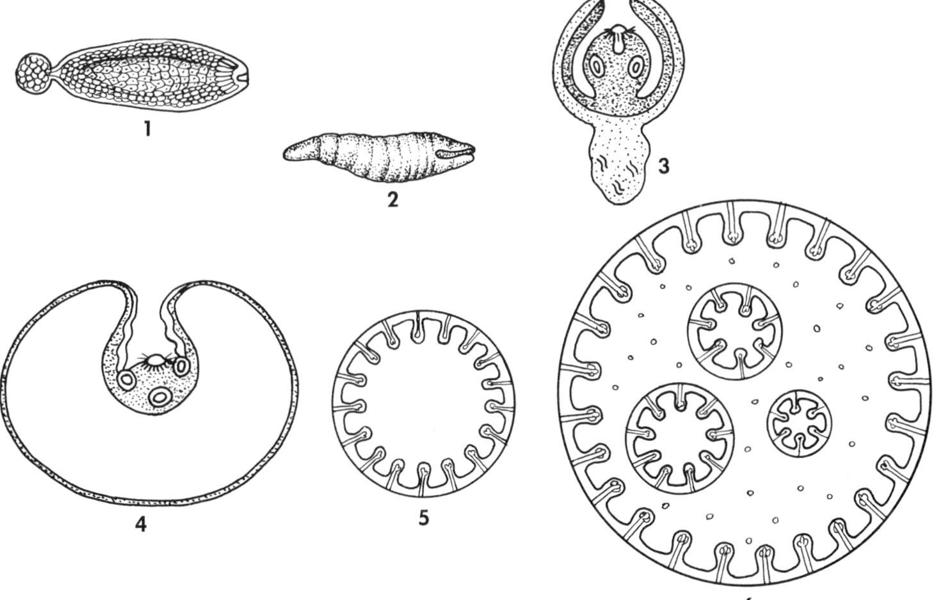

1. Procercoid larva (It develops in a crustacean [*Cyclops* or *Diaptomus* species] after ingestion of a *Dyphyllobothrium* species coracidium.)
2. Sparganum (plerocercoid) larva (It develops from a procercoid larva in the muscle of fish.)
3. Cysticercoid larva (It develops in tissues of the intermediate host in *Hymenolepis* and *Dipylidium* species and lacks a bladder.)
4. Cysticercus larva, *Taenia* species in intermediate host (The larval head is invaginated into the bladder.)
5. Coenurus (multiceps) larva, *Multiceps* species in intermediate host (Multiple invaginated heads are in a single bladder.)
6. Hydatid larva, *Echinococcus* species in intermediate host (The bladder contains multiple attached invaginated heads and secondary bladders with multiple attached invaginated heads.)

■ **Comment on the sensitivity of serologic tests for echinococcosis when the cysts are located in the lungs and when they are in the liver. What related condition can produce high cross-reacting titers, and what unrelated diseases cause low cross-reacting titers?**

Over 80% of patients with hepatic echinococcosis are identified by serologic methods (IHA, bentonite flocculation [BF]), but the sensitivity for pulmonary disease is only 33% to 50%. Cysticercosis sera cross-react in high titers, and sera from patients with collagen diseases and cirrhosis may have low levels of cross-reacting antibodies.[8]

■ **List six tapeworms inhabiting man as the definitive host.**

Diphyllobothrium latum, Taenia solium, Taenia saginata, Hymenolepis nana, Hymenolepis diminuta, and *Dipylidium caninum* all inhabit man as the definitive host.

■ **List four tapeworms infesting man as an intermediate (accidental) host, and give the names of the diseases these infestations represent.**

1. *Diphyllobothrium* species: sparganosis acquired by ingesting infected crustaceans or by application of infected frog muscle to lacerations as poultice
2. *Taenia solium:* cysticercosis
3. *Multiceps multiceps:* coenurosis
4. *Echinococcus granulosus:* echinococcosis (hydatid disease)

■ **How are the pork tapeworm and cysticercosis acquired?**

The tapeworm is acquired by eating pork containing the cysticercus larva. Cysticercosis is acquired by eating the ova of *T. solium* from pig or human feces. Autoinfection is a great danger in individuals infested with this tapeworm.

■ **What is *Cysticercus cellulosae?***

It is the cysticercus larva of *T. solium.*

■ **Does *T. saginata* infest the tissues of man?**

No.

■ **How are the adult tapeworms of *T. solium* and *T. saginata* distinguished?**

Proglottids of *T. solium* have thirteen or fewer lateral uterine branches on each side, whereas *T. saginata* shows fifteen or more. The scolex of *T. solium* has an armed rostellum, but that of *T. saginata* lacks both rostellum and hooklets.

■ **Describe the life cycle of *T. solium*.**

A pig eats the ova in human feces; the cysticercus larva forms in pig tissues and is eaten by man. The larva matures in the small intestine of man.

■ **Describe the life cycle of *T. saginata*.**

It is the same as *T. solium*, but with cattle substituted for the pig.

■ **Identify these two ova.**

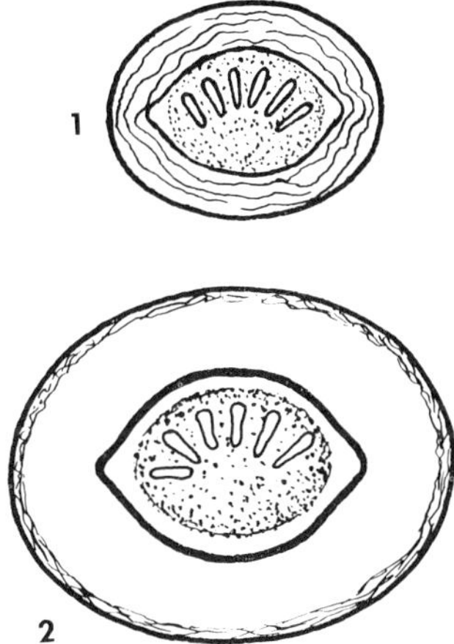

1. The ovum of *H. nana* (It is 30 to 47 μm in diameter, and four to eight slender filaments arise from each pole of the embryophore to envelop the hexacanth embryo.)
2. *H. diminuta* (Note its larger size and the absence of polar filaments.)

■ **Describe the life cycle of *Hymenolepis nana*.**

The adult worm lives in the small intestine of rats, mice, and men. Ova are infective to the definitive host, and no intermediate host is necessary, but fleas and other insects can serve as intermediate hosts experimentally. The egg hatches in the small intestine, and the oncosphere enters a villus where it becomes a cysticercoid larva. The cysticercoid larva reenters the small intestinal lumen, attaches, and it matures into an adult tapeworm. Hyperinfection is possible but has not been demonstrated in man.

■ **What are the natural definitive hosts of *H. diminuta,* and how are human beings infected?**

Rats and mice are the ordinary definitive hosts. Most infections in man have been in children less than 3 years old. An intermediate host is always required. It may be a larva or adult of several insects: meal moths, earwigs, fleas, or beetles. They may be ingested with food (precooked breakfast cereal, etc.). The cysticercoid larva of the tapeworm develops in these intermediate hosts.

■ **How does man become infected with the dog tapeworm, *Dipylidium caninum?***

He becomes infected by ingesting fleas containing the cysticercoid larvae. The ova are ingested by larval fleas, and the oncospheres bore through the intestinal wall to develop within the hemocele.

■ **Identify this tapeworm.**

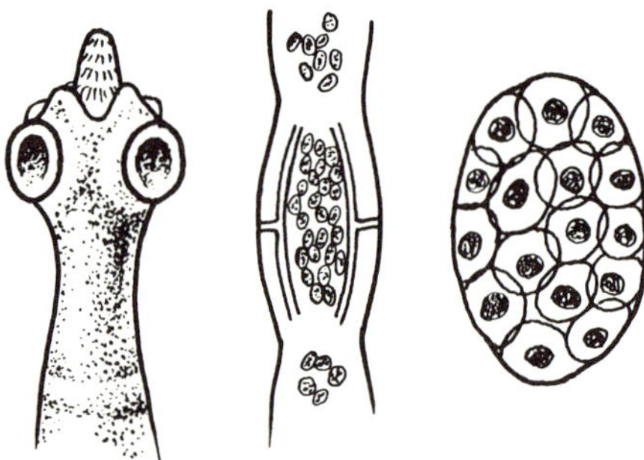

It is *D. caninum.* The scolex has four suckers and a prominent armed rostellum with hooks arranged in three or four circles. The proglottid has a gonopore on each side (hence the generic term *Dipylidium*). The ova resemble those of *H. diminuta* but occur in clusters.

■ **What is the normal life cycle of *Echinococcus granulosus,* and how does man become infected?**

The adult worm lives in the small intestine of the dog. Mature eggs passed in feces are ingested by sheep or cattle. The oncosphere bores through the intestinal wall and is carried to distant organs by the circulation. Hydatid larvae in tissues of sheep or cattle are ingested by the dog and mature in its intestine. Man is infected by ingesting eggs passed by the dog. The eggs resemble those of *Taenia* species.

■ **What is the most sensitive and specific test for echinococcosis?**

It is the intradermal (Casoni) test. Complement fixation and precipitin tests are of less value except in old and complicated cases.

- **Identify the six ova.**
    1. *T. saginata* or *T. solium*
    2. *D. caninum* (single ovum separated from packet)
    3. *C. sinensis*
    4. *O. felineus*
    5. *H. heterophyes*
    6. *M. yokogawai*

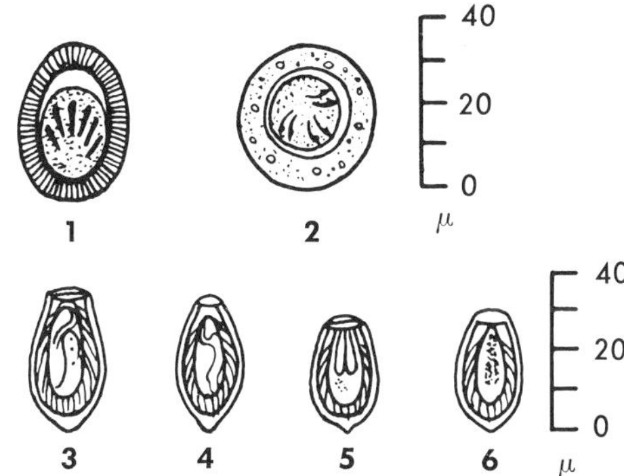

- **Identify these ova.**

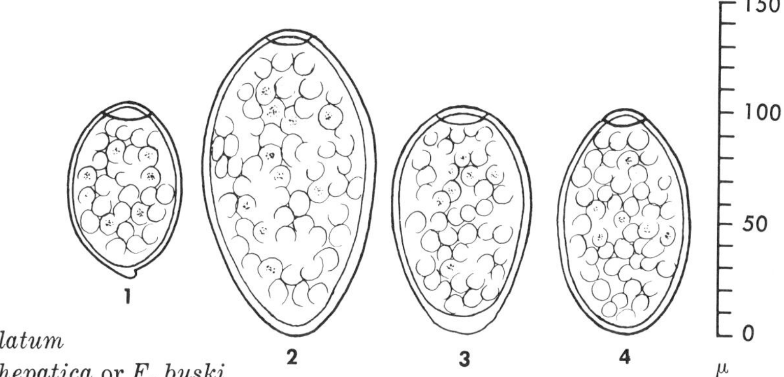

    1. *D. latum*
    2. *F. hepatica* or *F. buski*
    3. *P. westermani*
    4. *E. ilocanum*

- **State the possible identities of the ova shown below found in the stool.**

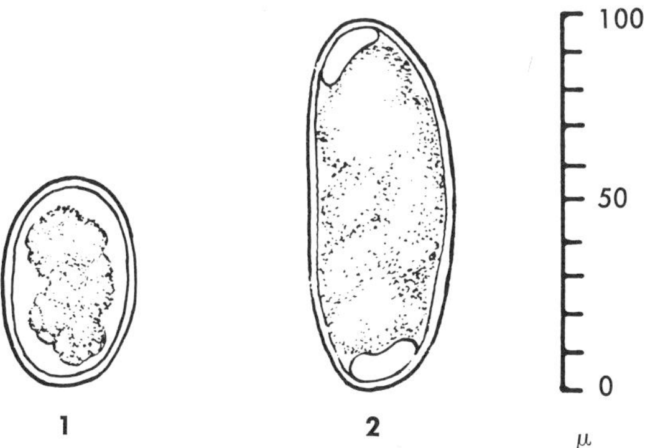

    1. Any of the hookworms (*A. duodenale*, *A. braziliense*, or *N. americanus*), or *S. stercoralis* (found unhatched in the stool in presence of diarrhea)
    2. *Heterodera marioni*, a harmless plant parasite (The ova of *H. marioni* pass through the digestive tract unchanged.)

■ **What is *Pneumocystis carinii?***

Pneumocystis carinii is an organism that is found in the lungs. The merozoites are 1 to 2 μm long and resemble those of *T. gondii* but are smaller. Cysts form in the alveoli. They are 4 to 8 μm in diameter and contain eight merozoites.

■ **What disease is caused by *P. carinii*, and what is its epidemiology?**

P. carinii causes interstitial pneumonia with a mixed cellular infiltrate that includes many plasma cells. It occurs in debilitated infants and in individuals with congenital or acquired (chemotherapeutically induced) immunologic defects.

■ **How can *P. carinii* pneumonitis be diagnosed?**

It can be diagnosed by finding organisms in fluid aspirated from the lungs or in lung biopsies. The cysts are best recognized after staining with the Gomori methenamine sliver technic, and the merozoites are recognized by the Giemsa stain.[4]

■ **What is the significance of the presence of these microscopic, highly refractile particles of round, triangular, and axially symmetrical shapes in the lungs postmortem? What is their significance if found in the liver, in bone marrow, or in the feces?**

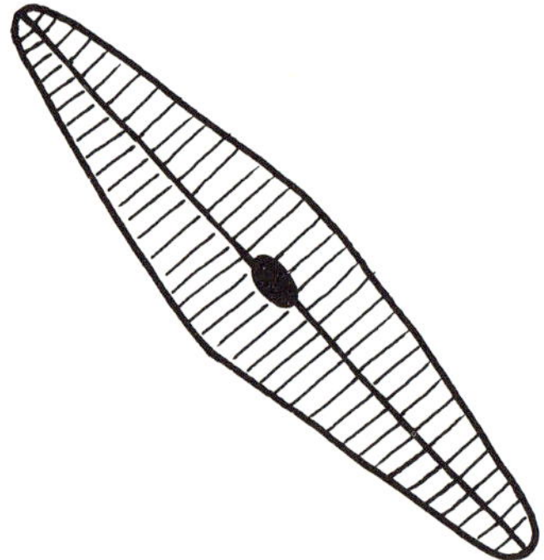
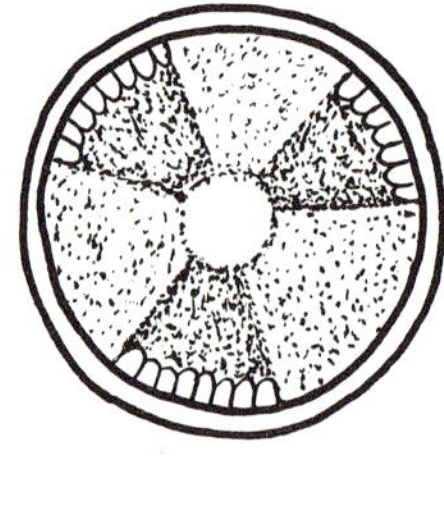

The structures are diatoms (unicellular algae with silicaceous exoskeleton). If found in the lungs, they are consistent with drowning or postmortem immersion in salt or fresh water. If found in bone marrow and other nonpulmonary internal organs, they indicate drowning. If found in feces, they indicate recent ingestion.

ENTOMOLOGY

■ **Name and define briefly the four classes of Arthropoda.**

1. Chilopoda: the centipedes and millipedes, composed of many similar segments
2. Crustacea: aquatic with true gills
3. Arachnida: lacking antennae, body composed of dissimilar segments—head, thorax (or cephalothorax), and abdomen (example: ticks and mites)

4. Insecta: dissimilar segments—head, thorax, and abdomen; one pair of antennae

■ **Identify the three inherently dangerous arachnids illustrated below.**

1. Scorpion (*Centruroides* species of Arizona)
2. *Latrodectus mactans* (black widow spider)
3. *Loxosceles reclusa* (brown recluse spider)

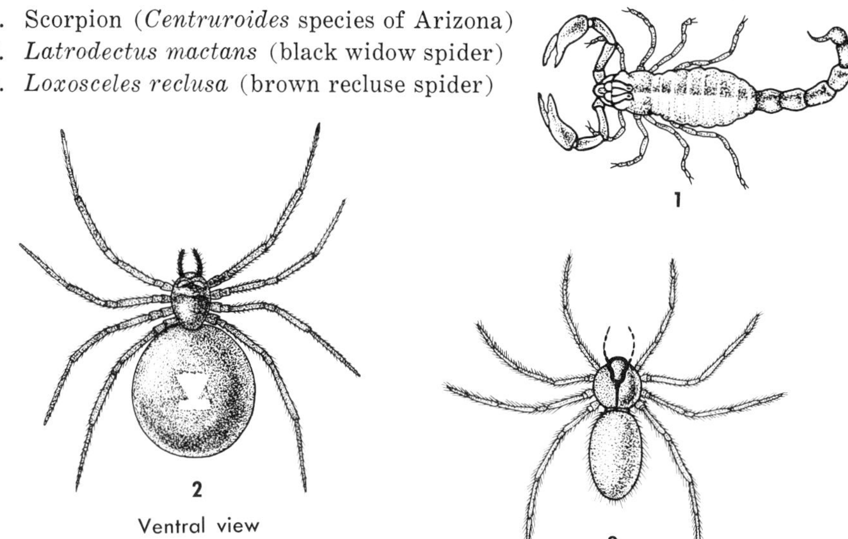

Ventral view

■ **Describe the reaction to a bite of *L. reclusa*.**

The reaction is initially pain, formation of hemorrhagic bleb after 8 hours, then gradual formation of eschar. Systemic effect of poison may cause hemolysis with jaundice and hemoglobinuria, arthralgia, and fever up to 103° F. Tissue necrosis results in an ulcer that forms over 3 to 5 weeks.

■ **Name these arachnids.**

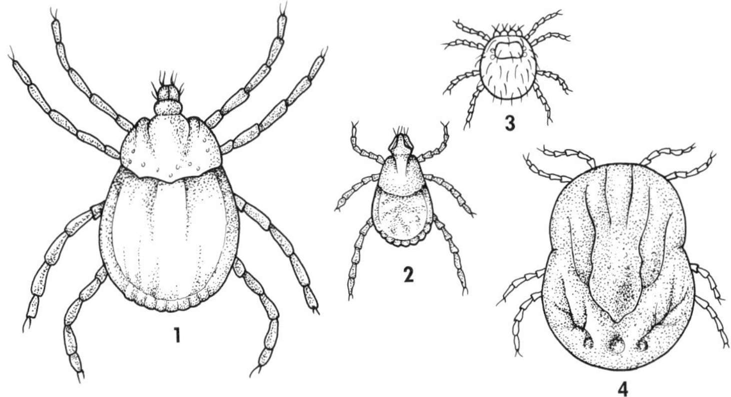

1. Family Ixodidae (hard tick)
2. Larval tick (note three pairs of legs contrasted with four pairs of the adult)
3. Mite
4. Family Argasidae (soft tick)

■ **How do Ixodidae (hard ticks) differ from Argasidae (soft ticks)?**

Soft ticks lack the scutum (dorsal shield).

■ **Describe tick paralysis, and name the responsible tick.**

Tick paralysis is caused by venom injected with a bite of the female *Dermacentor* tick and is an ascending motor paralysis that may regress after removal of the tick.

■ **Name five diseases transmitted by *Dermacentor andersoni*.**

Rocky Mountain spotted fever, Q fever, tularemia, Colorado tick fever, and encephalomyelitis are transmitted by *D. andersoni*.

■ **Name three diseases transmitted by the American dog tick, *Dermacentor variabilis*.**

Rocky Mountain spotted fever ("Eastern spotted fever"), tularemia, and St. Louis encephalitis are transmitted by *D. variabilis*.

■ **Name three diseases transmitted by *Dermacentor occidentalis* (Pacific Coast tick).**

Spotted fever, tularemia, and Q fever are transmitted by *D. occidentalis*.

■ **Name four diseases transmitted by *Amblyomma americanum*, the lone star tick.**

Spotted fever, tularemia, Q fever, and Bullis fever (Camp Bullis, Texas) are transmitted by *A. americanum*.

■ **What disease is transmitted by the bite of Argasidae (soft ticks)?**

Relapsing fever (Borrelia) is transmitted by the bite of soft ticks.

■ **What diseases are transmitted through feces of soft ticks?**

Tularemia and Q fever are transmitted through feces of soft ticks.

■ **What is this arachnid?**

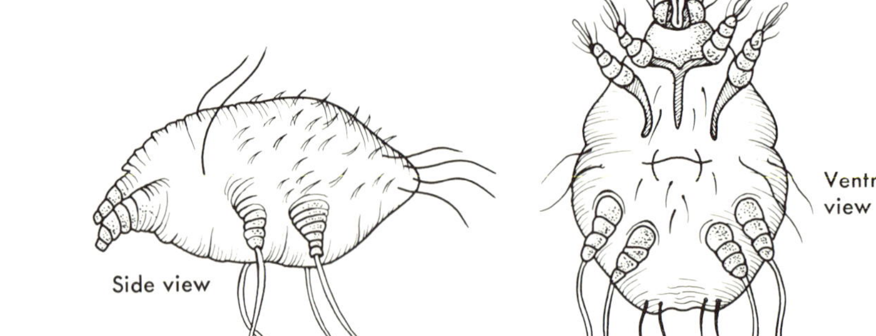

It is *Sarcoptes scabiei*, a mite.

- **How large is *Sarcoptes scabiei?***

  It is 0.4 mm long.

- **How long does it live?**

  It lives 2 months.

- **Where does it live? Describe its life cycle.**

  It lives in epidermal burrows especially on interdigital webs, the wrists, penis, scrotum, buttocks, axillae. The male and female wander about, meet, and copulate. Ova are laid in burrows at a rate of two to three a day. They hatch in the burrows, and larvae leave them to enter hair follicles, where they develop into nymphs and adults. Palms and soles are spared except in children.

- **What is this creature, and what is its significance?**

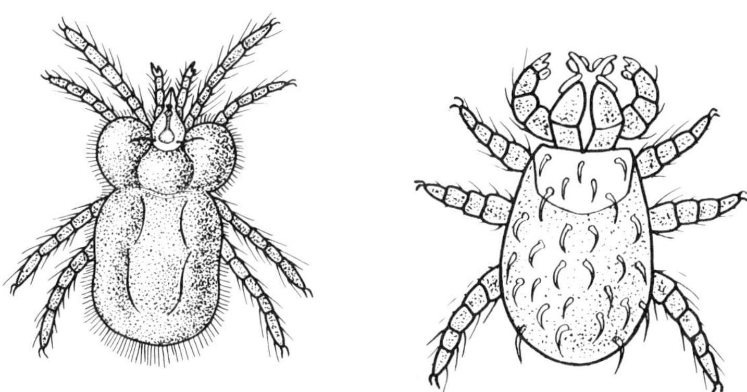

  It is *Trombicula irritans.* An adult is on the left, six-legged larva on right. It is the larva that parasitizes. It attaches to skin, sucks lymph, and injects an irritating fluid. Within a day or two after itching begins, it drops off or is scratched off and matures on vegetation, especially blackberry bushes. The larva is identified by three pairs of legs and scutum with seven hairs.

- **What is *Trombicula akamushi*, and what is its medical importance?**

  It is a mite, and its orange-red larva transmits Tsutsugamushi fever.

- **What is this arachnid, and what is its clinical significance?**

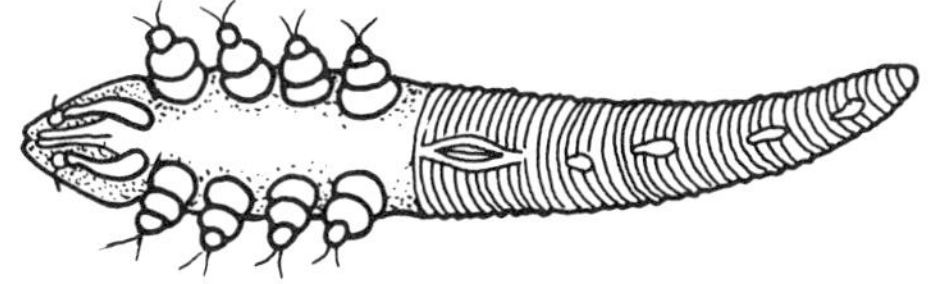

  It is *Demodex folliculorum,* a mite with rudimentary legs. It lives in hair follicles and sebaceous glands, particularly on the face, but usually does not cause symptoms.

■ **Identify this insect.**

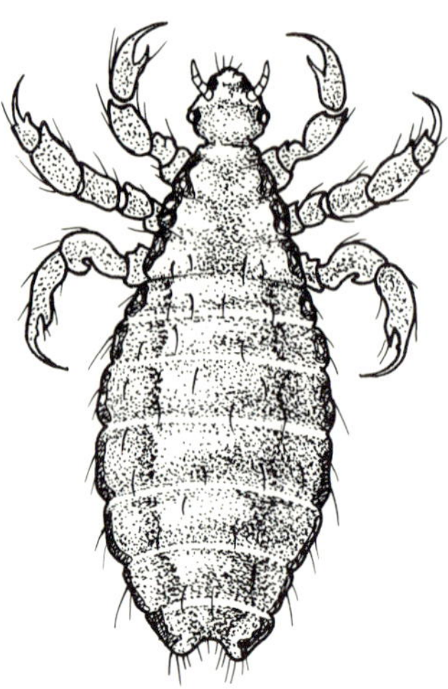

It is *Pediculus humanis* (body louse).

■ **Which diseases are transmitted by fleas?**

Fleas transmit plague, endemic typhus *(R. mooseri)*, and tularemia.

■ **What is this insect? Give its life cycle, life expectancy, and habits.**

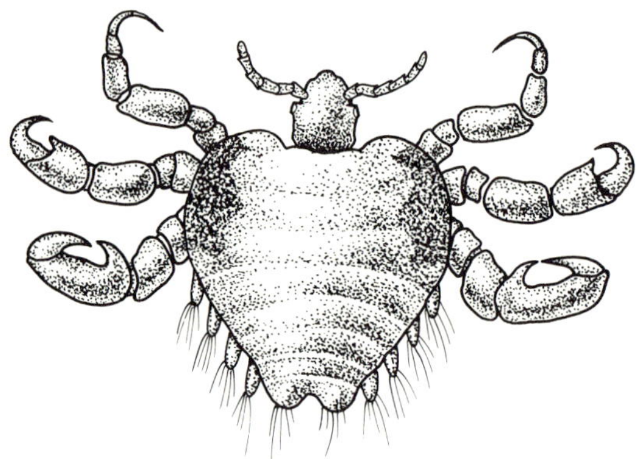

It is *Phthirus pubis*. It is 1 to 2 mm long, clings to hairs, and inserts mouth parts into a capillary. This louse (anopluran) moves little and is transmitted by prolonged contact. The egg-to-adult cycle is 25 days. Its adult life expectancy is about 30 days. Eggs, in groups cemented to hairs, are known as nits.

■ **Identify these ova. Ova *1* and *2* are illustrated at ×40 magnification; ova *3* are shown at ×5 magnification.**

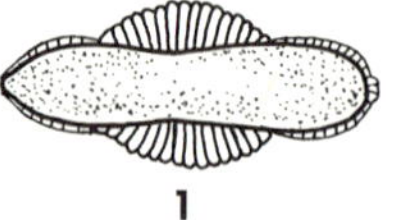

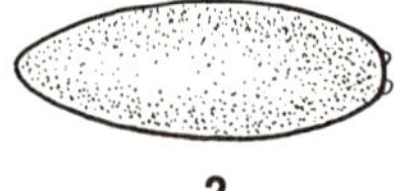

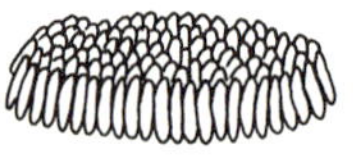

1   2   3

1. *Anopheles* species, single ovum (Note floats.)
2. *Aedes* species, single ovum
3. *Culex* species, multiple ova forming raft

- **Identify these larvae. Each is magnified approximately ×3.**

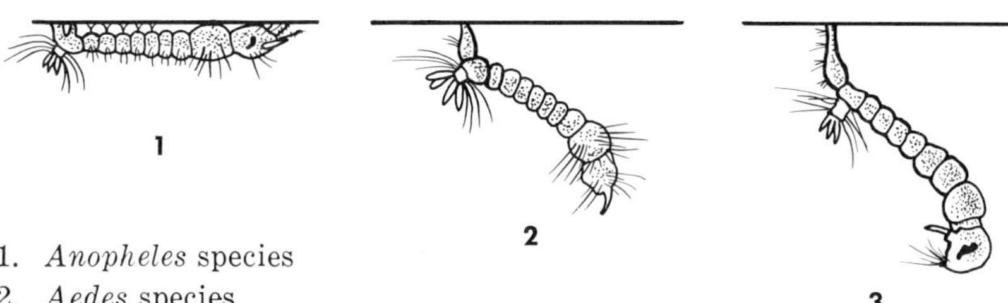

1. *Anopheles* species
2. *Aedes* species
3. *Culex* species

- **Identify these heads as anopheline and culicine, male and female.**

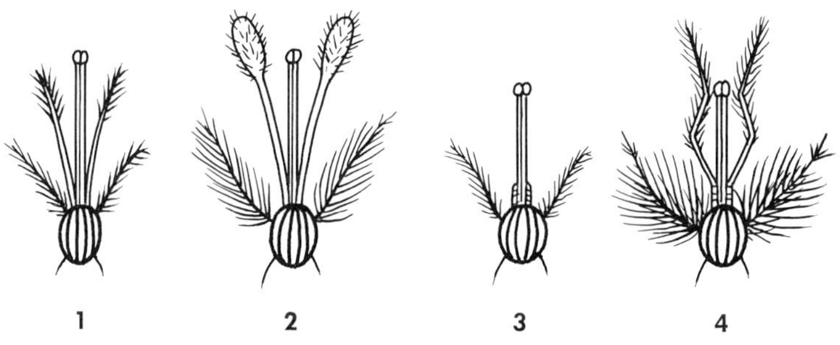

1. Anopheline, female (Note long palps.)
2. Anopheline, male (Note bushy antennae and swollen palps.)
3. Culicine, female (Note short palps.)
4. Culicine, male (Note bushy antennae without swollen palps.)

- **Which sex of *Anopheles* mosquitoes transmits malaria?**

The female *Anopheles* mosquito transmits malaria.

- **Which parasites do culicine (genera *Culex, Aedes,* and *Mansonia*) mosquitoes transmit?**

Culicine mosquitoes transmit *Wuchereria bancrofti* and *Brugia malayi.*

- **Which virus diseases do culicine mosquitoes transmit?**

Culicine mosquitoes transmit yellow fever, dengue fever, St. Louis encephalitis, eastern equine encephalitis, and western equine encephalitis.

■ **Identify these two dipterous insects. What diseases do they transmit?**

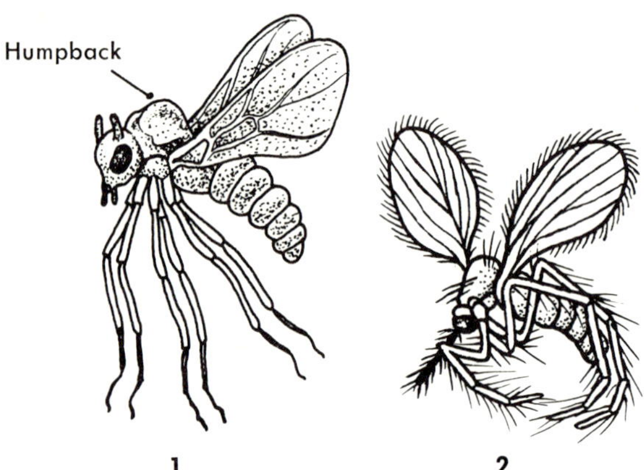

1. *Simulium* species (The female transmits onchocerciasis.)
2. *Phlebotomus* species (The female transmits leishmaniasis and bartonellosis.)

■ **What is this tiny crustacean that is found in fresh water? Name two parasites for which it serves as an intermediate host.**

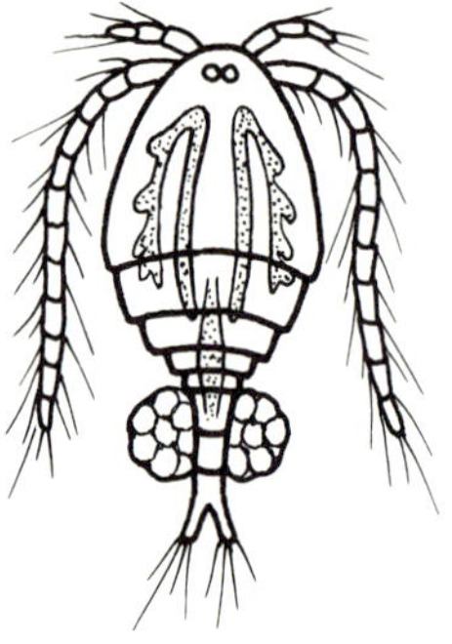

It is a *Cyclops* species. It is an intermediate host for *Diphyllobothrium latum* and *Dracunculus medinensis*.

■ **Identify the hemipterous insect illustrated, and state the disease that it transmits.**

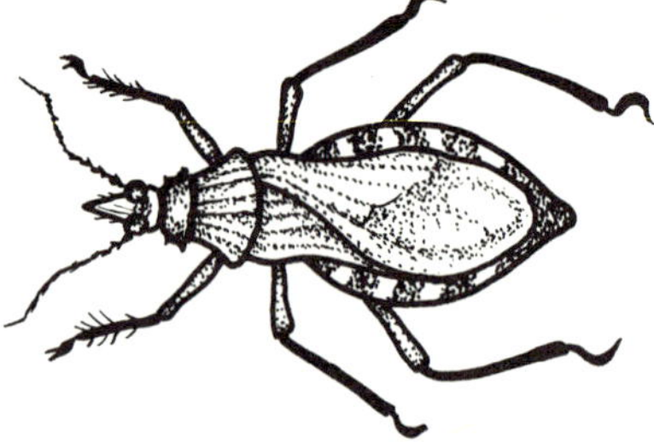

It is a *Triatoma* species (reduviid or cone-nosed bug). It transmits Chagas' disease (South American trypanosomiasis).

■ **Describe the life cycle of the screwworm, *Cochliomyia hominivorax,* and describe the disease caused by its larvae.**

C. hominivorax is a fly three times as large as the common housefly. The female deposits eggs at the margins of wounds. Sixteen hours later the eggs hatch, and the maggots enter the tissues with resultant bacterial inflammation. The disease is called myiasis. The mature larvae, 15 to 16 mm long, drop to the ground, pupate, and emerge as adult flies.[10]

■ **What parts of the body may be affected by myiasis caused by various flies?**

The skin, genitourinary tract, intestines, and stomach may be affected by myiasis.

■ **How is gastrointestinal myiasis contracted?**

It is contracted by ingestion of eggs or larvae of flies on food.

■ **How is genitourinary myiasis acquired?**

Fannia canicularis (lesser housefly) and *Fannia scalaris* (latrine fly) lay eggs on an unclean perineum, and maggots migrate into the anus, vagina, and urethra.

■ **What is the name of the common housefly? Can its larvae be parasitic?**

The common housefly is *Musca domestica.* Ingestion of food contaminated with eggs or maggots causes gastrointestinal myiasis.

■ **What is this?**

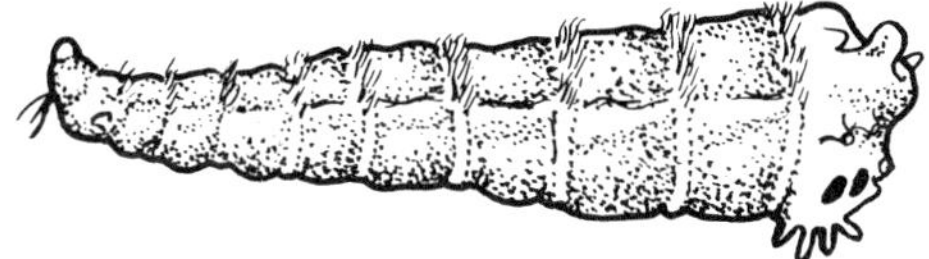

It is a housefly larva (maggot).

REFERENCES

1. Ambroise-Thomas, P., and Truang, T. K.: Fluorescent antibody test in amebiasis, Am. J. Trop. Med. Hyg. 21:907, 1972.
2. Ament, M. E., and Rubin, C. E.: Relation of giardiasis to abnormal intestinal structure and function in gastrointestinal immunodeficiency syndrome, Gastroenterology 62:216, 1972.
3. Denham, D. A., Ridley, D. S., and Voller, A.: Immunodiagnosis of parasitic diseases, Practitioner 207:191, 1971.
4. Dutz, W.: *Pneumocytis carinii* pneumonia. In Sommers, S. C., editor: Pathology annual, vol. 5, New York, 1970, Appleton-Century-Crofts.
5. Fife, E. H., Jr.: Advances in methodology for immunodiagnosis of parasitic disease, Exp. Parasitol. 30:132, 1971.
6. Frankel, J. K., Dubey, J. P., and Miller, N. L.: *Toxoplasma gondii* in cats: fecal stages identified as coccodian cocysts, Science 167:893, 1970.
7. Healy, G. R.: Laboratory diagnosis of amebiasis, Bull. N. Y. Acad. Med. 47:478, 1971.
8. Kagan, K. G.: Current status of serologic testing for parasitic diseases, Hosp. Pract. 9:157, 1974.
9. Krogstad, D. J., Juranek, D. D., and

Walls, K. W.: Toxoplasmosis, with comments on risk of infection from cats, Ann. Intern. Med. 77:773, 1972.

10. Macias, E. G.: Cutaneous myiasis in South Texas, N. Engl. J. Med. 289:1239, 1973.

11. Scholten, T.: An improved technique for the recovery of intestinal protozoa, J. Parasitol. 58:633, 1972.

12. Scholten, T. H., and Yang, J.: Evaluation of unpreserved and preserved stools for the detection and identification of intestinal parasites, Am. J. Clin. Pathol. 62:563, 1974.

13. Sheffield, H. G., and Melgon, M. L.: *Toxoplasma gondii:* the oocyst, sporozoite, and infection of cultured cells, Science 167:892, 1970.

14. Stamm, W. P.: Amoebic aphorisms, Lancet 2:1355, 1970.

CHAPTER 18

Pregnancy tests

■ **Describe the pattern of elevation of human chorionic gonadotropin (HCG) levels in pregnancy.**

Elevations are noted in the urine 4 to 10 days after the first missed period, depending on the sensitivity of the test used. The peak levels are reached approximately 7 weeks after conception. They persist to 12 weeks and then decline to approximately one tenth of the peak level, at which they remain from 15 weeks until term.

■ **What type of urine specimen should be collected for pregnancy tests, and what precaution should be taken in its handling?**

The best specimen is the first morning specimen (it has the highest HCG content, as it is usually the most concentrated). It should either be examined quickly or stored at $-20°$ C because HCG is not stable at room temperature.

■ **Explain the principle of the Gravindex test.**

This test is based on latex particle agglutination inhibition. The patient's urine is incubated with antihuman chorionic gonadotropin. Latex particles coated with HCG are then added. If the patient is pregnant, the HCG in the urine will neutralize the anti-HCG, and no agglutination will take place. In a nonpregnant patient the anti-HCG will clump the latex particles covered with HCG.

■ **Explain the principle of the urinary chorionic gonadotropin (CGH) hemagglutination test.**

The CGH test is based on the hemagglutination inhibition principle. The patient's serum (or urine) is incubated with anti-HCG serum. Red cells coated with HCG are added. In the pregnant female, hemagglutination caused by reaction between the anti-HCG and HCG-coated red cells is inhibited. The erythrocytes settle at the bottom of the test tube in a doughnut pattern. In the nonpregnant female, hemagglutination takes place, and the cells settle in a diffuse mat.

■ **Why may a false positive result of an immunologic pregnancy test occur in the postmenopausal female?**

Pituitary gonadotropins (which may be increased postmenopausally) can react immunologically with antibodies to HCG and therefore result in a false positive result of an immunologic pregnancy test.

■ **What other factors may produce a significant number of false positive HCG results?**

Proteinuria in excess of 1 gm/24 hr, gross hematuria in urine specimens, and presence of certain phenothiazine drugs can cause false positive tests. The exact mechanism whereby this interference is accomplished has not been fully determined.

■ **What is the sensitivity of the Gravindex and CGH tests?**

The Gravindex test measures as little as 5 international units (IU) of HCG per milliliter. The CGH test measures as little as 1 IU of HCG per milliliter. The Gravindex test usually shows positive results 7 to 10 days after a missed period, and few false negative results occur after 20 days. The CGH test shows positive results 4 to 7 days after the first missed period with few false negative results after 14 days.

■ **How might one diagnose threatened abortion or ectopic pregnancy during the first trimester by using an immunologic pregnancy test?**

During the peak HCG level (7 to 12 weeks past the last menstrual period), a finding of less than 3000 IU per 24-hour urine is associated with inevitable abortion. Ectopic pregnancy is also associated with abnormally low HCG levels (less than 10 IU/ml).

■ **How might pregnancy tests be used to determine the efficiency of therapy of a patient with choriocarcinoma or hydatidiform mole?**

If the patient has expelled a mole completely, HCG should disappear from the urine within 7 days. If HCG persists in the urine, then residual trophoblastic disease is present. HCG may occasionally persist for extended periods (6 months or more) in patients with benign disease, but a rising titer is suggestive of choriocarcinoma. A negative assay result for HCG is strong evidence against persistence of trophoblast, but negative assay results have been reported, although rarely, in presence of choriocarcinoma.

■ **In addition to placental abnormalities, what diseases or conditions have been associated with high urinary HCG levels?**

High urinary HCG levels may be found in twin pregnancies, polyhydramnios, eclampsia, and erythroblastosis fetalis in the third trimester of pregnancy.

■ **Does the absence of HCG in the urine rule out trophoblastic malignancy in a patient?**

It does not. There have been a few reported cases without detectable HCG.

■ **How might sequential HCG assays help in the diagnosis of trophoblastic disease?**

During normal pregnancy sequential assays tend to follow the normal pregnancy curve. In patients with trophoblastic disease, irregular fluctuations of HCG levels will be noted.

■ **In what other disease or diseases may the determination of HCG levels be useful?**

Ovarian and testicular tumors (teratomas, seminoma, dysgerminoma, embryonal carcinoma, choriocarcinoma) occasionally show elevated HCG levels.

CHAPTER 19

Semen

■ **What proportions of the seminal volume are provided by (1) the prostate gland and (2) the seminal vesicles?**

1. 20%
2. 60%

■ **After how long a period of continence should the seminal sample be collected?**

The sample should be collected after approximately 3 days. Longer periods may result in decreased motility.

■ **Approximately how long do sperm survive in the seminal vesicles?**

The sperm survive about a month.

■ **After collection, at what temperature should the specimen be maintained, and what is the maximum time that should elapse before examination?**

The specimen should be maintained at 37° C. Not more than 3 hours should elapse before examination.

■ **What is the significance of a low seminal pH (7.0, for example)?**

It indicates a relative preponderance of prostatic secretion, which is acid because of high content of citric acid. This condition may indicate hypoplasia of the seminal vesicles.

■ **What sequence of events occurs normally in semen after ejaculation?**

1. Coagulation (action of prostatic clotting enzyme on fibrinogen-like substrate secreted by seminal vesicles)
2. Liquefaction within 30 minutes of ejaculation because of prostatic fibrinolysin
3. Proteolysis of fibrin fragments

■ **What is the normal volume of semen in the ejaculate?**

It is 1.5 to 5 ml (average 3.5 ml).

■ **How is a sperm count performed?**

The same procedure is used as for WBC. Draw semen to the 0.5 mark in WBC pipet and dilute to the 11 mark with 1% formalin USP and 5% Na_2CO_3 in distilled water. This procedure immobilizes the sperm. Unusually viscous semen may first be diluted 1:1 with Alevaire, and the count is multiplied by 2.

■ **What is the significance of semen that is unusually viscous?**

Occasionally this condition has been associated with poor invasion of the cervical mucous and may be the only demonstrable defect in an infertile couple.

■ **What is the normal range of sperm counts?**

The normal range is 60 to 150 million/ml (average 100 million/ml).

■ **Infertility is usually associated with sperm counts below what level?**

Sperm counts below 20 million/ml will usually result in infertility. (This is not an absolute rule.)

■ **What is the normal proportion of motile sperm?**

The normal proportion is 60% or more (when examined within 3 hours or less of collection).

■ **Why is semen fluorescent?**

A high content of flavins causes greenish-white fluorescence.

■ **What is the proportion of abnormal sperm in normal seminal fluid?**

The proportion is 30% or less.

■ **How are agglutinating antibodies to sperm detected?**

Place 0.5 ml of undiluted serum and 0.5 ml of 1:4 diluted serum from the woman in two serology tubes. Add 0.05 ml of semen diluted to contain 50 million sperm per milliliter. Incubate for 4 hours at 37° C. Strong agglutination is indicated by agglutination of ten to twelve sperm per high-power field.

■ **Does presence of agglutinating antibodies in the woman correlate with infertility?**

Yes. Antibodies to sperm can be demonstrated in 75% of all women in whom no other cause of infertility is found.

■ **What can be done to decrease agglutinating antibodies in the woman?**

They decrease during 6 months of nonexposure to sperm.

■ **What is the acid phosphatase content of semen and of other body fluids?**

The content of semen is 2500 KA units per milliliter. The content in other body fluids is less than 5 KA units per milliliter.

■ **What is the incidence and importance of blood group substances in semen?**

Water-soluble A, B, or H blood group substances are present in about 80% of semens. By testing for neutralization of agglutinating activity of antisera, it may be possible to exclude a suspect in rape.

CHAPTER 20

Sputum

■ **How can one be sure that one is examining sputum rather than saliva?**

Sputum contains histiocytes (frequently containing pigment) and ciliated columnar epithelium, whereas saliva does not.

■ **List four diseases or conditions commonly associated with bloody sputum.**

Primary or metastatic neoplasms, congestive heart failure, pulmonary infarct, and tuberculosis and other progressive pulmonary infections are associated with bloody sputum.

■ **List six ordinarily saprophytic oropharyngeal organisms that occasionally may be pulmonary pathogens.**

Staphylococcus aureus, Streptococcus pneumoniae, Haemophilus influenzae, Klebsiella pneumoniae, Candida albicans, and *Actinomyces israelii* may be pulmonary pathogens.

■ **Which of the following organisms, if demonstrated in sputum by microscopy and culture, indicates disease caused by that organism with a high degree of certainty: *Aspergillus fumigatus, Candida albicans, Blastomyces dermatitidis, Cryptococcus neoformans, Histoplasma capsulatum, Coccidioides immitis, Actinomyces israelii, Nocardia asteroides,* and *Mycobacterium tuberculosis?***

B. dermatitidis, C. neoformans, H. capsulatum, C. immitis, and *M. tuberculosis* are usually pathogenic. The other organisms frequently are present as saprophytes.

■ **How may the diagnosis of pulmonary alveolar proteinosis be made by sputum examination?**

Sections of formalin-fixed sputum may contain amorphous eosinophilic, granular, periodic acid-Schiff (PAS)–positive alveolar casts with laminated bodies similar to those seen in lung biopsies.

■ **What are Curschmann spirals and what is their significance?**

Curschmann spirals are mucous casts of bronchi or bronchioles. They occur in sputum from patients with asthma.

■ **List three diseases or conditions in which the sputum usually contains large numbers of eosinophils.**

Large numbers of eosinophils occur in asthma, Löffler's pneumonia, and parasitic pneumonitis (visceral larval migrans, pulmonary phase of ascariasis, and other roundworm infestations).

■ **Comment on the diagnostic significance of the structures shown in the illustration below when found in sputum.**

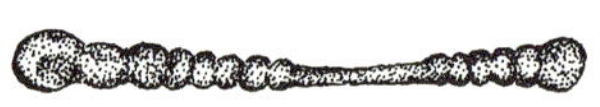

On the left is an asbestos body, indicative of pulmonary asbestosis. In the center are Charcot-Leyden crystals, which are eosinophilic, are derived from granules of eosinophils, and usually indicate a diagnosis of asthma. On the right are elastic fibers, which occur in association with pus and indicate lung abscess.

■ **What stain may be helpful in delineating asbestos bodies in sputum?**

The Prussian blue reaction, which stains the iron present in the asbestos bodies, may be helpful.

■ **Describe the usual characteristics of sputum of a patient with bronchiectasis.**

The sputum is mucopurulent with a "pea soup" appearance and has a sickly sweet odor. It initially settles into three and finally into two layers as the upper frothy layer subsides. The upper layer is watery saline, and the lower layer is mainly pus containing Dittrich's plugs.

■ **Describe the usual characteristics of sputum of a patient with *Klebsiella* pneumonia.**

The sputum is dark brown or red with "currant jelly" consistency and is thick and tenacious.

■ **What stains should be used to demonstrate *Pneumocystis carinii* in sputum?**

Gormori's methenamine silver nitrate, which stains the cysts of *Pneumocystis carinii*, and Giemsa stain, which reveals the merozoites, should be used.

■ **What is the significance of pleomorphic gram-negative rods and gram-positive cocci in a smear of foul-smelling sputum?**

These findings are virtually diagnostic of anaerobic lung abscess.

CHAPTER 21

Statistics and quality control

The calculations necessary in clinical chemistry are basically those of quantitative chemical analysis. Brief sections on quality control in the clinical laboratory can be found in several texts, including Henry and associates' *Clinical Chemistry: Principles and Technics, Todd-Sanford Clinical Diagnosis by Laboratory Methods,* and *Chemistry for Medical Technologists* by White, Erickson, and Stevens. The text by Hoel is an excellent introductory text to statistical methods intended for those with a limited mathematical background.

Henry, R. J., Cannon, D. C., and Winkelman, D. W.: Clinical chemistry: principles and technics, ed. 2, New York, 1974, Harper & Row, Publishers.

Hoel, P. G.: Elementary statistics, New York, 1960, John Wiley & Sons, Inc.

White, W. L., Erickson, M. M., and Stevens, S. C.: Chemistry for medical technologists, ed. 3, St. Louis, 1970, The C. V. Mosby Co.

■ **The molecular weight of Na_2SO_4 is 142.044. How can a 1 molar solution with a volume of 1 L be prepared?**

Dissolve 142.044 gm of Na_2SO_4 in water in a 1 L volumetric flask, add water to the 1 L mark, and mix.

■ **How would 1 L of Na_2SO_4 solution 1 normal with respect to Na^+ be prepared?**

Dissolve 71.022 gm of Na_2SO_4 in water and bring to 1 L volume.

■ **Describe how to prepare a 1 molal solution of Na_2SO_4.**

Dissolve 142.044 gm of Na_2SO_4 in 1 kg of water.

■ **Give a formula for computing the mean from original sample values, using the following symbols:**

X = Original sample value

$\overline{X}$ = Sample mean calculated from original sample values

i = Any one sample

n = The final sample or the total number of samples

$\sum$ = Sum of terms that follow

$\sum\limits_{i=1}^{n}$ = Sum of all samples

s = Standard deviation calculated from original sample values

C.V. = Coefficient of variation

$$\overline{X} = \frac{\sum\limits_{i=1}^{n} X_i}{n}$$

Explanation: Let there be five determinations of serum potassium as follows: 4.2, 4.4, 4.3, 4.2, and 4.4 mEq/L. X_i is any one of the determinations. $n = 5$.

$$\sum\limits_{i=1}^{n} X_i = 21.5 \qquad \overline{X} = 4.3$$

- **Give a formula for determining the standard deviation from original sample values.**

$$s = \sqrt{\frac{\sum\limits_{i=1}^{n} (X_i - \overline{X})^2}{n-1}}$$

- **Define the coefficient of variation (relative standard deviation, coefficient of error).**

$$\text{C.V.} = \frac{s}{\overline{X}}\ (100\%)$$

This is the standard deviation divided by the mean times 100%.

- **In the clinical chemistry laboratory, taking serum glucose measurement as an example, how might the precision of a test be determined?**

It might be determined by repeating the measurement a number of times on a pooled serum specimen and determining standard deviation and coefficient of variation. Determine the glucose level twenty times on daily or twice-daily runs, and from these data calculate s and C.V. Standard deviation and C.V. are measurements of precision.

- **How can accuracy of a measurement be determined?**

Accuracy can be determined by comparing the technic in use with another technic for performing the same measurement. Agreement of the two measurements by differing technics suggests accuracy. In practice, automated and hand methods can be assessed against each other, newly introduced methods against older, established methods and a method of one laboratory against the same or different method of another laboratory. The latter often involves use of commercial standards. Testing for recovery of known amounts of added material to the sample analyzed is another way of determining accuracy.

- **Is it possible to have excellent precision and yet have inaccurate results?**

It is possible if improper standards or improper reagents are used even though the technic is excellent and the results are highly reproducible.

- **Describe how to construct a quality control chart for daily use in serum glucose determination.**

Prepare a frozen pooled serum control by addition of leftover serum specimens until sufficient volume has accumulated to last for several months. Determine the glucose concentration on twenty or more successive runs, and calculate the mean and standard deviation. Indicate the mean as a horizontal line on graph paper with milligrams of glucose per deciliter on the vertical axis and date of analysis on the horizontal axis. Draw horizontal lines above and below the mean separated from it by 2 or 3 standard deviations. (Whether to use 2 or 3 standard deviations is a matter of individual preference.) A glucose value determined on the pooled serum that falls outside the area enclosed by the two horizontal lines indicates that the analysis is probably out of control.

■ **For a computation of standard deviation to be valid, what must be true of the population studied and the sampling method?**

The population must be normally distributed, and the sampling must be random.

■ **In a normal (gaussian) distribution, what percentages of the population are included within the following limits: (1) ±1 standard deviation, (2) ±2 standard deviations, (3) ±3 standard deviations?**

1. 68%
2. 95%
3. 99.7%

■ **When the concentration of hydrogen ion is 40 nEq/L (nanoequivalents per liter), what is the pH?**

$$\text{pH} = \log_{10} \frac{1}{40(10^{-9})} = \log_{10} 2.5(10^7) = 7.40$$

■ **The concentration of H_2CO_3 in plasma as milliequivalents per liter equals 0.03 times the plasma P_{CO_2} as millimeters of mercury. The ionization constant of carbonic acid in plasma is 794 nmol/L (nanomoles per liter). When the plasma bicarbonate concentration is 26 mEq/L and the P_{CO_2} is 40 mm Hg, what is the hydrogen ion concentration?**

$$H^+ = 794 \frac{0.03 \times 40}{26} = 36.6 \text{ nEq/L}$$

■ **Use the Hassalbalch equation to calculate the pH from the above data.**

$$\text{pH} = \text{pK}_a + \log \frac{[HCO_3^-]}{[H_2CO_3]}$$

$$= 6.10 + \log \frac{26}{0.03 \times 40}$$

$$= 7.44$$

■ **In a serum glucose procedure, Beer's law is followed from a concentration of 0 to 400 mg/dl. After appropriate adjustment for a blank reading, the percent transmissions at the appropriate wavelength for the unknown** serum and a standard containing 100 mg of glucose per deciliter are 56.2% and 75.0%, respectively. What is the concentration of glucose in the unknown serum?

$$\text{Optical density (OD)} = -\log_{10} \frac{\%\ \text{transmission}}{100}$$

The OD of the unknown is 0.250, and the OD of the standard is 0.125. The concentration of glucose in the unknown is 200 mg/dl.

■ **Define mean, mode, and median.**

The mean is the average of a set of measurements. The mode is the most frequently occurring value in a set of measurements. The median is the middle measurement after all measurements have been arranged in order of magnitude.

■ **Why is it frequently not possible to use published "normal ranges" in actual practice?**

Significant interlaboratory differences caused by different methods, instruments or reagents may occur. Furthermore, possible population differences, such as those due to climate, age, or ethnic background may also affect "normal ranges."

■ **If the normal range for each test is defined as the mean ±2 standard deviations determined by testing a large population of normal individuals, what percentage of individuals drawn from the same normal population would be expected to have one result or more outside the limits of normal when screened with a battery of twelve tests?**

One can expect 46% (computed from binomial distribution).

■ **What percentage of individuals in the situation defined in the previous question might be expected to have (1) two or more, (2) three or more, and (3) four or more abnormal results of the tests?**

1. 9.8%
2. 2.0%
3. 0.31%

■ **Eleven replicate determinations on aliquots of pooled serum yield the following potassium concentrations in milliequivalents per liter: 4.2, 3.6, 4.8, 3.9, 4.5, 4.1, 4.3, 4.0, 4.4, 3.7, and 4.7. Calculate the mean and the standard deviation.**

1. Mean: 4.2 mEq/L
2. Standard deviation: 0.38 mEq/L

■ **What are the 95% confidence limits of the above mean?**

The limits are 4.2 ± 2(0.38) or 3.44 to 4.96 mEq/L.

■ **Do the above results for replicate potassium determinations show sufficient precision?**

No. The standard deviation for serum potassium determination should not exceed 0.15 mEq/L.

■ **What is the "significant change limit" for laboratory measurements? For example, if the serum bicarbonate concentration is 24.6 mEq/L on day 1 and 21.2 mEq/L on day 2 after therapy with acetazolamide (Diamox), and the standard deviation for bicarbonate measurement in the laboratory is 0.8 mEq/L, has the bicarbonate concentration changed significantly?**

The "significant change limit" is a given value ±3 standard deviations. In the example, a significant drop in serum bicarbonate concentration occurred.

■ **How many measurements of a constituent of pooled serum should be made for calculation of the mean and standard deviation?**

One should make fifteen to twenty-five measurements.

■ **Define ionic strength.**

The ionic strength of a solution is half the sum of the molar concentrations of the ions, each multiplied by the square of its valence.

■ **Calculate the ionic strength (μ) of a 1 molar solution of Na_2HPO_4.**

Ionic strength $\mu = \frac{1}{2}\Sigma cZ^2$, where c is the molarity and Z is the charge on the ion. For the above solution:

$$\mu = \frac{2\ (1^2) + 1\ (1^2) + 1\ (3^2)}{2} = 6$$

CHAPTER 22

Toxicology

The field of medical toxicology has received marked impetus from the proliferation of a variety of drugs—depressants, stimulants, and perception-alter-
ing drugs—together with increasing traffic in narcotics and ever-present
ethanol. The chemical industry has produced a formidable array of new poisons
that include the halogenated insecticides, herbicides, and anticholinesterases;
and the environment is increasingly polluted by industrial wastes ranging from
gases, such as oxides of nitrogen and carbon monoxide, to heavy metals such as
mercury and lead. Clinical toxicology is a rapidly developing subspecialty in
which the clinical pathologist should play an important role.

Sections on toxicology can be found in several clinical pathology texts. For a
more comprehensive introduction to the field, one should refer to *Handbook of
Emergency Toxicology* by S. Kaye and to *Essentials of Toxicology* by T. A.
Loomis.

Bauer, J. D., Ackermann, P. G., and Toro, G.: Clinical laboratory methods, ed. 8,
St. Louis, 1974, The C. V. Mosby Co.
Kaye, S.: Handbook of emergency toxicology: a guide for the identification, diag-
nosis, and treatment of poisoning, ed. 3, Springfield, Ill., 1970, Charles C Thomas,
Publisher.
Loomis, T. A.: Essentials of toxicology, ed. 2, Philadelphia, 1974, Lea & Febiger.

INTRODUCTORY QUESTIONS

- **What is the principle of the Reinsch test?**

Certain elements are deposited on a copper wire spiral to produce a silver
or black coating when boiled after acidification with HCl.

- **Which elements are detectable by the Reinsch test?**

Arsenic, antimony, bismuth, sulfur, selenium, and tellurium are detectable.

- **What is the desirable amount of material necessary for performing the
Reinsch test?**

At least 20 gm (40 gm for arsenic) is desirable.

■ **What is the principle of the Gutzeit test?**

Generation of arsine (AsH_3) or stibine (SbH_3) results in yellow to brown discoloration of a paper strip impregnated with 5% mercuric bromide in ethanol.

■ **Is there a general procedure for an unknown poison?**

There is not an efficient, inexpensive one. Consequently, the history and clinical findings are most important in narrowing the area of search.

■ **What tissue is the principal storage depot for chlorinated hydrocarbon insecticides and herbicides (DDT, DDD, aldrin, dieldrin, endrin, 2,4-D)?**

Adipose tissue is the principal storage depot. (These substances are highly fat soluble.)

ANTICHOLINESTERASES

■ **What class of poisons cause depression of serum cholinesterase activity?**

Such depression is caused by the organic phosphates (insecticides and "nerve gases" such as diisopropylfluorophosphate, tetraethyl pyrophosphate, parathion, and malathion).

■ **In organic phosphate poisoning, what is the status of the pupils?**

The pupils are constricted. The victim shows signs of general parasympathetic hyperactivity (excessive salivation, lacrymation, and gastrointestinal hyperactivity).

■ **How is serum cholinesterase determined?**

It is determined by measuring pH change resulting from release of acetic acid by hydrolysis of acetylcholine. Methods include use of pH meter and spectrophotometric technics with methyl red or *m*-nitrophenol.

■ **What conditions other than poisoning with phosphate esters affect serum acetylcholinesterase levels?**

The levels are decreased in pregnancy, parenchymatous liver disease, malnutrition, anemias, metastatic carcinoma, acute infections, myocardial infarction, and dermatomyositis. Elevation of the acetylcholinesterase level occurs in the nephrotic syndrome.

ARSENIC

■ **What is (1) the normal plasma arsenic level and (2) the normal urine arsenic excretion?**

1. Less than 10 μg/dl
2. Less than 100 μg/24 hr

■ **In what internal organ is arsenic content highest?**

The arsenic content is highest in the liver (normal content up to 4 μg/100 gm).

■ **What proportion of blood arsenic is contained in the red blood cells?**

Over 94% is in RBC.

■ **What is the normal arsenic content of human hair?**

The normal content is up to 32 μg/100 gm. Arsenic has a particular affinity for hair, and in chronic arsenic poisoning the level in hair is four to six times that in the liver. The arsenic content of hair is not elevated in victims dying within 6 to 8 hours after ingestion, but it may be elevated in hair of survivors after excessive levels have disappeared from other organs.

■ **Does the presence of high concentrations of arsenic in hair and finger-nails always indicate arsenic poisoning?**

No. Arsenic in solution (as in insecticides) is readily bound to keratin via direct contact.

■ **After a single injection, how long are blood and urine arsenic levels elevated?**

Blood levels are essentially normal after 24 hours. Most of the arsenic excreted by the kidneys appears in the urine within 4 days, but urine levels may be elevated for 10 days.

BARBITURATES

■ **What are the principles for quantitative determination of barbiturates by ultraviolet spectrophotometry?**

Absorbance at specific wavelengths is affected by pH. Peak absorbance occurs at 255 nm at pH 13 (NaOH) with low absorbance at 240 nm. At pH 10.5 (NH_4Cl added), peak absorbance is at 240 nm, and minimal absorbance is at 255 nm.

■ **How are barbiturates extracted from serum?**

They are extracted with CCl_4 at acid pH (H_2SO_4).

■ **How are barbiturates identified and quantitated by ultraviolet absorbances?**

1. Determine absorbance curve 220 to 300 nm. From this information, pentobarbital, amobarbital, secobarbital, phenobarbital, and barbituric acid can be identified.
2. Determine absorbance differences at pH 13 and 10.5. Absorbance differences of equal quantities in milligrams of the various barbiturates are proportionately as follows: barbital 48, amobarbital 40, pentobarbital 39, secobarbital 36, phenobarbital 36.

■ **What are protein-binding properties of barbiturates?**

Long-acting barbiturates are bound but little (5%), pentobarbital and amobarbital 37%, secobarbital 44%, and pentothal 90% at low concentration and 50% at high concentration.

■ **After oral dosage, when are peak plasma levels of barbiturates reached?**

Peak plasma levels are reached in 3 to 12 hours.

■ **What is the distribution of barbiturates in tissues?**

Most tissues other than fat have approximately the same concentration as blood. RBC contain little of most barbiturates.

■ **Which barbiturates are selectively concentrated by fat?**

The ultrashort-acting barbiturates (thiobarbiturates) are selectively concentrated by fat.

■ **How rapidly are barbiturates eliminated from blood?**

Fast-intermediate barbiturates (pentobarbital, secobarbital) are eliminated at a rate of about 2.5% per hour, and long-acting barbiturates (barbital, phenobarbital) are eliminated at about 0.7% per hour.

■ **Where and how are barbiturates detoxified?**

They are detoxified in the liver by oxidation of side chain to alcohol, ketone, or carboxylic acid, and by glucuronide conjugation. Thiobarbiturates are detoxified by desulfuration.

■ **What are the lethal blood levels of barbiturates?**

They are approximately 3.5 mg/dl for short- and intermediate-acting, and 8 mg/dl for long-acting barbiturates.

BROMIDE

■ **At what level in serum does bromide cause central nervous system depression?**

Central nervous system depression occurs when the bromide level is 100 mg/dl (12.5 mEq/L) or higher.

■ **What is the effect of ingestion of bromide on plasma electrolytes?**

The plasma chloride concentration is decreased in proportion to the bromide concentration. Chloride is replaced by bromide, milliequivalent for milliequivalent.

■ **By ordinary methods of measurement of serum chloride, would a decreased apparent chloride level be noted in a patient with severe bromide intoxication?**

The apparent serum chloride level would probably be normal, because the methods used to measure chloride do not distinguish it from bromide.

■ **How much time is required for return of serum bromide concentration to normal (3 mg/dl or less) after ingestion of bromide?**

Up to 3 weeks is required.

■ **What color results when gold chloride is added to deproteinized serum to measure bromide concentration?**

The color is brown-orange.

ETHANOL

■ **How rapidly is alcohol absorbed, and when do peak blood levels occur after ingestion?**

About 90% is absorbed within an hour, and peak blood levels occur within about 30 minutes of ingestion.

■ **How do levels in the brain and urine compare with blood levels?**

The levels in the brain are slightly higher than in the blood; the urine level is 1.3 times that of the blood.

■ **How rapidly is alcohol eliminated, and by what pathways?**

About 10 ml/hr is eliminated, of which 90% is oxidized by the liver and 10% is eliminated via urine and breath.

■ **What are the intoxicating, stupefying, and lethal doses of pure alcohol taken acutely?**

One hundred milliliters produces symptoms; 300 ml produces stupor; and 350 to 600 ml is lethal.

■ **At what blood levels will nonalcoholics be euphoric, show severe defects in mentation, and be comatose?**

1. 100 to 150 mg/dl: euphoria, slow reaction time
2. 150 to 200 mg/dl: severe effects on mentation, slight disturbances in equilibrium and coordination
3. 350 to 400 mg/dl: coma, possibly fatal

■ **What is the expected rate of alcohol catabolism in subjects who have not had recent chronic intake of alcohol, and how is the rate of catabolism affected by recent chronic intake of alcohol?**

Subjects without recent chronic intake of alcohol catabolize it at the rate of approximately 14 mg/dl of plasma per hour, whereas recent chronic intake increases the rate of catabolism to 18 to 24 mg/dl of plasma per hour.[5]

■ **What precautions must be observed in collecting samples of breath and blood for alcohol analysis?**

1. Breath: no alcohol in mouth, no belching
2. Blood: skin cleansed with soap, not alcohol

■ **How should blood be preserved for alcohol analysis, and for how long is preservation effective?**

When preserved with 150 mg of NaF plus 0.5 mg of heparin sodium per 10 ml of blood, alcohol contents are stable for at least 18 days without refrigeration, for over a month at 5° C, and indefinitely at −20° C.

■ **What is Anstie's reagent? Is it a specific test for ethanol?**

Anstie's reagent is potassium dichromate in sulfuric acid. Oxidation of ethanol by dichromate yields the green Cr^{+++} ion. Other oxidizable substances including methanol and isopropanol also react with Anstie's reagent.

■ **Describe two methods for determination of ethanol in blood serum.**

1. Diffusion methods will determine the presence of ethanol in blood serum. Conway microdiffusion cells or the aeration apparatus of Bogen can be used. Ethanol and other diffusable, oxidizable substances reduce the Anstie's reagent used as the indicator in these methods.
2. The alcohol dehydrogenase method with measurement of $NADH_2$ absorbance at 340 nm can also be used. This method is not entirely specific for ethanol; other primary and secondary aliphatic alcohols and acetaldehyde interfere.

LEAD

■ **What is the normal 24-hour lead excretion in the urine?**

It is less than 150 μg/24 hr.

■ **At what blood lead levels do symptoms of plumbism appear?**

Symptoms and signs of plumbism are unusual when blood lead levels are less than 50 μg/dl. They are likely to be present when levels exceed 80 μg/dl.[4]

■ **What is the maximum permissible daily intake of lead?**

It is 0.6 mg/24 hr. The average urban adult takes in about 0.4 mg/24 hr.

■ **How is lead transported in the blood?**

Nearly all is bound to RBC.

■ **What proportion of ingested lead is absorbed?**

Approximately 8% is absorbed.

■ **What abnormality of amino acid metabolism often occurs in chronic lead poisoning?**

Aminoaciduria often occurs.

■ **What are the RBC abnormalities induced by lead poisoning?**

Decreased osmotic fragility, increased mechanical fragility, shortened life span, and basophilic stippling are induced by lead poisoning.

■ **Name three ways in which lead poisoning interferes with RBC production.**

1. It blocks condensation of glycine with succinate to form delta-aminolevulinic acid, and it blocks conversion of delta-aminolevulinic acid to porphobilinogen.
2. It blocks incorporation of iron into protoporphyrin.
3. It inhibits synthesis of globin in RBC precursors.

■ **What precursor of heme is elevated in urine in lead poisoning?**

The delta-aminolevulinic acid level is elevated.

■ **What urinary porphyrin is excreted in excessive amounts in lead poisoning?**

A large amount of coproporphyrin III is excreted.

MERCURY

■ **After ingestion of inorganic mercury, what organ contains the highest concentration, and how rapidly does the mercury level fall?**

The kidney contains the highest concentration; 60% to 80% of the peak level remains after a week after exposure. Mercury disappears rapidly from other organs.

■ **By which routes is mercury eliminated from the body?**

About twice as much is eliminated in urine as in feces.

■ **What is the upper limit of normal for whole blood mercury?**

Whole blood mercury should not be in excess of 100 parts per billion.

■ **What is the maximum safe concentration of mercury in food?**

Levels of mercury in food of 0.5 parts per million or less are considered safe.

■ **What are the symptoms of acute poisoning with inorganic mercury?**

Acute poisoning with inorganic mercury causes vomiting, bloody diarrhea, fever, leukocytosis, shock, and anuria.

■ **Are the symptoms of organic mercury poisoning (after ingestion of methyl mercury in fish, for example) principally oculocerebral, renal, or gastrointestinal?**

The symptoms of organic mercury poisoning are principally oculocerebral.[3]

METHANOL

■ **What are the lethal and blinding doses of methanol?**

Death can result from a dose of 30 to 100 gm. Blindness can result from a series of small doses.

■ **How is methanol metabolized?**

It is evenly distributed in body fluids (slightly higher in CSF than in blood) and is excreted in urine largely unchanged. It is oxidized to formic acid, but oxidation is at only one seventh the rate of that of ethanol, and therefore only about 1 ml/hr. Excretion and oxidation require several days.

■ **What sort of sample should be drawn, and how is methanol determined?**

One should draw 5 ml of blood in a fluoride-heparin tube. One should then analyze for methanol by gas chromatography or by oxidation to formaldehyde and distillation into chromotropic acid.

SALICYLATES

■ **Describe a urine screening test for salicylates.**

Add 10% ferric chloride drop by drop to several milliliters of urine until no further precipitation occurs. A violet to Bordeaux red color indicates a positive reaction. False positive reactions caused by acetoacetic acid in diabetes are eliminated by boiling. Phenacetin may also give a positive reaction. False positive reactions caused by phosphates are eliminated by using excess $FeCl_3$.

■ **Name a spectrophotometric method for salicylates in blood.**

The method is that of Natelson, using ferric nitrate.

■ **What are toxic levels of salicylate?**

Toxic levels are over 30 mg/dl. Death occurs in adults at serum levels of 47 to 75 mg/dl after absorption of 12 to 30 gm of salicylate.

■ **What is the initial metabolic derangement after onset of salicylate intoxication?**

It is respiratory alkalosis caused by stimulation of the respiratory center.

■ **What is the next metabolic event in salicylate intoxication?**

It is increased production of ketone bodies with metabolic acidosis.

MISCELLANEOUS

■ **In what form is the greater part of morphine or heroin excreted in the urine?**

Both morphine and heroin are excreted predominantly as morphine glucuronide. Heroin (diacetyl morphine) is rapidly hydrolyzed to morphine after injection or ingestion.[2]

■ **Are immunoassays performed on urine or serum specific for metabolites of morphine and heroin?**

The immunoassays are usually unable to distinguish among metabolites of morphine, heroin, codeine, and other chemically similar narcotics.[2]

■ **Compare the efficiency of radioimmunoassay (RIA), hemagglutination inhibition (HI), automated spectrofluorometry (SPF), and thin-layer chro-**

matography (TLC) for detection of heroin metabolites in urine within 24 hours of the last injection of the drug.

RIA and HI methods are nearly 100% effective and are sensitive enough to give positive results when more than 25 ng/ml of morphine equivalent is present. SPF and TLC methods are considerably less sensitive, and detection rates fall to 30% to 40% by 24 hours after injection.[2]

■ **Why is glutethimide (Doriden) overdosage serious and difficult to treat?**

It is rapidly taken up by adipose tissue and gradually released into the blood. It is relatively insoluble so that it is difficult to remove from the blood.

■ **What is the generally accepted toxic level of lithium?**

The toxic level is 1.5 mEq/L.

■ **What is the preferred method of measuring lithium levels and why?**

Atomic absorption spectrophotometry is more accurate than emission (flame) photometry. Furthermore, in most laboratories the latter is used to measure sodium and potassium as well. The internal standard, lithium, must be totally washed out of the system.

■ **What effect does lithium, in therapeutic doses, have on the white blood cell count, blood urea nitrogen (BUN), sodium, and potassium levels?**

The white blood cell count and BUN are increased, and the sodium and potassium levels are decreased.

■ **What are the principal toxic effects of low doses of ^{239}plutonium?**

Low doses (0.1 to 1.0 microcurie per kilogram injected or 2 to 12 nanocuries per gram lung deposited by inhalation) produce high rates of osteosarcoma and pulmonary neoplasia.[1]

■ **What are the principal sites of deposition of plutonium in the body?**

When inhaled, the sites are lungs and regional lymph nodes. When injected or ingested, the sites are bone and liver. Inhaled plutonium is gradually translocated to bone and liver. In bone, it is strikingly localized to the surfaces of bone spicules.[1]

REFERENCES

1. Blair, W. J., and Thompson, R. C.: Plutonium: biomedical research, Science 183:715, 1974.
2. Catlin, D. H.: Urine testing: a comparison of five current methods for detecting morphine, Am. J. Clin. Pathol. 60:719, 1973.
3. Eyl, T. B.: Organic-mercury food poisoning, N. Engl. J. Med. 284:706, 1971.
4. Lin-Fu, J. S.: Undue absorption of lead among children—a new look at an old problem, N. Engl. J. Med. 286:702, 1972.
5. Rubin, E., and Lieber, C. S.: Alcoholism, alcohol, and drugs, Science 172:1097, 1971.

CHAPTER 23

Urinalysis

Urinalysis is covered in standard texts of laboratory medicine and renal disease. The book by Freeman and Beeler thoroughly covers clinical microscopy of urine sediment and is illustrated with color plates. The monograph by Free and Free is a programmed text, and the Medcom monograph presents urinalysis against a background of simplified physiology and pathophysiology.

Free, A. H., and Free, H. M.: Urodynamics: concepts relating to urinalysis, Elkhart, Ind., 1974, Ames Co.
Freeman, J. A., and Beeler, M. F.: Laboratory medicine—clinical microscopy, Philadelphia, 1974, Lea & Febiger.
MEDCOM: Urinalysis in the 70s, Elkhart, Ind., 1973, Ames Co.
Relman, A. S., and Levinsky, N. G.: Clinical examination of renal function. In Strauss, M. B., and Welt, L. G., editors: Diseases of the kidney, ed. 2, Boston, 1971, Little, Brown & Co.

■ **What is the normal daily urine volume for adults?**

The normal volume is 1000 to 1500 ml.

■ **Name three substances that produce a brown color in the urine.**

Hemoglobin, myoglobin, and sometimes porphyrins produce a brown color.

■ **Name two conditions that produce dark brown or black urine when the urine is alkaline and is allowed to stand.**

Alkaptonuria (homogentisic acid) and metastatic malignant melanoma (melanin) produce a dark brown or black color.

■ **Name four causes of red urine.**

Hemoglobin, erythrocytes, porphyrins, and the urinary antiseptic-analgesic pyridium will cause red urine.

■ **What is the cause of the pungent odor that urine acquires on standing?**

It is the liberation of ammonia by bacterial hydrolysis of urea.

■ **What disorder would one suspect in an infant who fails to thrive and whose urine smells like maple syrup?**

The problem is probably a defect in oxidative decarboxylation of branched chain alpha-keto acids, called maple syrup urine disease, in which plasma and urine levels of valine, leucine, and isoleucine are grossly elevated.

■ **The dinitrophenylhydrazine (DNPH) screening test is of value in looking for which rare metabolic disorders?**

Phenylketonuria, histidinemia, Oasthouse syndrome, isovaleric acidemia, and various glycogen storage diseases are detected.

■ **What other screening tests are also of value in screening for inborn errors of metabolism?**

The ferric chloride test (phenylketonuria, maple syrup disease, histidinemia, and tyrosinosis) and the nitroprusside-cyanide test (homocystinuria, cystinuria, hyperglycinemia) are of value.

■ **How high should urine specific gravity and osmolality be after overnight restriction of fluids?**

Specific gravity should be 1.020 or more, and the osmolality should be 850 mOsm/kg or more.

■ **Describe a simple urine concentration test.**

For the test of Relman and Levinsky, deprive the patient of fluids after the evening meal. Discard the first voided urine specimen in the morning, and test the next specimen. The specific gravity should be 1.026 or greater.

■ **Name three conditions in which the overnight concentration test result may be abnormal despite the presence of normal kidneys.**

Congestive heart failure (nocturnal diuresis), third trimester of pregnancy (nocturnal diuresis), and diabetes insipidus (deficiency of antidiuretic hormone) will cause abnormal results.

■ **What is the normal range of total urine solids (determined refractometrically) after overnight fluid deprivation?**

The normal range is 5.4 to 8.5 gm/dl.

■ **The specific gravity of freshly voided urine is tested with a hydrometer calibrated at 24° C, and it registers 1.015. What is the true specific gravity?**

The true specific gravity is 1.019 if the urine was 37° C when measured. Specific gravity decreases by approximately 0.001 for each 3 degrees above 24° C.

■ **Why is a refractometer preferable to a hydrometer for determining the specific gravity of urine?**

It requires only a few drops of urine and is temperature compensated from 16° to 38° C.

- **The specific gravity of the urine of a diabetic patient is 1.024 but it contains 1.0 gm of glucose per deciliter. What would the specific gravity be if the glucose were not present?**

It would be 1.021. The specific gravity increases 0.003 unit for each gram of glucose per deciliter.

- **A patient has recently been in hypotensive shock and exhibits a fluid deficit (dehydration). The specific gravity of 50 ml of urine voided over a 4-hour period is 1.010. Is dehydration alone responsible for the oliguria?**

No. Renal tubular damage is present, otherwise the specific gravity would be much higher in the presence of a water deficit.

- **What is the effect of hypercalcemia on the ability of the kidneys to produce concentrated urine?**

With severe hypercalcemia, the kidneys can not produce concentrated urine.

- **What is the pH range of urine that the human kidney is capable of producing?**

The range is 4.5 to 8.0.

- **Under what condition or conditions is it possible for a patient to have metabolic alkalosis yet produce acid urine?**

This will occur in patients who are potassium depleted.

- **In a patient with pyuria, a urine colony count of more than 100,000 bacteria per milliliter of urine, and urine pH of 9.0, what is the likely identity of the bacteria present?**

It is probably a species of *Proteus*. *Proteus* species produce urease that alkalinizes the urine by hydrolyzing urea to produce ammonia.

- **What is the pH of urine in renal tubular acidosis?**

It usually is 6.5 or higher. (Systemic acidosis results from inability of the kidney to secrete acid urine.)

- **What is the Tamm-Horsfall mucoprotein?**

It is a high-molecular-weight mucoprotein that arises in the kidney and forms an important component of hyalin casts.

- **What is the upper limit of daily urinary protein excretion in normal adults?**

It is 150 mg/24 hr.

- **Give six causes of proteinuria in the presence of normal kidneys.**

The causes are orthostatic proteinuria, congestive heart failure, severe anemia, hyperthyroidism, acute febrile illness, and Bence Jones proteinuria.

■ **What concentrations of protein in the urine will give trace, light precipitation, and 4+ flocculation reactions with heat and acetic acid?**

A concentration of 5 mg/dl will give a trace reaction; 10 to 30 mg/dl will give light precipitation; and 500 mg/dl will give heavy flocculation.

■ **What is the principle of the bromphenol blue (dipstick) test for protein in urine?**

Bromphenol blue is an indicator that changes from yellow to blue from pH 3.0 to 4.6. A citrate buffer in the dipstick provides a pH of 3.0. Protein causes a "pH error" of the indicator so that the more protein present, the bluer it will be at pH 3.0.

■ **In most cases of proteinuria, does albumin or globulin predominate in the urine?**

Albumin predominates because of its relatively low (69,000) molecular weight.

■ **What solubility characteristics of Bence Jones protein lead to a simple test for its identification in urine?**

It precipitates at 45° to 55° C and redissolves at higher temperatures.

■ **How can Bence Jones protein be detected in urine when other proteins are also present?**

Filter the urine at the boiling point to remove the other proteins, and cool to 50° C to precipitate Bence Jones protein.

■ **What are the electrophoretic characteristics of Bence Jones protein at pH 8.6?**

It migrates with the gamma globulins.

■ **List five diagnostic or therapeutic agents that will cause false positive test results for urine protein by sulfosalicylic acid precipitation. Which of them will give false positive results by the heat and acetic acid method?**

Para-aminosalicylic acid (PAS), penicillin (massive doses), sulfisoxazole (Gantrisin), tolbutamide metabolites, and x-ray contrast media will cause false positive results. All but sulfisoxazole metabolites give false positive results with heat and acetic acid.

■ **Which of the above agents will give false positive urine protein test results with bromphenol blue dipsticks?**

None will give such results.

■ **What will give a false positive test result for protein in urine with

bromphenol blue dipsticks, and what is its effect on other urine protein tests?

Highly buffered alkaline urine will give such a result. It may cause a false negative result for protein with either heat and acetic acid or with sulfosalicylic acid precipitation tests.

■ **To which is the bromphenol blue test more sensitive, albumin or globulin?**

It is more sensitive to globulin.

■ **What is the normal amount of reducing substances (measured by alkaline cupric solution) in the urine per 24 hours expressed as glucose?**

It is 100 to 200 mg/24 hr.

■ **List five sugars that may occur as reducing substances in urine.**

The five sugars are glucose, pentose, fructose, galactose, and lactose.

■ **Will sucrose added to urine produce an increase in reducing substances?**

It will not, because the molecule contains no aldehyde groups.

■ **What is the significance of reducing substances in the urine during pregnancy?**

Moderate increases in reducing substances commonly occur as a result of increased glomerular filtration of glucose, large amounts of glucuronic acid conjugated to estriol, and lactosuria. Lactosuria persists after parturition.

■ **In what conditions other than diabetes mellitus is glycosuria not uncommonly present?**

Glycosuria may be present with renal glycosuria, pancreatitis, thyrotoxicosis, acromegaly, Cushing's syndrome, alpha cell tumors of the pancreas, after head injuries and general anesthesia, and during conditions with elevated epinephrine production (pheochromocytoma, stress or excitement).

■ **False negative glucose oxidase tests are most frequent under what two conditions?**

Patients taking vitamin C and patients excreting a large amount of ketones may have false negative tests.

■ **What is the principle of the glucose oxidase method of determining urine glucose?**

Glucose oxidase oxidizes glucose to gluconic acid, producing hydrogen peroxide. The latter produces a blue color when combined with orthotolidine.

■ **What are the effects of large amounts of ascorbic acid in the urine on copper reduction and glucose oxidase (dipstick) methods for determination of glucose?**

Ascorbic acid will give false positive results for glucose by the copper reduction technics, but it may interfere with the glucose oxidase test and give false negative results in the presence of glucose.

■ **Which of the following substances in urine will cause false positive results when testing for glucose by the copper-reduction and the glucose oxidase (dipstick) methods: fructose, pentose, galactose, lactose, maltose, homogentisic acid, large amounts of creatinine or uric acid, salicylates, penicillin, chloral hydrate, and para-aminosalicylic acid (PAS)?**

All may give false positive reactions by copper reduction, but none will give positive reactions with glucose oxidase.

■ **Which of the ketone bodies are detected by nitroprusside tests (Rothera test or Acetest tablets)?**

Acetoacetic acid and acetone are detected by nitroprusside tests. These tests do not detect beta-hydroxybutyric acid.

■ **List several causes of nondiabetic ketonuria.**

Caloric undernutrition (starvation, chronic vomiting, malabsorption), fever, and severe exercise cause nondiabetic ketonuria.

■ **What is the sensitivity of the Acetest tablet for acetoacetic acid?**

As little as 10 mg/dl is detectable.

■ **In which of the following disorders would one expect to find bile in the urine: extrahepatic and intrahepatic obstructive jaundice, virus hepatitis, decompensated Laennec's cirrhosis, Dubin-Johnson, Rotor's, Crigler-Najjar, and Gilbert's syndromes, and hemolytic jaundice?**

Bile occurs in the urine in all but the Crigler-Najjar and Gilbert's syndromes and hemolytic jaundice.

■ **What accounts for the appearance of bile in the urine in some types of jaundice but not in others?**

Only conjugated bilirubin (bilirubin diglucuronide) is excreted by the kidney because unconjugated bilirubin is insoluble and strongly bound to protein.

■ **What is the principle of the Harrison spot test for bilirubin?**

It is oxidation of bilirubin to biliverdin (green) by the ferric chloride in Fouchet's reagent.

■ **If a Schwartz-Watson test shows a red-brown color in the top layer, how would one interpret it?**

The result is positive for porphobilinogen. The reaction product of porphobilinogen and Ehrlich's reagent is soluble in water that layers above the chloroform.

■ **What are the normal ranges for urine urobilinogen by the semiquantita-**

tive method of Wallace and Diamond and by quantitative measurement in 24-hour urine specimens?

A positive reaction (indicating the presence of urobilinogen) will occur in dilutions of 1:8 to 1:32 by the method of Wallace and Diamond. The normal range by quantitative measurement is 0.05 to 4.0 mg/24 hr.

- **What are the effects of biliary obstruction, hepatocellular disease without obstruction, and hemolytic disease on urine urobilinogen excretion?**

Urine urobilinogen excretion is decreased or absent in biliary obstruction, and it is increased in hepatocellular disease and hemolysis.

- **Where is urobilinogen formed?**

It is formed in the intestine by bacterial reduction of bilirubin.

- **How are uroporphyrins and coproporphyrin III detected in the urine?**

They are detected by fluorescence under ultraviolet light.

- **Which two precursors or byproducts of heme synthesis are excreted in the urine in excessive amounts in lead poisoning?**

Delta-aminolevulinic acid and coproporphyrin III are excreted in excessive amounts.

- **Name three inherited disorders of amino acid metabolism that result in a positive reaction to a ferric chloride test on urine.**

Phenylketonuria, maple syrup urine disease, and histidinemia will show a positive reaction. The reaction is also positive in some patients with tyrosinemia.

- **Patients with the carcinoid syndrome have an increase in what substance in the urine?**

They have an increase in 5-hydroxyindoleacetic acid.

- **What is the normal daily urinary excretion of 5-hydroxyindoleacetic acid?**

The normal excretion is 1 to 5 mg/24 hr.

- **In what diseases or conditions is an increase in the urine creatine excretion found?**

Myopathies, febrile and wasting diseases, testosterone administration, hyperthyroidism, pregnancy, and bone fractures will increase urine creatine excretion.

- **What is alkaptonuria?**

It is a congenital metabolic disease in which there is a lack of homogentisic acid oxidase and a corresponding increase in the homogentisic acid excretion in the urine. The urine darkens on standing if the pH is sufficiently alkaline.

■ **What is the site of formation of casts that appear in the urine sediment?**

Casts form in the renal tubules.

■ **What are the maximum numbers of blood cells and casts present in centrifuged sediment from normal urine?**

Three red blood cells and five white blood cells per high-power field and occasional hyaline casts (fewer than one per high-power field) are present.

■ **A brown, refractile pigment present in cells or in casts in the urine sediment should be subjected to what test?**

It should be subjected to the Prussian blue reaction for iron. A positive reaction indicates hemosiderin.

■ **In what conditions is hemosiderin found in the urine?**

It is found in intravascular hemolysis of any cause and in hemochromatosis.

■ **What are glitter cells?**

They are large, pale polymorphonuclear leukocytes seen with the Sternheimer-Malbin stain usually in patients with pyelonephritis. They show brownian movement and streaming of their granules when the osmolality of the urine is relatively low (less than 600 mOsm/kg).

■ **How can the Gram stain be used to screen urines for significant bacteriuria?**

It can be used by staining uncentrifuged urine. If bacteria are readily visible in such preparations, the microbial colony count will probably be in excess of 100,000/ml. However, the culture should never be omitted.

■ **What is the significance of broad casts in the urine sediment?**

Broad casts originate in the collecting tubules and indicate advanced renal disease.

■ **In what condition are renal tubular epithelial cells numerous in the urine sediment?**

They are numerous in acute renal tubular necrosis.

■ **What type of casts occur in simple fluid deficit (dehydration)?**

Hyaline casts occur in dehydration.

■ **What finding in the urine sediment is particularly characteristic of the nephrotic syndrome?**

Oval fat bodies are characteristic.

■ **What simple microscopic technic should be used to confirm the presence of oval fat bodies?**

Polarized microscopy should be performed. The oval fat bodies are bire-fringent and resemble Maltese crosses.

- **What are the origins of granular casts?**

They are degenerate red or white blood cell casts or aggregates of albumin and globulins from the plasma in a matrix of Tamm-Horsfall mucoprotein.

- **Identify these cells.**

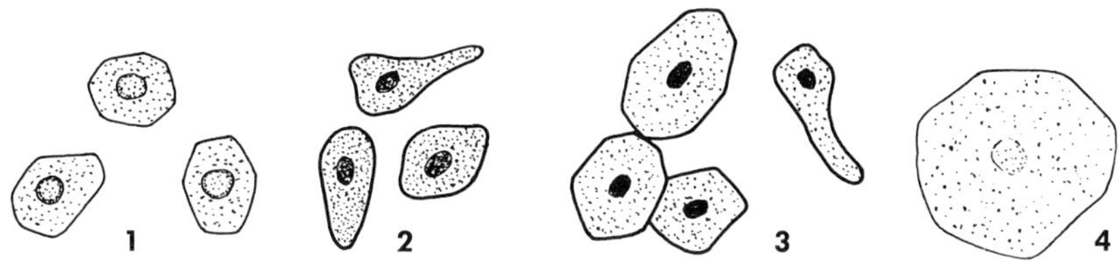

1. Renal tubular epithelial cells
2. Caudate cells from renal pelvis
3. Transitional epithelium from urinary bladder
4. Squamous cell from vagina or urethra

- **Identify these crystals, and state whether they occur in acid, alkaline, or either acid or alkaline urine.**

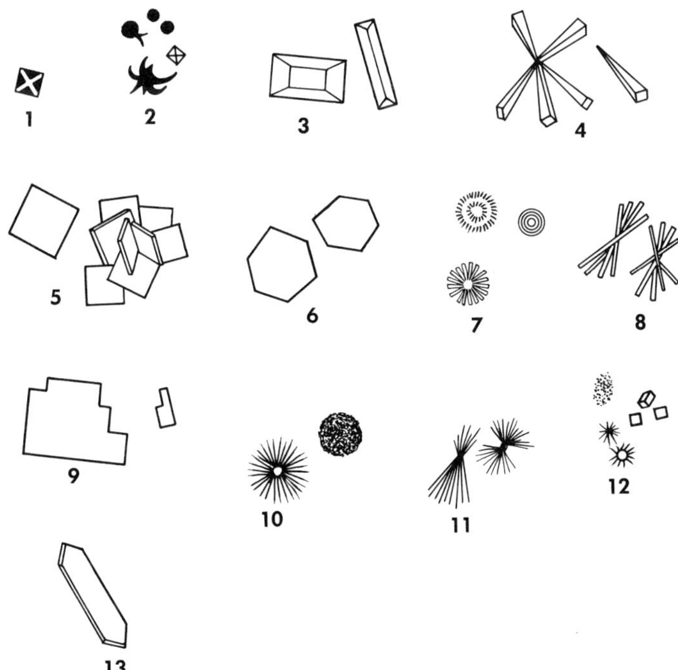

1. Calcium oxalate, either acid or alkaline
2. Ammonium urate, alkaline
3. Ammonium magnesium phosphate, alkaline or neutral
4. Calcium phosphate, alkaline or neutral
5. Uric acid, acid
6. Cystine, acid
7. Leucine spheres, acid or neutral
8. Tyrosine needles, acid or neutral
9. Cholesterol, acid or neutral
10. Sulfadiazine, acid or neutral
11. Acetyl sulfadiazine, acid
12. Bilirubin, acid or neutral
13. Hippuric acid, acid or alkaline

■ **What color are bilirubin crystals?**

They are red-brown.

■ **What colors are uric acid and ammonium urate crystals?**

They are brown, red-brown, or yellow. Small uric acid crystals may be colorless.

■ **What solubility characteristic distinguishes sulfonamide crystals?**

They are highly soluble in acetone.

■ **Give thermal and pH solubility characteristics of urates and uric acid.**

Both are soluble at 60° C and in alkali, but they are insoluble in acid.

■ **Give pH solubility characteristics of phosphates.**

They are soluble in dilute acetic acid and insoluble in alkali.

■ **In what three conditions may large numbers of oxalate crystals be seen in urine?**

They may be seen in oxalosis, ethylene glycol poisoning, and vitamin B_6 deficiency.

■ **What metabolic diseases should be suspected in children who form urinary calculi?**

Cystinuria and oxalosis should be suspected.

INDEX

Heparin—cont'd
  excess of, bleeding from, differentiation of, from bleeding from other causes, 123-124
  injected, anticoagulant effect of, half-life of, 123
  mode of action of, 123
Hepatic; *see also* Liver
Hepatic coma, diagnostic indications of, 216
Hepatitis
  active chronic, laboratory findings in, 217
  chronic or slowly resolving indicator of, 217-218
  elevated serum acid phosphatase level in, 100
  posttransfusion, due to hepatitis B, proportion of total cases, 61
  risks of, from transfusion from volunteer vs. commercial donors, 59
  severe, abnormal serum cholesterol levels in, 216
  transmission of, by factor VIII concentrates, 128
  type B, appearance of anti-HB_sAg in, 217
  viral
    bile in urine in, 280
    HB_sAg-positive acute, persistence of HB_sAg in, 217
Hepatocellular disease
  glutamic-pyruvic transaminase elevation in, 95
  without obstruction, effect of, on urinary excretion of urobilinogen, 281
Hepatocellular injury, elevation of serum aldolase activity in, 100
Hepatocellular jaundice
  Bromsulphalein retention in, 214
  laboratory findings in, 215
  and obstructive jaundice, distinguishing between, parenteral administration of vitamin K in, 215
  parameters in, 213-214
Hepatocellular necrosis, elevated serum transaminase levels in, 95
Herbicides, chlorinated hydrocarbon, principal storage depot for, 267
Hereditary ovalocytosis, seriousness of, 174
Hereditary spherocytosis, results of laboratory procedures in, 174
Herellea vaginicola, characteristics of, 32

Heroin, excretion of, in urine, 273
Herpesvirus hominis, characteristics of cerebrospinal fluid in, 70
Heterophyes heterophyes, ova of, appearance of, 243
Hip joint, fluid in, 144
Histalog, 158
Histamine stimulation, maximal, in pernicious anemia, 157
Histamine test, augmented, 158
Histamine-fast achlorhydria in pernicious anemia, 171
Histidinemia
  dinitrophenylhydrazine screening test for, 276
  positive reaction to ferric chloride test on urine in, 281
Histoplasma capsulatum
  appearance of, 152
  morphology of, 151
  in sputum as indication of disease, 259
  yeast phase of, lowest significant titer of, 154
Histoplasmosis
  acute, latex agglutination test for diagnosis of, 154
  disseminated, white blood cell count in, 152
  immunologic test in diagnosis of, 152
HL-A antibodies, lymphocytotoxicity tests for, principle of, 60
HL-A antigen associated with rheumatoid spondylitis, 60
HL-A antigen system, description of, 60
HL-A system, 60
Hollander test for vagotomy, 159-160
Homologous chromosomes, 131
Homologous translocation, 135
Homovanillic acid (HVA), excretion of increased, conditions causing, 77
Hookworm
  adult
    daily blood consumption of, 230
    size of, 230
  infestation by, anemia resulting from, 231
  life cycle of, 230
  ova of
    confusion of, with decorticate *Ascaris lumbricoides*, 231
    identification of, 233
Hormone(s)
  adrenal cortical, 73-77

Ixodidae and Argasidae, difference between, 246

J

Jaffe chromogens, noncreatinine, 110

Jaundice

"breast milk," 212

cholestatic, drug-induced parameters in, 214

hemolytic, Bromsulphalein retention in, 214

hepatocellular, 213-215; *see also* Hepatocellular jaundice

hyperbilirubinemias due to, 212-213

nonhemolytic, BSP excretion test in, indications for, 214

obstructive; *see* Obstructive jaundice

Jockey itch, dermatophytes causing, 150

Joint(s)

Charcot's, cell count in synovial fluid from, 145

degenerative disease of, synovial fluid from, results of Rope test in, 145

fluid of, normal, appearance of, 144

hip, fluid normally present in, 144

knee, fluid normally present in, 144

osteoarthritic, cell count in synovial fluid from, 145

and serous cavities, fluids of, 142-147

K

K antigen slide agglutination test for enteropathogenic *E. coli*, technic for, 21

Kala-azar, 223

Karyosome, 220

Karyotyping

metaphase figures counted in, 134

technic of, 133

Katayama's test, 163

Kell blood group, 45

Kernicterus, definition of, 212

Ketoacidosis, diabetic, cerebrospinal pH in, 70

17-Ketogenic steroid, measurement of, in urine, conditions for, 75

Ketone bodies detected by nitroprusside tests, 280

Ketonuria, nondiabetic, causes of, 280

17-Ketosteroids, urinary, 74-75

Ki capsular polysaccharide antigen in isolates from neonatal meningitis, 21

Kidd blood group antigens, percentage distribution of, in black and white Americans, 45

Kidney(s), 202-209

concentration of inorganic mercury in, 272

damaged, secondary to chronic glomerulonephritis, maintenance of low blood urea nitrogen level in, 206

diseases of, associated with proteinuria, 207

failure of

acute, effect of, on radioactive iodine uptake, 117

chronic, abnormal glucose tolerance test in, 85

in hemolytic transfusion reaction, 48

function of

parameter of, measured by phenolsulphonphthalein test, 205

serum creatinine as indicator of, 110, 203-204

infarcts of

LDH isoenzymes elevated in, 97

normal, proteinuria in, causes of, 277-278

osteodystrophy of, biochemical abnormalities in, 81

plasma flow in, normal range of, 205

resection of, for hypertension, 208

sodium reabsorption by, effect of aldosterone on, 203

Kinetoplast, 220

King-Armstrong method in measurement of acid phosphatase, 99

Klebsiella

characteristics of, on brilliant green agar, 18

nonmotility of, 20-21

pneumonia, sputum in, characteristics of, 260

Klebsiella rhinoscleromatis as cause of rhinoscleroma, 23

Klebsiella species, characteristics of, 22

Klinefelter's syndrome

Barr bodies in, 137

characteristics of, 137

decreased testosterone production in, 112

FSH and LH levels in, 105

mental deficiency in, incidence of, 137

Knee joint, fluid normally present in, 144

Renal tubular necrosis—cont'd
LDH isoenzymes elevated in, 97
Renal tubular reabsorption of phosphorus, 79
Renal tubule, potassium excretion and absorption by, 203
Renin, 207-208
Resection, gastric and intestinal, malabsorption after, effect of, on fecal organic anion output, 141
Respiratory acidosis, major causes of, 93
Respiratory alkalosis due to salicylate intoxication, 273
Respiratory distress syndrome, conditions disposing toward, 5
Reticulocytes, polychromatophilic staining of, with Wright's stain, 166
Reticuloendothelial system, breakdown of hemoglobin in, 210
Reticuloendotheliosis, leukemia, lymphocytes in, acid phosphatase isoenzymes predominant in, 183
Rh antibodies, titer of, significance of, 51
Rh genotypes, frequency of, in Americans, 54
Rh immune globulin, 51-52
Rh incompatibilities in pregnancy, screening procedures for, 50-51
Rh-compatible platelets, uses of, 58
Rh-negative women, proportion of, susceptible to $Rh_o(D)$ sensitization by transplacental transfusion of Rh-positive blood, 49
Rh_o variant (D^u), 55
Rheumatic fever
group A streptococci in, 38
synovial fluid in, 145
Rheumatoid arthritis
antinuclear factor in, 193
antinuclear immunofluorescent pattern association with, 194
joint effusions associated with, complement levels of, 146
sera of, antinuclear factor in, 193
synovial fluid counts in, 145
synovial fluid from
polymorphonuclear leukocytes in, 146
results of Ropes test in, 145
variants of, giving negative results to tests for rheumatoid factor, 188
Rheumatoid factor (RF)
definition, 146
serologic tests for, principle of, 187

Rheumatoid factor (RF)—cont'd
testing for, euglobulin fraction of serum in, 187
tests for, 188
titers of, significant, 188
Rheumatoid spondylitis, HL-A antigen associated with, 60
Rhinorrhea, cerebrospinal fluid test for, 66
Rhinoscleroma, causes of, 23
Rickettsial diseases, serodiagnosis of, *Proteus* OX 19 antigen in, 187
Rocky Mountain spotted fever, ticks transmitting, 246
Ropes test
definition, 144
results of, in various conditions, 145
Rothera test, ketone bodies detected by, 280
Rotor's syndrome, bile in urine in, 280
Roundworms
intestinal
propagating in free-living state, 229
reproducing repeatedly in man, 230
larval forms of, 228
tissue, 233
causing solitary pulmonary nodules, 235
intermediate host for, 234
reproductive characteristics of, 233
Wuchereria bancrofti, size of adult, 234
Rubella, clinical, diagnosis of, rubella hemagglutination-inhibition test for, 196
Rubella hemagglutination-inhibition (HI) test, 196

S

St. Louis encephalitis, transmission of
by culicine mosquitoes, 249
by ticks, 246
Salicylates in, screening test for, 273
Saliva
differentiating of, from sputum, 259
organisms in, most abundant, 15
Salmonella paratyphi, characteristics of, on brilliant green agar, 18
Salmonella-Shigella (SS) agar, 19
Salmonella typhi
characteristics of, on brilliant green agar, 18
infection with, negative agglutination test after, 186-187